GASTRITIS AND GASTRIC CANCER – NEW INSIGHTS IN GASTROPROTECTION, DIAGNOSIS AND TREATMENTS

Edited by **Paola Tonino**

Gastritis and Gastric Cancer – New Insights in Gastroprotection, Diagnosis and Treatments
Edited by Paola Tonino

Published by InTech
Janeza Trdine 9, 51000 Rijeka, Croatia

Publishing Process Manager Martina Blecic

Technical Editor Teodora Smiljanic

Cover Designer InTech Design Team

Additional hard copies can be obtained from orders@intechopen.com

Gastritis and Gastric Cancer – New Insights in Gastroprotection, Diagnosis and Treatments, Edited by Paola Tonino
p. cm.
ISBN 978-953-307-375-0

For EU product safety concerns:
IN TECH d.o.o., Prolaz Marije Krucifikse Kozulić 3, 51000 Rijeka, Croatia,
info@intechopen.com or visit our website at intechopen.com.

Meet the editor

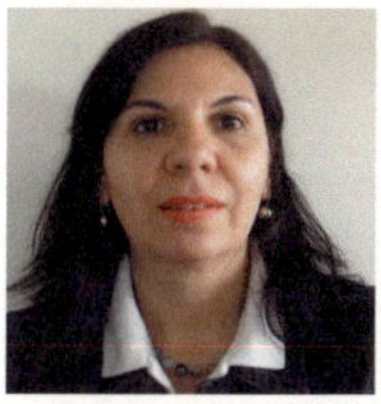

Dr. Paola Tonino holds a Doctoral Degree in Cell Biology from the Universidad Central de Venezuela (Caracas, 1999), where she studied tumor angiogenesis in different regions of human gastrointestinal carcinomas. She currently works as an Associate Professor at the Universidad Central de Venezuela and has 15 years of experience teaching at undergraduate and graduate level. Her post doctoral work in the United States includes the study of the structure and function of myosin smooth muscle and nebulin skeletal muscle in a knockout mouse model. She has published her work in several peer reviewed journals and given oral and poster presentations at national and international conferences. In addition she has authored Venezuelan grants and participated in grants from the National Institute of Health. She was also awarded for the most outstanding programs in Venezuela in the past 16 years. Her fields of special expertise include cancer biology and angiogenic factors as biomarkers of diagnosis and prognosis in gastrointestinal carcinomas.

Contents

Preface

In the last two decades, the research on gastritis, gastroduodenal ulcers and gastric carcinoma focused on the *Helicobacter pylori* infection process, but the mechanisms leading to these diseases are not completely understood. Gastritis is an inflammatory disease of the gastric mucosa in response to several intrinsic and extrinsic factors. Diet antigens, extracellular pollutants and pathogenic infections trigger the inflammatory process in the gastrointestinal tract. Thus, the disruption of the intestinal barrier results in intestinal inflammation by pro-inflammatory reactions of immune cells. The inflammatory progression into the gastric lining depends on environmental factors, host state and *H. pylori*-specific virulence factors. Albeit the stomach is frequently exposed to hazardous agents, several gastroprotective mechanisms exist to response to this harsh environment. Furthermore, a better understanding of the mechanisms of gastric mucosal defense system might provide new insights into potential therapeutic targets. The modification of functional capsaicin-sensitive afferent nerves also offers new opportunities in gastroprotective therapy. The severity of gastric inflammation has also been related to high concentration of free radicals. Chronic inflammation of the gastric mucosa may predispose susceptible cells to neoplastic transformation. The reactive oxygen species (ROS, e.g. nitric oxide and superoxide) are key regulatory factors in molecular pathways linked to carcinogenesis. *H. pylori* infection increases the oxidative DNA damage by ROS in epithelial cells as a causal factor in malignant transformation. Two distinct molecular pathways for gastric carcinogenesis by *H. pylori* infection has been proposed; the direct action of the bacterial proteins such as Cag A on gastric epithelial cells, and the accumulation of genetic and epigenetic changes in tumor-related genes of the gastric epithelial cells caused by prolonged bacterial infection and chronic inflammation. Then the identification of novel genes regulated by *H. pylori* (cagA, cagT, vacA and dupA) in early stages of gastric cancer might help to understand the differential susceptibility to this pathogen. Recent studies have demonstrated the phenotypic and genotypic diversity of *H pylori* isolates that may engender differential host inflammatory responses with influence in the clinical outcome. New strategies for control of *H. pylori* infection involve the disruption of the interaction between the bacteria and target cells via downregulation of apoptosis and upregulation of autophagy.

Besides, the integral analysis of immunohistopathology and overexpression of specific tumor suppressor genes (e.g. p53 and p73) or a protein secreted by antrum mucosa (gastrokine 1), might be important to the identification of possible biomarkers for the gastric carcinogenesis. DNA methylated genes have been detected not only in gastric mucosa but also in the plasma of gastric cancer patients (e.g. Reprimo, RPRM) as a cell-free DNA, which can be considered a diagnostic tool for non-invasive detection of premalignant gastritis and gastric cancer. It is also worth to mention that proper chronic gastritis classification considering both, clinical and histopathological aspects is fundamental for the diagnosis and successful therapy. Current classification of gastritis is the 1994 Houston-updated Sydney System. It has been suggested that digital morphometric evaluation of the inflammatory and epithelial cells of the gastric mucosa, and the density of neuroendocrine cells in association with chronic gastritis type, and clinicopathological factors may also be valuable in diagnosis.

The treatment of gastritis depends on the specific cause. In the present, not only several drugs are in use, but also phytotherapy compounds including tannins and flavonoids (phenolic compounds) have been associated with healing properties attributed to the inhibition of cytokine-mediated inflammatory mechanism, suppression of inducible nitric oxide synthase and antioxidants activities. In addition, probiotic lactic acid bacteria and probiotic foods might promote beneficial effects on the gastric mucosa.

Untreated chronic gastritis and other host factors could progress to gastric carcinogenesis. The model postulated by Correa and Houghton (2007) shows the combination of *H. pylori* factors, environmental insults, and the host immune response involved in the initiation and progression of mucosal atrophy, metaplasia, and dysplasia toward gastric cancer. It is known that *H. pylori* eradication changes the cellular phenotype of gastric intestinal metaplasia, which may be an important factor in the reduction of cancer incidence.

Recently, *H. pylori* lipopolysaccharide (LPS) was associated with the enhancement of the inflammatory reaction and upregulation of the growth rate of epithelial cells via activation of the MEK1/2-ERK1/2 MAP kinase cascade.

All these aspects are considered in this book, as a comprehensive overview of invited contributions about gastroprotection, gastritis and gastric carcinogenesis and new approaches in diagnosis and treatments. The first part of the book covers topics related to the pathophysiology of gastric mucosal defense system and gastritis including the gastroprotective function of the mucus, the importance of capsaicin-sensitive afferent nerves and the oxidative stress pathway involved in inflammation, apoptosis and autophagy in *Helicobacter pylori* related gastritis. The next chapters deal with molecular pathogenesis and treatments, which consider the role of neuroendocrine cells in gastric disease, DNA methylation in *H. pylori* infection, the role of antioxidants and phytotherapy in gastric disease. The final part presents the effects of cancer risk factors associated with *H. pylori* infection. These chapters discuss several factors such as, the serum pepsinogen test, K-ras mutations, cell kinetics, and *H. pylori* lipopolysaccharide, as well as the roles of several bacterial genes (cagA, cagT, vacA and dupA) as virulence factors in gastric cancer, and the gastrokine-1 protein in cancer progression. The topics presented in this book are suggested to all clinicians and researchers interested in gastroprotection, gastritis and gastrointestinal cancer diagnosis and treatments.

I would like to thank the In Tech Publishing team for this opportunity and especially to all the authors for their contribution to the better understanding of gastritis and gastric cancer.

August 2011

Dr. Paola Tonino
Associate Professor (UCV),
Venezuela

Part 1

Pathophysiology of Gastric Mucosal Defense System and Gastritis

1

Protective Effects of Gastric Mucus

Takafumi Ichikawa and Kazuhiko Ishihara
Kitasato University Graduate School of Medical Sciences
Japan

1. Introduction

The gastric mucosa is continuously exposed to many noxious factors and substances. How the gastric mucosa maintains structural integrity and resists auto-digestion by substances such as acid and pepsin puzzled clinicians and investigators for more than 200 years. The gastric epithelium must also resist damage from extrinsic agents, including *Helicobacter pylori* (*H. pylori*) and noxious ingestions such as ethanol and nonsteroidal anti-inflammatory drugs (NSAIDs). The luminal surface of the stomach is covered by a viscoelastic mucus gel layer that acts as a protective barrier against the harsh luminal environment. The structural characteristics of this barrier are primary indicators of its physiological function and changes of its composition have been identified in gastrointestinal pathologies. This chapter presents recent insights into the implication of the gastric mucus barrier as "no mucus, no protection".

While acid, pepsin, and *H. pylori* are thought to be major factors in the pathophysiology of gastritis, the importance of the mucosal defense system has also been emphasized. Gastric 'cytoprotection' refers to a reduction or prevention of chemically induced acute hemorrhagic erosions by compounds such as prostaglandin (PG) and SH derivatives without inhibiting acid secretion in rodents (Robert, 1979; Szabo et al., 1981). Since the concept of 'cytoprotection' was introduced, increasing attention has been paid to the effect of medications on the gastric mucosal defensive mechanisms. Although the exact mechanisms of the mucosal defense system are unknown, it involves one or more of the naturally occurring gastric mucosal defensive factors such as mucus metabolism. For estimation of the gastroprotective function, many drugs have been investigated for their activity to protect the gastric mucosa from a variety of necrotizing agents such as ethanol and HCl. Considerable information has accumulated about the gastroprotective function of the mucus that covers the mucosal surface of the stomach.

2. Fundamental aspects of gastric mucus

2.1 Constituent of gastric mucus

Mucus is produced in mucus-producing cells, secreted and extensively covers the surface layer of the mucosa by forming a mucus gel layers. As shown in Figure 1, mucus is a complex mixture containing mucin, water electrolytes, sloughed off cells, enzymes and various other materials, including bacteria and bacterial products depending on the source and location of the mucus (Hotta, 2000).

Gastric mucus is present in the mucus granules of the mucus-producing cells, the insoluble mucus gel layer adhering to the mucosal surface and the gastric lumen in a solubilized

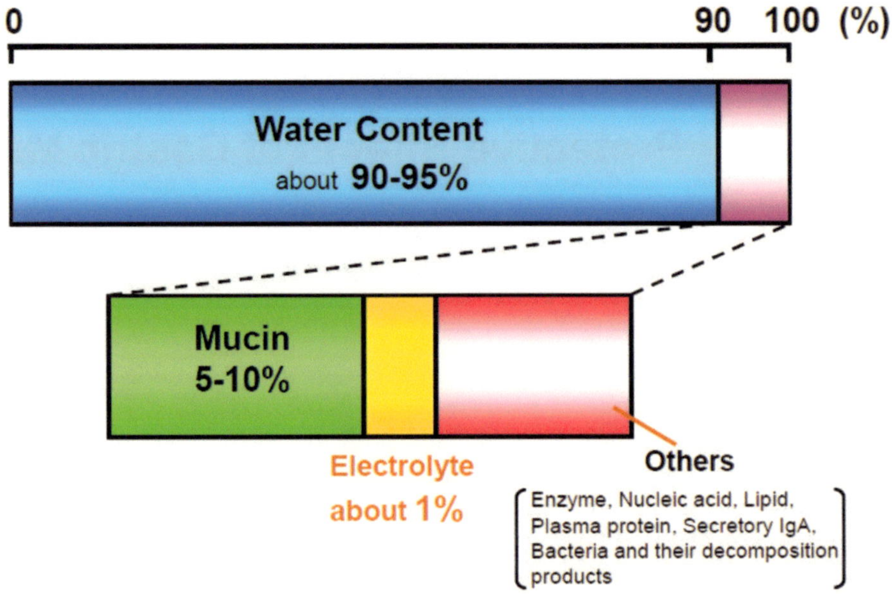

Fig. 1. Composition of gastric mucus.

condition. Mucus rapidly responds to pathological and physiological changes in the stomach. Moreover, mucus present in the stomach exhibits various actions such as maintaining lubrication of the mucosal surface, covering ingested foods to mix them, helping digestion, and protecting the surface epithelium from irritation by forming a thick mucus gel layer.

Mucin, the major constituent of the mucus, is biosynthesized by the mucus-producing cells and secreted from them. Mucus-producing cells of the mammalian gastric mucosa are classified mainly as surface mucus or gland mucus cells (Fig. 2) and respective mucins differ in their peptide sequences and chemical composition of the carbohydrate moieties. The core peptides of the mucins from the surface and gland mucus cells of the human stomach are characterized as MUC5AC and MUC6, respectively. Mucins from these two types of cells have distinct roles in the physiology of the gastric mucosa. In the studies using experimental animals, the appearance of specific mucin was observed in the regenerating epithelia during the healing process from gastric mucosal damage (Hayashida et al., 2001; Ikezawa et al. 2004).

2.2 Outline of gastric mucin

Electron microscopy has indicated 200 to 4000 nm fibers to be present in a gastric mucin molecule. Mucins are composed of glycoprotein subunits (monomer molecular weight : 3 to 5 x 10^5) joined by disulfide bridges, to form high-molecular-weight polymers (having a molecular weight of millions). Each glycoprotein subunit consists of a central peptide core, with many closely packed carbohydrate side chains attached (Fig. 3). Each carbohydrate chain is composed of several sugar residues (up to 19 in length) in gastric mucus, and many will carry a negative charge because of the presence of ester sulfate and sialic acid residues. It is these negatively charged carbohydrate chains that give the mucin its acidic-staining

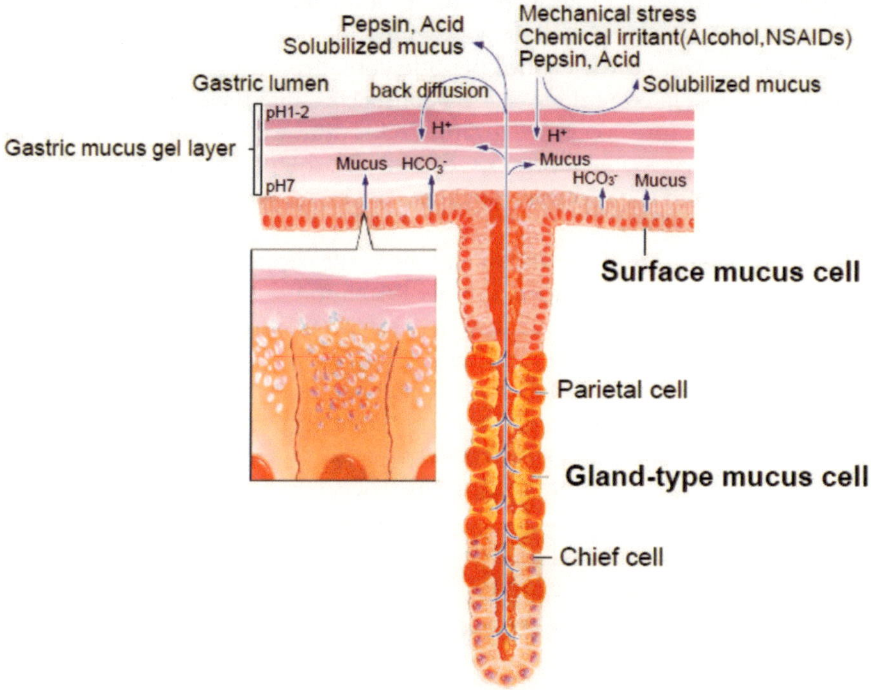

Fig. 2. Distribution of cells constituting the oxyntic gland.

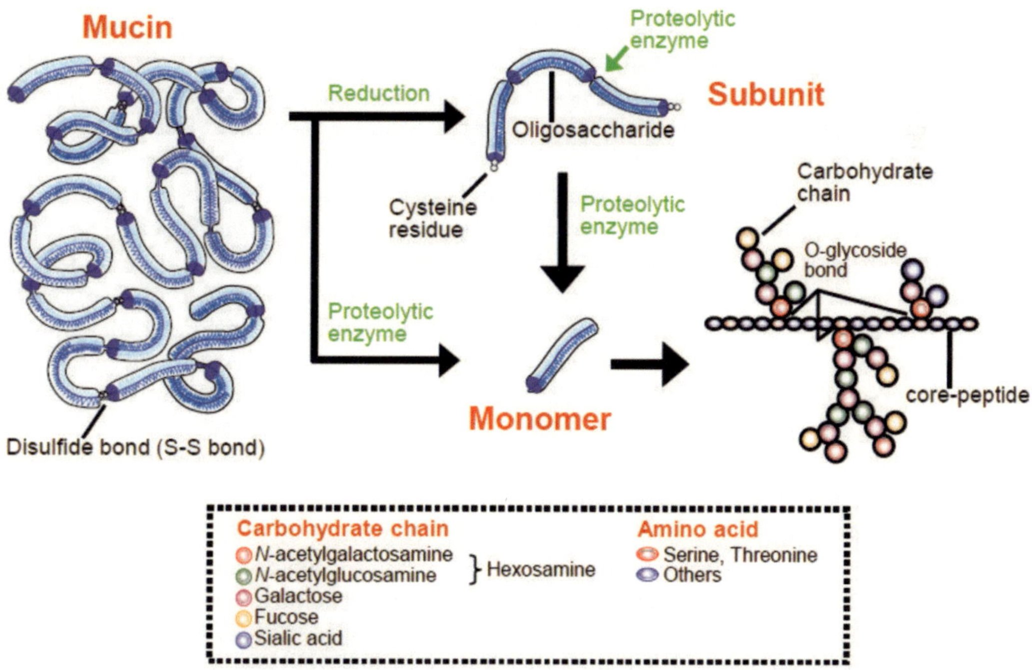

Fig. 3. Polymeric structure of mucin molecules.

properties. Each glycoprotein subunit can be divided into two functional regions on the basis of the peptide core: (1) glycosylated regions in which carbohydrate chains form a closely packed sheath around the central peptide core, protecting it from proteolytic attack; and (2) other nonglycosylated regions of the peptide core that have little or no carbohydrate attached, which are therefore accessible to proteolytic attack by pepsin and other proteolytic enzymes. These nonglycosylated regions of the peptide core are also the site of the disulfide bridges that join the glycoprotein subunits together to form the polymeric mucin structure.

Gel formation between intact polymeric mucin molecules occurs at high concentration (15 to 50 mg/ml) by noncovalent interactions. For gel formation to take place, the mucin must be in its polymeric form. This is the reason why proteolytic enzymes such as pepsin, which degrades the mucin polymeric structure, will dissolve mucus gels. Proteolysis digests the nonglycosylated regions of the peptide core, hence that part containing the disulfide bridges that join the glycoprotein subunits together. The resulting proteolytically degraded subunit consists of the glycosylated region, which is resistant to further proteolytic digestion. There is no detectable loss of carbohydrate during proteolysis and, since it is more than 80% by weight of the glycoprotein subunit, the proteolytically degraded glycoprotein is still quite large.

3. Method and tools for mucus research

3.1 Biosynthesis of mucin

Mucin is produced within mucus-producing cells. To serine or threonine in the polypeptide core synthesized in ribosomes, sugars are transferred one after another in the Golgi complex. Dekker & Strous (1990) have indicated the biosynthesis of gastric mucin to occur as follows. A polypeptide (molecular weight: about 270,000) is synthesized in ribosome and the mucin precursor is synthesized in the rough endoplasmic reticulum (RER). A small portion of an *N*-glycoside sugar chain is connected to each end of the peptide in the RER and is required for efficient oligomerization of the precursor. Three to 4 molecules of this precursor are polymerized in an ATP-unrelated manner in the RER to form an oligomer. *N*-acetylgalactosamine is subsequently transferred to serine and threonine in the late RER compartment (transitional elements) or in cisternae of the Golgi complex. The three-dimensional structure of the polypeptide core changes to an elongated random coil as a result of this transfer. The other sugars are transferred to mucin intermediates before they can reach the trans-cisternae of the Golgi complex and the mucin intermediates form mature mucin. Following biosynthesis in mucus-producing cells, mucin accumulates as mucus granules in the cells and is subsequently secreted through exocytosis. Consequently, a mucus gel layer is formed, which is degraded or directly secreted (Fig. 4).

3.2 Methods for isolation of gastric mucus

The distribution in the stomach, localization and composition of mucus were mainly determined by histochemical methods. By virtue of the development of new staining methods, it has become possible to determine the histochemical characteristics of the produced mucus. However, this method is not suitable for a quantitative assay to grasp the disposition of mucus as a whole. To continue our mucus research, the development of some biochemical assay methods was needed. Gastric mucus is a mixture with a complicated

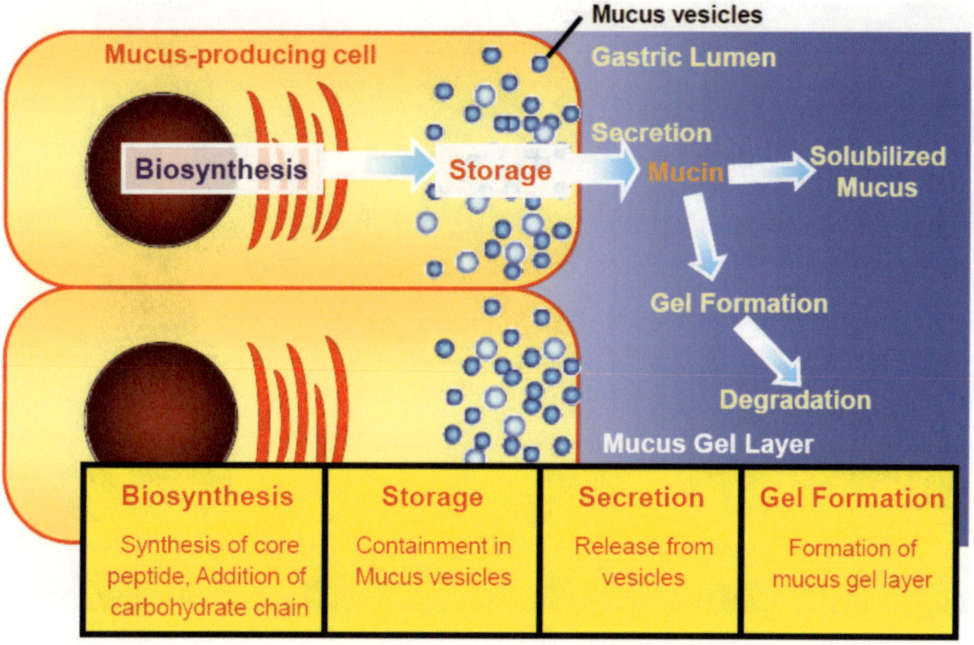

Fig. 4. Biosynthesis and secretion of mucin on mucus-producing cell.

composition. It is not easy to quantify this substance. To overcome this difficulty, we decided to determine the major constituent of mucus, mucin, alone for quantitative evaluation of the gastric mucus. As mucin is a highly glycosylated macromolecule, we developed a method to efficiently extract and isolate mucin from the gastric mucus and established the method to quantify its constituent sugars.

Mucus is isolated from corpus and antral mucosa of rat stomach (Fig. 5). To determine mucus content, lyophilized tissues are subjected to extraction with Tris-HCl buffer containing 2% Triton X-100 and separated by gel filtration. The first peak eluted with the void volume is characterized as mucin and the change in mucin content is determined by measurement of hexose (Azuumi et al., 1980). The amount of hexose per dry tissue weight is calculated and the results expressed relative to the control. To investigate the biosynthetic activity of mucin, 2 x 2 mm tissue samples are incubated in a medium containing a labelled precursor and the mucin fraction is isolated. The radioactivity is determined and given as levels per tissue protein (Ichikawa et al., 1993).

These biochemical methods are suitable for quantification of the total mucin content in the entire mucosal layer. With the use of these methods, it became possible to quantify the amount of mucus and the extent of biosynthesis in each portion of the stomach (corpus and antrum). Moreover, it became possible to determine the physiological changes and also changes in the amount of mucus and qualitative changes due to pathological changes such as an experimental ulcer. However, when using this described method, it was impossible to determine the disposition of mucin in the mucus gel layer which is important for the gastric defense mechanism. We normally mechanically scraped the gel layer from the mucosa, and therefore, it was impossible to make a precise determination due to the loss of surface epithelial cells. To solve this problem, various methods for removal of the gel layer were

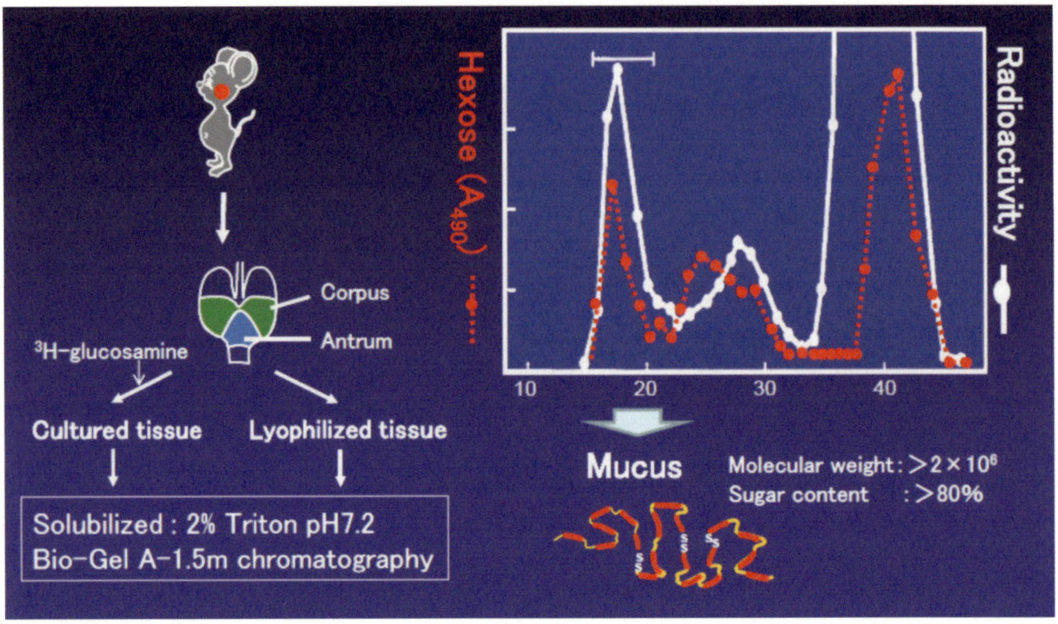

Fig. 5. Preparation of labeled and unlabeled mucus.

tried. As a result, it was confirmed that the mucus gel layer alone can be separated without damaging the surface epithelium when *N*-acetylcysteine is used as a mucolytic agent (Komuro et al., 1991). At present, it has become possible to remove the gel layer, to scrape the surface mucosa and deep mucosa, and then to determine the mucin content in the mucus for each region and each layer (Komuro et al., 1992a, 1992b). Our scraping method enables us to biochemically assess the mucin content of the gel layer by separating it from the deep mucosa of the stomach, and we have demonstrated that quantitative changes in the gastric mucin are closely related to mucosal protective activity (Kojima et al., 1992, 1993; Ichikawa et al., 1994a; Komuro et al., 1998).

3.3 Development of monoclonal antibody against gastric mucin

Previous studies have shown that different types of mucin, differing in their carbohydrates and core protein structure, are expressed in different regions of the gastrointestinal tract. In the stomach, the corpus mucin differs from the antral mucin, and in each region the surface-type mucins (surface mucus cell-type mucins) differ from the gland-type mucins, synthesized in deeper layers of the gastric mucosa (Corfield et al. 2000). Histochemical studies revealed that surface-type mucins have different carbohydrate chains from gland-type mucins in the stomach. For instance, surface-type mucins were stained by galactose oxidase-cold thionine Schiff (GOTS) staining, while glandular mucins were stained by paradoxical concanavalin A staining (PCS) (Ota et al., 1991; Ota & Katsuyama, 1992). On the other hand, studies using gene technology revealed that, in the stomach, the mucin bearing MUC5AC core protein was expressed in the surface mucosa, while MUC6 was expressed in the glandular mucosa (De Bolos et al., 1995; Ho et al., 1995a, 1995b; Buisine et al, 2000). The biochemical characterization of individual mucin molecules is important to understand their functions, and specific tools to recognize particular mucin species are essential. For these purposes, many monoclonal antibodies (mAbs) against mucins have been developed and used in our laboratory (Ishihara et al., 1993). Representative anti-mucin monoclonal antibodies are shown in Figure 6. The mAbs RGM21 and HIK1083, which recognize a specific carbohydrate portion of rat gastric surface- and gland-type mucins, respectively (Ishihara et al., 1996a, 1996b), are frequently used to characterize the different mucin molecular structures. From histological studies and epitope analyses, the characteristics of each antibody have been elucidated (Goso et al., 1999, 2003, 2009; Tsubokawa et al., 2007, 2009).

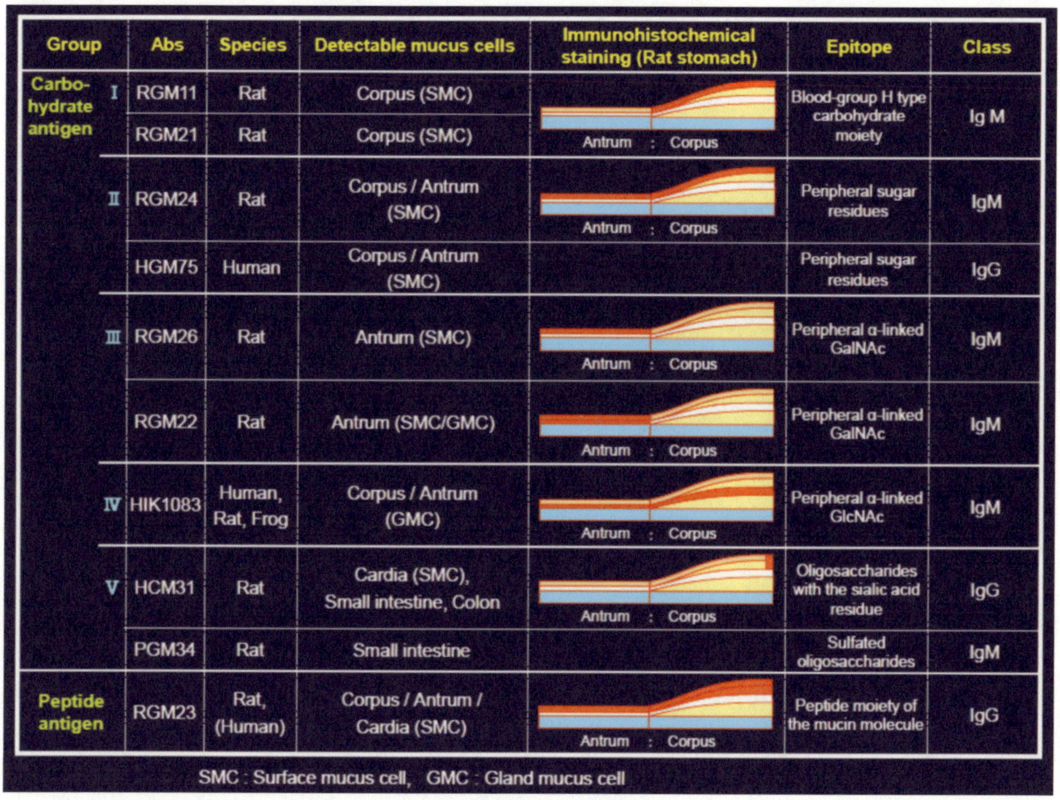

Group		Abs	Species	Detectable mucus cells	Immunohistochemical staining (Rat stomach)	Epitope	Class
Carbo-hydrate antigen	I	RGM11	Rat	Corpus (SMC)	Antrum : Corpus	Blood-group H type carbohydrate moiety	Ig M
		RGM21	Rat	Corpus (SMC)			
	II	RGM24	Rat	Corpus / Antrum (SMC)	Antrum : Corpus	Peripheral sugar residues	IgM
		HGM75	Human	Corpus / Antrum (SMC)		Peripheral sugar residues	IgG
	III	RGM26	Rat	Antrum (SMC)	Antrum : Corpus	Peripheral α-linked GalNAc	IgM
		RGM22	Rat	Antrum (SMC/GMC)	Antrum : Corpus	Peripheral α-linked GalNAc	IgM
	IV	HIK1083	Human, Rat, Frog	Corpus / Antrum (GMC)	Antrum : Corpus	Peripheral α-linked GlcNAc	IgM
	V	HCM31	Rat	Cardia (SMC), Small intestine, Colon	Antrum : Corpus	Oligosaccharides with the sialic acid residue	IgG
		PGM34	Rat	Small intestine		Sulfated oligosaccharides	IgM
Peptide antigen		RGM23	Rat, (Human)	Corpus / Antrum / Cardia (SMC)	Antrum : Corpus	Peptide moiety of the mucin molecule	IgG

SMC : Surface mucus cell, GMC : Gland mucus cell

Fig. 6. Representative anti-mucin monoclonal antibodies.

4. Changes of gastric mucus and mucosal protection

4.1 Gastric mucosal protection

The gastric mucosa acts to maintain homeostasis through the physiological mechanism naturally given to it in the presence of endogenous irritants such as gastric acid, pepsin, and exogenous irritants such as NSAIDs, stress, and alcohol (Fig. 7). During the protection of the mucosa, various factors such as bicarbonate ion, mucosal blood flow and cell turnover are involved other than the mucus. In recent years, the roles played by indirect factors such as prostaglandin and superoxide dismutase have also been clarified. These factors interact with each other, and damage to the mucosa occurs through an imbalance between the aggressive factors and protective factors (Fig. 7).

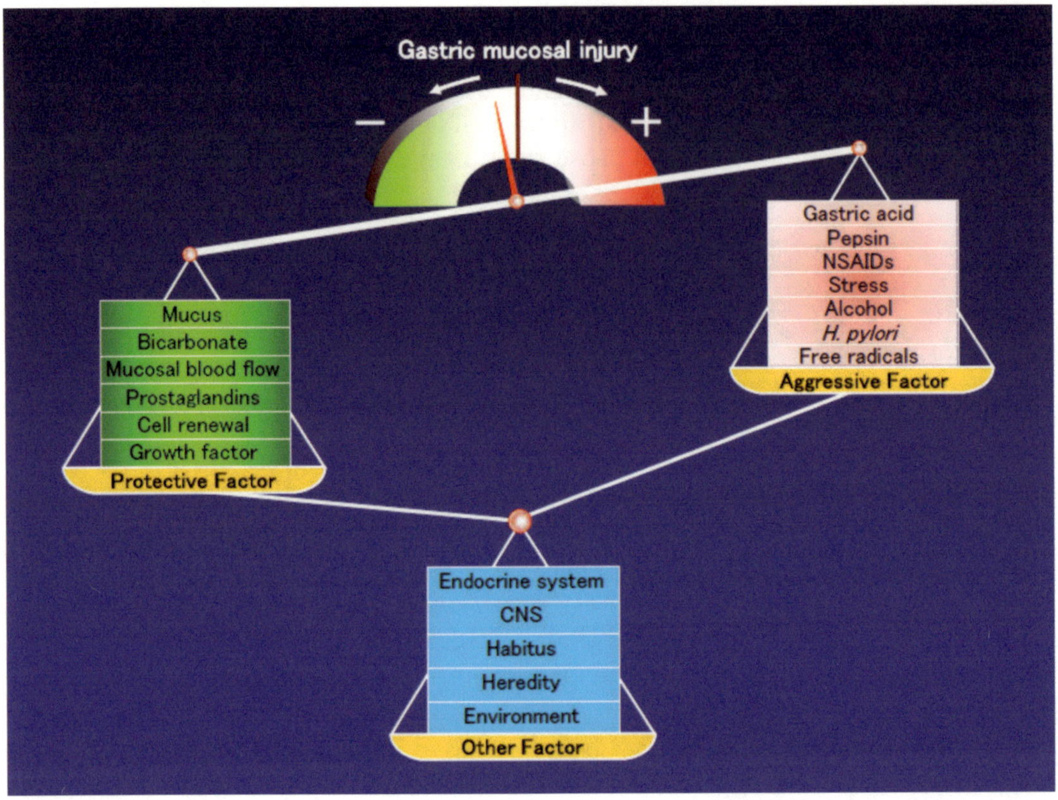

Fig. 7. Gastric protection: which is stronger, aggressive factor or protective factor?

4.2 Changes of gastric mucus

The response of the gastric mucosa to acute injury is uniform regardless of the damaging agent; it usually results in exfoliation of the surface epithelium and injury of deeper mucosal layers. Deep mucosal injury is most likely caused, at least in part, by injury to the gastric mucosal microvasculature. Acute injury is most often produced by alcohol, aspirin, indomethacin, and other NSAIDs.

Figure 8 shows the changes of rat gastric mucosa after orally administration of aspirin (100 mg/kg in 0.15N HCl). In the control rat, after fasting for 24 hr, surface mucus cells of the corpus were strongly stained by RGM21 (Fig. 8a). After the administration of aspirin, the immunohistochemical reactivity of RGM21 in the corpus of the rat stomach had decreased when compared with the control situation (Fig. 8b). Figure 8c shows the gastric mucosa treated with teprenone (geranylgeranylacetone) 3 hr after aspirin administration. Teprenone is a gastric mucosal protective drug without affecting gastric acid secretion and clinically used in Japan for treatment of gastritis. This drug has been reported to reveal various pharmacological actions including the promotion of gastrointestinal mucus (Iwai et al., 2011; Rokutan et al., 2000).

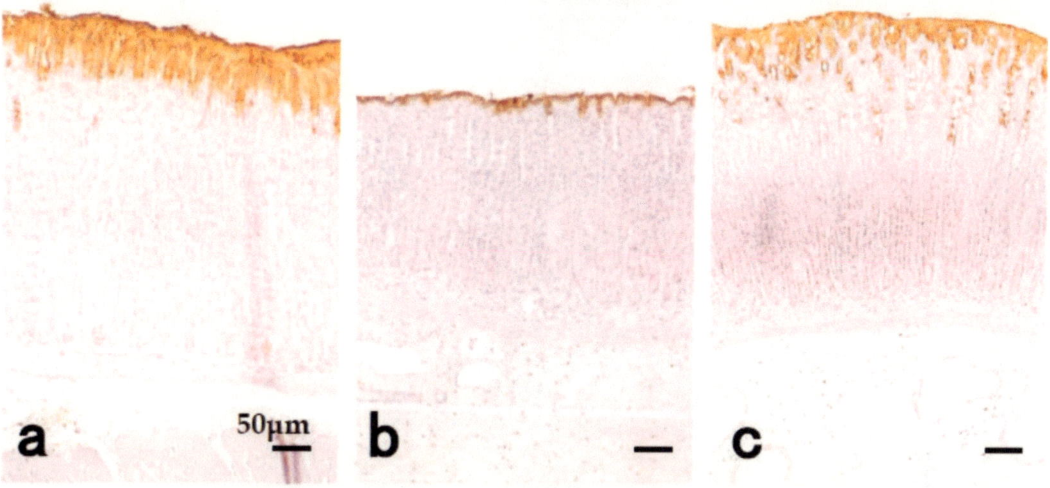

Fig. 8. Immunohistochemical staining with RGM21 in the gastric mucosa. (a) Normal control rat. (b) Aspirin (100 mg/kg) was administered orally and lesion formation was assessed 3 hr later. (c) Rat treated with teprenone (200 mg/kg) after aspirin administration.

4.3 Regulatory mechanism of gastric mucus metabolism

It has been elucidated that various factors are involved in the regulation of the mucus metabolism and each of these factors acts on some specific kind of mucus cells (Fig. 9). Among the endogenous regulatory factors of the stomach, gastrin, histamine and carbachol, which have an acid secretory action, EGF and HGF, which are growth factors and PG, which is an autacoid, are all able to increase the biosynthesis of the gastric mucin. However, a difference is seen in the mucin synthetic reactions based on these factors. Thus, the increase in mucin biosynthesis induced by gastrin among these acid secretagogues can be observed in the surface mucus cells of the gastric oxyntic mucosa, indicating that it occurs by way of specific gastrin receptors independent of the acid secretion mechanism (Ichikawa et al., 1993). Moreover, gastrin stimulates the process of glycosylation without any change in the backbone peptide elongation, and the stimulation is mediated by nitric oxide (NO). Histamine activates the peptide biosynthesis process of mucin, but this process is not mediated by NO. On the other hand, carbachol stimulates the biosynthesis of the mucin peptide as well as the glycosylation step, both in the corpus and the antrum (Ichikawa et al., 1998). As shown in Figure 9, EGF and HGF have distinct effects on the mucin biosynthesis in a specific region of gastric mucosa without their trophic effects (Ichikawa et al., 2000a, 2000b). In other words, endogenous regulatory factors act on the mucus-producing cells through different modes of action, thus regulating their biosynthesis. It has also been indicated that different regulatory mechanisms are present at various sites in the stomach, and that NO and neuropeptides are involved in part of the regulatory process (Ichikawa et al., 2000c).

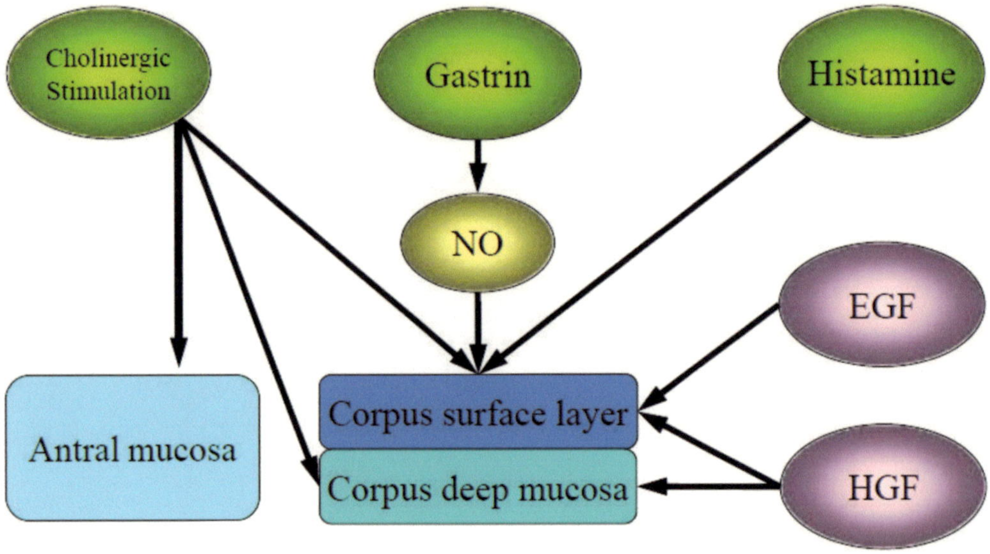

Fig. 9. Regulation of gastric mucin biosynthesis.

5. Second-generation H_2-blockers

5.1 Structure of second-generation H_2-blockers

The H_2-blockers are widely used these days in the treatment of gastritis. The chemical structures of some frequently used H_2-blockers are shown in Figure 10. All the known H_2-blockers comprise an aromatic ring with a flexible chain joined to a polar group. Despite considerable diversity, these compounds can be grouped into two main series according to the nature of the aromatic rings, namely five-membered and six-membered aromatic ring series. Cimetidine and ranitidine belong to the conventional group characterized by a five-membered aromatic ring. Recently, some of the newer H_2-blockers (so-called second-generation H_2-blockers) have been reported to promote the gastric mucosal defense mechanisms (Fukushima et al., 2006; Harada et al., 2007; Marazova et al. 1998; Murashima et al., 2009; Saegusa et al., 2008; Ichikawa et al., 2009a). Second-generation H_2-blockers contain a six-membered aromatic ring, instead of a five-membered heterocyclic ring.

Of the four H_2-blockers shown in Figure 10, lafutidine and roxatidine have a stimulant effect on mucin biosynthesis in the rat gastric mucosa. In contrast, first-generation H_2-receptor antagonists such as cimetidine, ranitidine and famotidine, failed to stimulate mucin biosynthesis (Ichikawa et al., 1994b, 2009b). Second-generation H_2-blockers, lafutidine and roxatidine, have been reported to prevent the formation of gastric mucosal lesions induced by necrotizing agents in rats (Fukushima et al., 2006; Shiratsuchi et al., 1988), and this effect may be due not only to the inhibition of aggressive factors such as acid, but also to the maintenance of defensive factors such as mucus. On the other hand, many reports have indicated that cimetidine and ranitidine lack a protective effect against necrotizing agent-induced gastric mucosal damage in the rat (Shiratsuchi et al., 1988; Tarnawski et al., 1985).

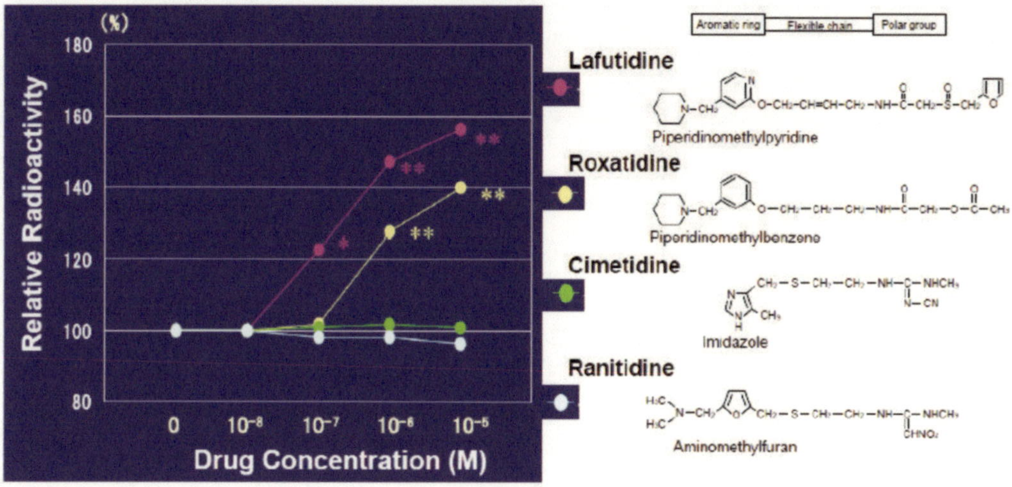

Fig. 10. Effects of representative H_2-blockers on mucin biosynthesis.

5.2 Structure-activity relationship for gastroprotective actions

The above findings have clarified that the second-generation H_2-blockers have a unique structure, and not only inhibit acid secretion but also enhance the protective mechanisms of the gastric mucosa. This should stimulate new interest in the chemical analysis of these drugs to determine the structural requirements for their gastroprotective actions.

Compared with the structural requirements of the acid-inhibitory mechanisms of the H_2-blockers, only a few detailed analyses have been reported of the structural aspects of their gastroprotective actions (Ichikawa et al., 1996, 1997; Sekine et al., 1998; Hirakawa et al., 1998) because of the complicated mechanisms of mucosal protection. However, the cardinal chemical features of lafutidine that determine its mucin biosynthetic activity, as a quantitative index of its gastroprotective action, were identified by considering the structural analogs (Fig. 11) of this drug using an rat stomach organ culture system (Ichikawa et al., 1996). As shown in Figure 11, compounds A, B and C bear the pyridine ring and compounds D and E bear the furan ring, which are commonly present in the structure of lafutidine. Mucin biosynthetic activity was increased by the addition of two pyridine derivatives, lafutidine and compound A. In contrast, compounds D and E, lacking a pyridine ring, failed to stimulate mucin biosynthesis. Similar results were obtained for compounds B and C, which have a pyridine ring but lack an amide structure. These results indicate that pyridine-based compounds containing an amide structure may be essential for activating the gastroprotective function. Furthermore, comparison with the H_2-receptor antagonistic activities of these compounds suggests that H_2-receptor antagonism is not directly correlated with lafutidine-induced stimulation of mucin biosynthesis.

A more detailed analysis has been performed using roxatidine and its structural analogs to reveal the structural requirements of second-generation H_2-blockers for the stimulant effect on rat gastric mucin biosynthesis, particularly with regard to whether the cardinal features of roxatidine are only the six-membered aromatic ring and amide structure, and its relation to H_2-receptor antagonism (Ichikawa et al., 1997). Of six compounds containing both a benzene ring and an amide structure, analogs A and B, but not C, stimulated mucin biosynthesis in a manner similar to that of roxatidine. These three compounds contain a

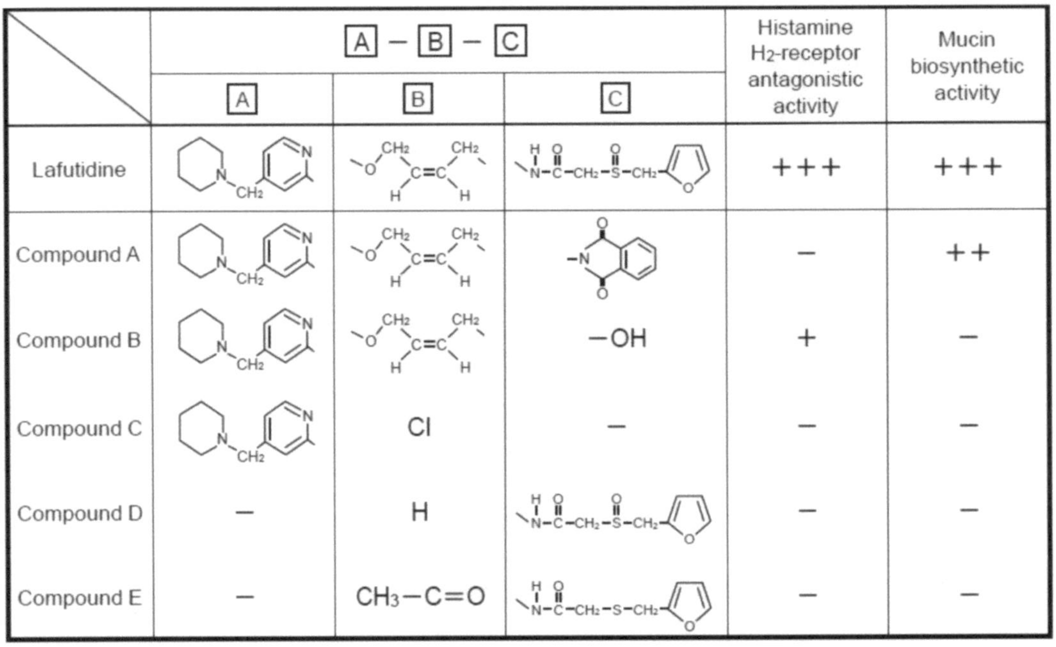

Fig. 11. Structures and pharmacological activities of lafutidine and its analogs. Mucin biosynthetic activity was evaluated in an organ culture system of the rat stomach. Score was divided into the following 4 groups: -, no effect at 1 x 10^{-6} M; +, under 20% increase from the baseline at dose of 1 x 10^{-6} M; ++, significant 20-30% increase of biosynthetic activity ($p < 0.05$) at 1 x 10^{-6} M; +++, significant over 30% increase of mucin biosynthesis ($p < 0.01$) at 1 x 10^{-6} M. Histamine H_2-receptor antagonistic activity was investigated on the histamine-induced positive chronotropic responses in the isolated guinea-pig right atria. Score was divided into the following 4 groups: -, no effect at 1 x 10^{-5} M; +, under 70% inhibition at 1 x 10^{-6} M; ++, 70-90% inhibition at 1 x 10^{-6} M; +++, over 90% inhibition at 1 x 10^{-6} M. Data are taken from the reference (Ichikawa et al., 1996).

piperidine ring (indicated by R_1 in Figure 12) attached to the benzene ring via a methylene bridge, but the length of the flexible chain (indicated by R_2 in Figure 12) of analog C differs from that of roxatidine. This means that the length of the flexible chain between the benzene ring and the amide structure is essential for this stimulation of mucin biosynthesis. Analogs D, E and F, having different ring structures or no ring structure at R_1 of the roxatidine molecule, failed to activate mucin biosynthesis. Analogs D, E and F contain the same flexible chain as roxatidine. Thus, the piperidine ring is also important for their activity. These results indicate that the structural requirements for the stimulant effect of roxatidine on mucin biosynthesis are not only the six-membered aromatic ring and amide structure, but the attachment of the piperidinomethyl group and the appropriate length of the flexible chain are also important for this function. With regard to their H_2-receptor antagonistic properties, the six analogs were investigated using competition with the binding of the radiolabeled H_2-receptor antagonist [^{125}I]iodoaminopotentidine to membranes of the guinea pig striatum (Leurs et al., 1994; Ruat et al., 1990). All compounds, except analog F in Figure 12, displaced the specific [^{125}I]iodoaminopotentidine binding to H_2-receptor sites. The relative potencies of these antagonists were: analog B > A > roxatidine > D > C > E. Compared with the IC_{50} value (concentration required to inhibit 50% of specific binding) for cimetidine obtained under similar experimental conditions, roxatidine and analogs A, B, C and D were 4.6, 9.5, 13.7, 1.6 and 2.7 times more potent than cimetidine, respectively (Ichikawa et al., 1997). These results suggest that H_2-receptor antagonism does not directly correlate with roxatidine-induced stimulation of mucin biosynthesis.

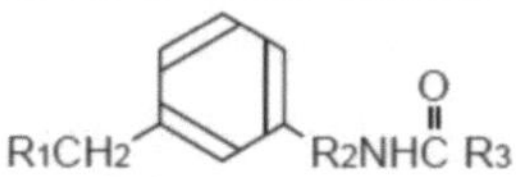

	R1	R2	R3	Histamine H_2-receptor antagonistic activity	Mucin biosynthetic activity
Roxatidine	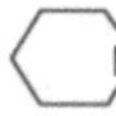 N−	$-OCH_2CH_2CH_2-$	$-CH_2OCOCH_3$	+++	+++
Analog A	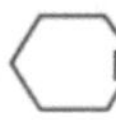 N−	$-OCH_2CH_2CH_2-$	$-CH_2OH$	+++	+++
Analog B	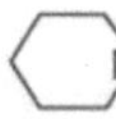 N−	$-OCH_2CH_2CH_2-$	$-CH_3$	++++	++
Analog C	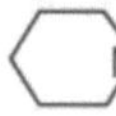 N−	$-OCH_2CH_2CH_2CH_2-$	$-CH_3$	++	−
Analog D	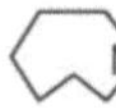 N−	$-OCH_2CH_2CH_2-$	$-CH_3$	++	−
Analog E	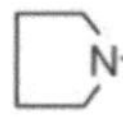 N−	$-OCH_2CH_2CH_2-$	$-CH_3$	+	−
Analog F	CH_3 CH_3 >N−	$-OCH_2CH_2CH_2-$	$-CH_3$	−	−

Fig. 12. Structures and pharmacological activities of roxatidine and its analogs. Mucin biosynthetic activity was evaluated in an organ culture system of the rat stomach. Score was divided into the following 4 groups: -, no effect at 1 x 10^{-6} M; +, under 20% increase from the baseline at dose of 1 x 10^{-6} M; ++, significant 20-30% increase of biosynthetic activity ($p <$ 0.05) at 1 x 10^{-6} M; +++, significant over 30% increase of mucin biosynthesis ($p < 0.01$) at 1 x 10^{-6} M. Histamine H_2-receptor antagonistic activity was investigated on the competition studies with [^{125}I]iodoaminopotentidine binding to membranes of the guinea-pig striatum. IC_{50} values (concentration required to inhibit 50% of specific binding) were determined and divided into the following 5 groups: -, IC_{50} > 4000 nM; +, 800 > IC_{50} > 500 nM (similar to cimetidine in the antagonism); ++, 500 > IC_{50} > 200 nM; +++, 200 > IC_{50} > 50 nM; ++++, 50 nM > IC_{50}. Data are taken from the reference (Ichikawa et al., 1997).

Taken together, these data indicate that the structural requirements for mucosal protective activity in the second-generation H_2-blockers are their amide structure and six-membered aromatic ring, such as benzene and pyridine derivatives. The cardinal chemical features of roxatidine for the activation of mucin biosynthesis are the appropriate length of the flexible chain between the amide structure and the aromatic ring system bearing the methylpiperidinyl group at the meta position. The thioether function can confer increased gastroprotective activity on lafutidine.

5.3 Effects of lafutidine on the mucus barrier

The adherent mucus gel layer is the functionally important component of the mucus barrier in the human stomach. However, it cannot be demonstrated by routine histological techniques because of its susceptibility to dehydration and shrinkage, which has hampered research. The developed method of stabilizing this layer with Carnoy's solution revealed that its laminated structure was composed of two types of mucin in alternating layers; one mucin is derived from the surface mucus cells and the other from the gland mucus cells. The surface mucus gel layer in Carnoy-fixed tissue sections is shown in the hematoxylin and eosin (HE) preparation (Figs. 13A, C) of the human gastric mucosa. This layer is well preserved and appeared as a thick eosinophilic band. The galactose oxidase/thionine Schiff reaction/paradoxical concanavalin A (GOTS-PCS) procedure stained surface mucus cells blue and gland mucus cells brown (Figs. 13B, D). The surface mucus gel layer consistently shows the laminated structure in the samples of gastric corpus mucosa from both the lafutidine positive and negative groups (Figs. 13B, D). The mucin produced by human gastric gland mucus cells appears to function as a natural antibiotic, protecting the host from *H. pylori* (Kawakubo et al., 2004). Figure 13 demonstrates that after administration of lafutidine there is thickening of the surface mucus gel layer. In other studies using experimental animals, lafutidine has been shown to possess gastroprotective properties, such as strengthening the mucus gel layer, apart from its antisecretory activity (Ichikawa et al., 1994a; Onodera et al., 1999a; Sato et al., 2003).

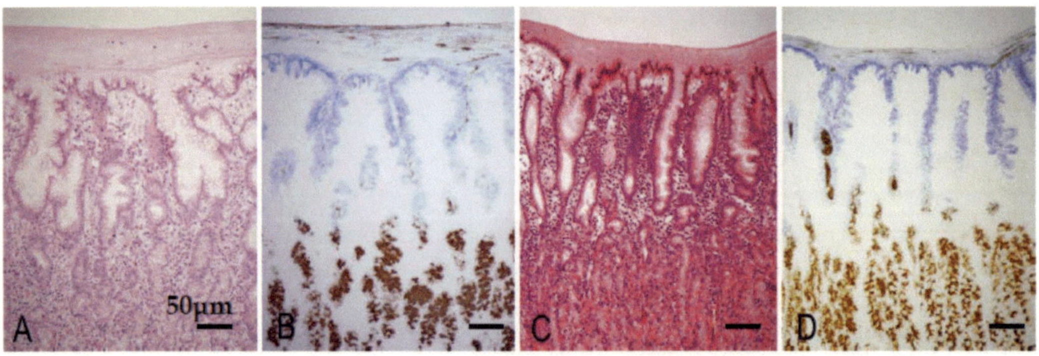

Fig. 13. Surface mucus gel layer of the human gastric mucosa from (A, B) lafutidine positive and (C, D) lafutidine negative groups stained with (A, C) HE and (B, D) GOTS-PCS.

5.4 Mechanisms of gastroprotective actions

Although the exact mechanisms that underlie the gastroprotective activity of the second-generation H_2-receptor antagonists are not well understood, recent findings suggest that the activation of capsaicin-sensitive sensory neurons is associated with their maintenance of gastric mucosal integrity (Fukushima et al., 2006; Harada et al., 2007; Murashima et al., 2009; Sugiyama et al., 2008). The gastrointestinal tract is known to possess a rich neural network, among which afferent neurons of extrinsic origin are reported to operate as the emergency protective system. The discovery of these sensory neuron functions was made possible by capsaicin, a pharmacological tool with which the activity of certain primary afferent neurons can be manipulated selectively. Capsaicin is an excitotoxin that acutely stimulates a group of afferent neurons with unmyelinated (C) or thinly myelinated (Aδ) nerve fibers. This excitotoxic action is restricted to neurons with C- and Aδ-fibers because only these cells express receptor-binding sites (vanilloid receptor type 1: VR1) for capsaicin and structurally related ligands. The mammalian stomach, particularly the submucosa, is densely innervated with capsaicin-sensitive afferent neurons. These neurons not only serve a sensory and afferent role, but also display a local effector function initiated by the release of neuropeptide transmitters, such as calcitonin gene-related peptide (CGRP) and substance P, from their peripheral nerve endings. CGRP is reported to exhibit significant mucosal protective roles in the gastrointestinal tract (Ichikawa et al., 2000c; Mizuguchi et al., 2005; Ohno et al., 2008). The action of CGRP is in part mediated by endogenous NO.

The gastroprotective action of lafutidine has been reduced or abolished by treatment with tetrodotoxin, $CGRP_{8-37}$, or chemical defunctionalisation of afferent nerves (Mimaki et al., 2002; Onodera et al., 1999a), indicating that capsaicin-sensitive nerves contribute significantly to the mechanisms underlying the actions of lafutidine (Nishihara et al., 2002). Moreover, lafutidine has been shown to significantly increase CGRP release in both experimental animal models and humans (Harada & Okajima, 2007; Nishihara et al., 2002; Ikawa et al., 2006; Shimatani et al., 2006). Several reports indicate that the VR1 of capsaicin-sensitive afferent nerves may not contribute the CGRP release by lafutidine, suggesting the existence of yet unidentified sites for lafutidine other than VR1 on these nerves (Fukushima et al., 2006; Nishihara et al., 2002). The gastroprotective effects of lafutidine are decreased by treatment with NO synthase inhibitors or NO antidotes (Nishihara et al., 2002; Ichikawa et al., 1998), indicating the involvement of NO generation in lafutidine function. Similar results have been obtained with another second-generation H_2-receptor antagonist, roxatidine (Ichikawa et al., 1997, 1999).

Lafutidine has been shown to enhance the healing of gastrointestinal mucosal lesions in a manner independent of its antacid secretory action (Kato et al., 2000; Onodera et al., 2004). However, lafutidine by itself does not have any direct effects on cell migration or proliferation. An earlier study demonstrated that lafutidine does not influence the impaired healing of epithelial wounds in RGM1 cells under *in vitro* conditions without neuronal innervations (Murashima et al., 2009), again confirming the importance of sensory neurons in the healing-promoting action of this agent. Several studies show that luminal lafutidine stimulates capsaicin-sensitive afferent nerves via presumably direct diffusion rather than after its absorption from intestine followed by via circulation, suggesting the rapid local diffusion reaching to the afferents before H_2-receptor blockade from the circulation (Onodera et al., 1999b; Nagahama et al., 2003). Second-generation H_2-receptor antagonists such as lafutidine are thought to facilitate capsaicin-sensitive sensory afferent nerves and exert gastroprotective effects through CGRP and in part via NO release in the stomach.

6. Summary and perspectives

The gastric mucus barrier constituted by the layer of viscous mucus is crucial to the defense of gastric mucosa. In this review, we have shown a new perspective on the ability of certain therapeutic agent for gastritis to strengthen gastric mucosal defense system. The development of mAbs against the carbohydrate moiety of gastric mucin with a different specificity is really a significant event. With the use of these mAbs, it would be possible to separately identify and determine the various mucins. Through the establishment of the mucus determining method, which utilizes mAbs, the roles of the mucus with different origins as protecting factors would be made clearer.

Second-generation H_2-blockers offer the possibility of more effective prevention of gastritis through the activation of mucosal defense mechanisms (Fig. 14). The structural requirements for mucosal protective activity in these antagonists were shown to be the amide structure and six-membered aromatic ring, such as benzene and pyridine derivatives. The cardinal chemical features of roxatidine for the activation of mucin biosynthesis are the appropriate length of the flexible chain between the amide structure and the aromatic ring system bearing the methylpiperidinyl group at the meta position. Although the exact mechanism underlying the gastroprotective action associated with these agents is unknown, capsaicin-sensitive nerves and CGRP/NO pathway are considered responsible for their anti-ulcer effects in experimental animal models of various gastric mucosal injuries. These mechanisms are also involved in the cytoprotective properties of gastrin, which is a physiologically important bioactive peptide (Ichikawa et al., 1998, 2000c). Taken together, these findings suggest the gastroprotective effects of second-generation H_2-blockers may be of physiological relevance.

Enhanced understanding of the mechanisms of gastric mucosal defense and injury provides new insight into potential therapeutic targets, which contributes towards the development of more well tolerated and more effective therapies.

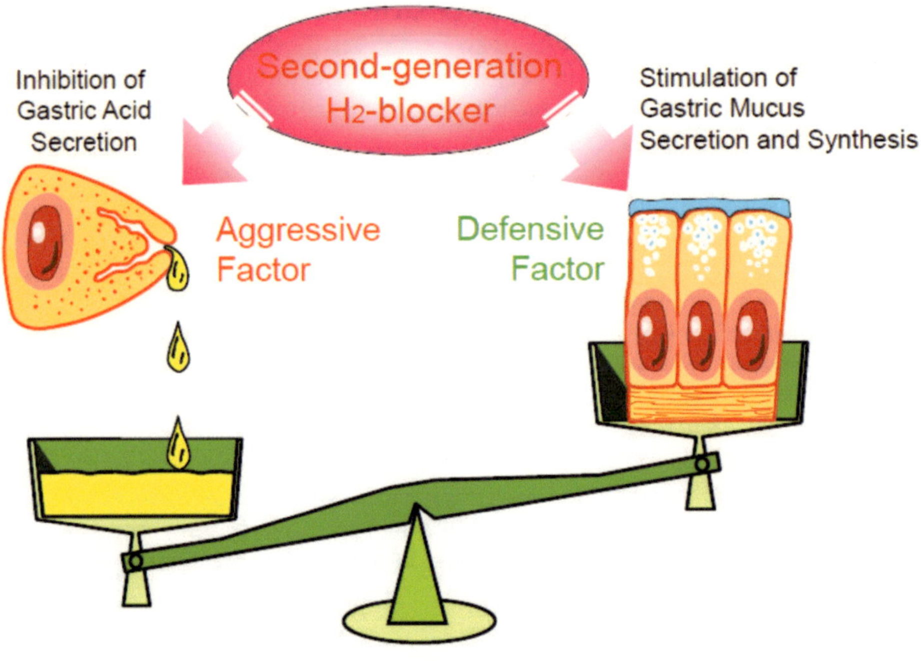

Fig. 14. Dual action of second-generation H_2-blockers.

7. References

Azuumi, Y.; Ohara, S.; Ishihara, K.; Okabe, H. & Hotta, K. (1980). Correlation of quantitative changes of gastric mucosal glycoproteins with aspirin-induced gastric damage in rats. *Gut* Vol.21, No.6, pp.533-536, ISSN 0017-5749

Buisine, M.P.; Devisme, L.; Maunoury, V.; Deschodt, E.; Gosselin, B.; Copin, M.C.; Aubert, J.P. & Porchet, N. (2000). Developmental mucin gene expression in the gastroduodenal tract and accessory digestive glands. I. Stomach. A relationship to gastric carcinoma. *J Histochem Cytochem* Vol.48, No.12, pp.1657-1666, ISSN 0022-1554

Corfield, A.P.; Myerscough, N.; Longman, R.; Sylvester, P.; Arul, S. & Pignatelli M. (2000). Mucins and mucosal protection in the gastrointestinal tract: new prospects for mucins in the pathology of gastrointestinal disease. *Gut* Vol.47, No.4, pp.589-594, ISSN 0017-5749

De Bolos, C., Garrido, M. & Real, F.X. (1995). MUC6 apomucin shows a distinct normal tissue distribution that correlates with Lewis antigen expression in the human stomach. *Gastroenterology* Vol.10, No.3, pp.723-734, ISSN 0016-5085

Dekker, J. & Strous, G.J. (1990). Covalent oligomerization of rat gastric mucin occurs in the rough endoplasmic reticulum, is *N*-glycosylation-dependent, and precedes initial *O*-glycosylation. *J Biol Chem* Vol.265, No.30, pp.18116-18122, ISSN 0021-9258

Fukushima, K.; Aoi, Y.; Kato, S. & Takeuchi, K. (2006). Gastro-protective action of lafutidine mediated by capsaicin-sensitive afferent neurons without interaction with TRPV1 and involvement of endogenous prostaglandins. *World J Gastroenterol* Vo.12, No.19, 3031-3037, ISSN 1007-9327

Goso, Y.; Ikezawa, T.; Kurihara, M.; Endo, M.; Hotta, K. & Ishihara, K. (2003). Characterization of rat gastric mucins using a monoclonal antibody, RGM23, recognizing surface mucous cell-type mucins. *J Biochem* Vo.133, No.4, pp.453-460, ISSN 0021-924X

Goso, Y.; Ishihara, K.; Kurihara, M.; Sugaya, T. & Hotta, K. (1999). Rat gastric mucins recognized by monoclonal antibodies RGM21 and HIK1083: isolation of mucin species characteristic of the surface and glandular mucosa. *J Biochem* Vol.126, No.2, pp.375-381, ISSN 0021-924X

Goso, Y.; Tsubokawa, D. & Ishihara, K. (2009). Evaluation of conditions for release of mucin-type oligosaccharides from glycoproteins by hydrazine gas treatment. *J Biochem* Vol.145, No.6, pp.739-749, ISSN 1756-2651

Harada, N. & Okajima, K. (2007). Inhibition of neutrophil activation by lafutidine, an H_2-receptor antagonist, through enhancement of sensory neuron activation contributes to the reduction of stress-induced gastric mucosal injury in rats. *Dig Dis Sci* Vo.52, No.2, 469-477, 0163-2116

Hayashida, H.; Ishihara, K.; Ichikawa, T.; Okayasu, I.; Kurihara, M.; Saigenji, K. & Hotta, K. (2001). Expression of a specific mucin type recognized by monoclonal antibodies in the rat gastric mucosa regenerating from acetic acid-induced ulcer. *Scand J Gastroenterol* Vol.36, No.5, pp.467-473, ISSN 0036-5521

Hirakawa, N.; Matsumoto, H.; Hosoda, A.; Sekine, A.; Yamaura, T. & Sekine, Y. (1998). A novel histamine 2 (H_2) receptor antagonist with gastroprotective activity. II. Synthesis and pharmacological evaluation of 2-furfuryl-thio and 2-furfurylsulfinyl acetamide derivatives with heteroaromatic rings. *Chem Pharm Bull (Tokyo)* Vol.46, No.4, pp.616-622, ISSN 0009-2363

Ho, S.B.; Roberton, A.M.; Shekels, L.L.; Lyftogt, C.T.; Niehans, G.A. & Toribara, N.W. (1995a). Expression cloning of gastric mucin complementary DNA and localization of mucin gene expression. *Gastroenterology* Vol.109, No.3, 735-747, ISSN 0016-5085

Ho, S.B.; Shekels, L.L.; Toribara, N.W.; Kim, Y.S.; Lyftogt, C.; Cherwitz, D.L. & Niehans, G.A. (1995b). Mucin gene expression in normal, preneoplastic, and neoplastic human gastric epithelium. *Cancer Res* Vol.55, No.12, pp.2681-2690, ISSN 0008-5472

Hotta, K. (2000). "Gastric mucus", a mysterious and interesting substance. *Trends in Glycoscience and Glycotechnology* Vol.12, No. 63, pp.59-68, ISSN 0915-7352

Ichikawa, T.; Endoh, H.; Hotta, K. & Ishihara (2000a). Hepatocyte growth factor region specifically activates mucin synthesis in rat stomach. *Eur J Pharmacol* Vol.392, No.1-2, pp.87-91, ISSN 0014-2999

Ichikawa, T.; Endoh, H.; Hotta, K. & Ishihara (2000b). The mucin biosynthesis stimulated by epidermal growth factor occurs in surface mucus cells, but not in gland mucus cells, of rat stomach. *Life Sci* Vol.67, No.9, pp.1095-1101, ISSN 0024-3205

Ichikawa, T.; Hotta, K. & Ishihara, K. (2009a). Second-generation histamine H_2-receptor antagonists with gastric mucosal defensive properties. *Mini Rev Med Chem* Vo.9, No.5, pp.581-589, ISSN 1389-5575

Ichikawa, T.; Ishihara, K.; Komuro, Y.; Kojima, Y.; Saigenji, K. & Hotta, K. (1994a). Effects of the new histamine H_2 receptor antagonist, FRG-8813, on gastric mucin in rats with or without acidified ethanol-induced gastric damage. *Life Sci* Vol.54, No.10, pp.PL159-164, ISSN 0024-3205

Ichikawa, T.; Ishihara, K.; Kusakabe, T.; Hiruma, H.; Kawakami, T. & Hotta, K. (2000c). CGRP modulates mucin synthesis in surface mucus cells of rat gastric oxyntic mucosa. *Am J Physiol* Vol.279, No.1, pp.G82-89, ISSN 0193-1857

Ichikawa, T.; Ishihara, K.; Kusakabe, T.; Kawakami, T. & Hotta, K. (1999). Stimulant effect of nitric oxide generator and roxatidine on mucin biosynthesis of rat gastric oxyntic mucosa. *Life Sci* Vol.65, No.4, pp.PL41-46, ISSN 0024-3205

Ichikawa, T.; Ishihara, K.; Kusakabe, T.; Kurihara, M.; Kawakami, T.; Takenaka, T.; Saigenji, K. & Hotta, K. (1998). Distinct effects of tetragastrin, histamine, and CCh on rat gastric mucin synthesis and contribution of NO. *Am J Physiol* Vol.274, No.1, pp.G138-146, ISSN 0002-9513

Ichikawa, T.; Ishihara, K.; Saigenji, K. & Hotta, K. (1993). Stimulation of mucus glycoprotein biosynthesis in rat gastric mucosa by gastrin. *Biochem Pharmacol* Vol.46, No.9, pp.1551-1557, ISSN 0006-2952

Ichikawa, T.; Ishihara, K.; Saigenji, K. & Hotta, K. (1994b). Effects of acid-inhibitory antiulcer drugs on mucin biosynthesis in the rat stomach. *Eur J Pharmacol* Vol.251, No.1, pp.107-111, ISSN 0014-2999

Ichikawa, T.; Ishihara, K.; Saigenji, K. & Hotta, K. (1997). Structural requirements for roxatidine in the stimulant effect of rat gastric mucin synthesis and the participation of nitric oxide in this mechanism. *Br J Pharmacol* Vol.122, No.6, pp.1230-1236, ISSN 0007-1188

Ichikawa, T.; Ishihara, K.; Shibata, M.; Yamaura, T.; Saigenji, K. & Hotta, K. (1996). Stimulation of mucin biosynthesis in rat gastric mucosa by FRG-8813 and its structural analogs. *Eur J Pharmacol* Vol.297, No.1-2, pp.87-92, ISSN 0014-2999

Ichikawa, T.; Ito, Y.; Saegusa, Y.; Iwai, T.; Goso, Y.; Ikezawa, T. & Ishihara, K. (2009b). Effects of combination treatment with famotidine and methylmethionine sulfonium chloride on the mucus barrier of rat gastric mucosa. *J Gastroenterol Hepatol* Vol.24, No.3, pp.488-492, ISSN 1440-1746

Ikawa, K.; Shimatani, T.; Azuma, Y.; Inoue, M. & Morikawa, N. (2006). Calcitonin gene-related peptide and somatostatin releases correlated with the area under the lafutidine concentration-time curve in human plasma. *J Clin Pharm Ther* Vol.31, No.4, pp.351-356, ISSN 0269-4727

Ikezawa, T.; Goso, Y.; Ichikawa, T.; Hayashida, H.; Kurihara, M.; Okayasu, I.; Saigenji, K. & Ishihara, K. (2004). Appearance of specific mucins recognized by monoclonal antibodies in rat gastric mucosa healing from HCl-induced gastric mucosal damage. *J Gastroenterol* Vol.39, No.2, pp.113-119, ISSN 0944-1174

Ishihara, K.; Kurihara, M.; Eto, H.; Kasai, K.; Shimauchi, S. & Hotta, K. (1993). A monoclonal antibody against carbohydrate moiety of rat gastric surface epithelial cell-derived mucin. *Hybridoma* Vol.12, No.5, pp.609-620, ISSN 0272-457X

Ishihara, K.; Kurihara, M.; Goso, Y.; Ota, H.; Katsuyama, T. & Hotta, K. (1996a). Establishment of monoclonal antibodies against carbohydrate moiety of gastric mucins distributed in the different sites and layers of rat gastric mucosa. *Glycoconj J* Vol.13, No.5, pp.857-64, 0282-0080

Ishihara, K.; Kurihara, M.; Goso, Y.; Urata, T.; Ota, H.; Katsuyama, T. & Hotta, K. (1996b). Peripheral alpha-linked N-acetylglucosamine on the carbohydrate moiety of mucin derived from mammalian gastric gland mucous cells: epitope recognized by a newly characterized monoclonal antibody. *Biochem J* Vol.318, No.2, pp.409-416, ISSN 0264-6021

Iwai, T.; Ichikawa, T.; Kida, M.; Goso, Y.; Kurihara, M.; Koizumi, W. & Ishihara, K. (2011). Protective effect of geranylgeranylacetone against loxoprofen sodium-induced small intestinal lesions in rats. *Eur J Pharmacol* Vol.652, No.1-3, pp.121-125, ISSN 1879-0712

Kato, S.; Tanaka, A.; Kunikata, T.; Umeda, M. & Takeuchi, K. (2000). Protective effect of lafutidine against indomethacin-induced intestinal ulceration in rats: relation to capsaicin-sensitive sensory neurons. *Digestion* Vol.61, No.1, pp.39-46, ISSN 0012-2823

Kawakubo, M.; Ito, Y.; Okimura, Y.; Kobayashi, M.; Sakura, K.; Kasama, S.; Fukuda, M.N.; Fukuda, M.; Katsuyama, T. & Nakayama, J. (2004). Natural antibiotic function of a human gastric mucin against Helicobacter pylori infection. *Science* Vol.305, No.5686, pp.1003-1006, ISSN 1095-9203

Kojima, Y.; Ishihara, K.; Komuro, Y.; Saigenji, K. & Hotta, K. (1993). Effects of the muscarinic receptor agonist carbachol and/or antagonist pirenzepine on gastric mucus secretion in rats. *Scand J Gastroenterol* Vol.28, No.7, pp.647-651, ISSN 0036-5521

Kojima, Y.; Ishihara, K.; Ohara, S.; Saigenji, K. & Hotta, K. (1992). Effects of the M1 muscarinic receptor antagonist pirenzepine on gastric mucus glycoprotein in rats with or without ethanol-induced gastric damage. *Scand J Gastroenterol* Vol.27, No.9, pp.764-768, ISSN 0036-5521

Komuro, Y.; Ishihara, K.; Ishii, K.; Ota, H.; Katsuyama, T.; Saigenji, K. & Hotta, K. (1992a). A separating method for quantifying mucus glycoprotein localized in the different layer of rat gastric mucosa. *Gastroenterol Jpn* Vol.27, No.4, pp.466-472, ISSN 0435-1339

Komuro, Y.; Ishihara, K.; Kojima, Y.; Saigenji, K. & Hotta, K. (1998). Distinct effects of tetragastrin in rat gastroduodenal mucosa on mucin content and mucosal protective action against histamine-induced injury. *Dig Dis Sci* Vol.43, No.5, pp.1050-1056, ISSN 0163-2116

Komuro, Y.; Ishihara, K.; Ohara, S.; Saigenji, K. & Hotta, K. (1991). A new method of separation and quantitation of mucus glycoprotein in rat gastric mucus gel layer and its application to mucus secretion induced by 16,16-dimethyl PGE_2. *Gastroenterol Jpn* Vol.26, No.5, pp.582-587, ISSN 0435-1339

Komuro, Y.; Ishihara, K.; Ohara, S.; Saigenji, K. & Hotta, K. (1992b). Effects of tetragastrin on mucus glycoprotein in rat gastric mucosal protection. *Gastroenterol Jpn* Vol.27, No.5, pp.597-603, ISSN 0435-1339

Leurs, R.; Smit, M.J.; Menge, W.M. & Timmerman, H. (1994). Pharmacological characterization of the human histamine H2 receptor stably expressed in Chinese hamster ovary cells. *Br J Pharmacol* Vol.112, No.3, pp.847-54, ISSN 0007-1188

Marazova, K.; Klouchek, E.; Popov, A.; Ivanov, C.; Krushkov, I.; Ichikawa, T.; Ishihara, K. & Hotta, K. (1998). Effect of roxatidine bismuth citrate (MX1) against acetylsalicylic acid- and indomethacin-induced gastric mucosal damage in rats. *Methods Find Exp Clin Pharmacol* Vol.20, No.8, pp.667-672, ISSN 0379-0355

Mimaki, H.; Kagawa, S.; Aoi, M.; Kato, S.; Satoshi, T.; Kohama, K. & Takeuchi, K. (2002). Effect of lafutidine, a histamine H_2-receptor antagonist, on gastric mucosal blood flow and duodenal HCO_3^- secretion in rats: relation to capsaicin-sensitive afferent neurons. *Dig Dis Sci* Vol.47, No.12, pp.2696-2703, ISSN 0163-2116

Mizuguchi, S.; Ohno, T.; Hattori, Y.; Kamata, K.; Arai, K.; Saeki, T.; Saigenji, K.; Hayashi, I.; Kuribayashi, Y. & Majima, M. (2005). Calcitonin gene-related peptide released by capsaicin suppresses myoelectrical activity of gastric smooth muscle. *J Gastroenterol Hepatol* Vol.20, No.4, pp.611-618, ISSN 0815-9319

Murashima, Y.; Kotani, T.; Hayashi, S.; Komatsu, Y.; Nakagiri, A.; Amagase, K. & Takeuchi, K. (2009). Impairment by 5-Fluorouracil of the Healing of Gastric Lesions in Rats: Effect of Lafutidine, a Histamine H_2 Receptor Antagonist, Mediated by Capsaicin-Sensitive Afferent Neurons. *Dig Dis Sci* Vol.54, No.1, ISSN 0163-2116

Nagahama, K.; Yamato, M.; Kato, S. & Takeuchi, K. (2003). Protective effect of lafutidine, a novel H2-receptor antagonist, on reflux esophagitis in rats through capsaicin-sensitive afferent neurons. *J Pharmacol Sci* Vol.93, No.1, pp.55-61, ISSN 1347-8613

Nishihara, K.; Nozawa, Y.; Nakano, M.; Ajioka, H. & Matsuura, N. (2002). Sensitizing effects of lafutidine on CGRP-containing afferent nerves in the rat stomach. *Br J Pharmacol* Vol.135, No.6, pp.1487-1494, ISSN 0007-1188

Ohno, T.; Hattori, Y.; Komine, R.; Ae, T.; Mizuguchi, S.; Arai, K.; Saeki, T.; Suzuki, T.; Hosono, K.; Hayashi, I.; Oh-Hashi, Y.; Kurihara, Y.; Kurihara, H.; Amagase, K.; Okabe, S.; Saigenji, K. & Majima, M. (2008). Roles of calcitonin gene-related peptide in maintenance of gastric mucosal integrity and in enhancement of ulcer healing and angiogenesis. *Gastroenterology* Vol.134, No.1, pp.215-225, ISSN 1528-0012

Onodera, S.; Nishida, K. & Takeuchi, K. (2004). Unique profile of lafutidine, a novel histamine H_2-receptor antagonist: mucosal protection throughout gastrointestinal tract mediated by capsaicin-sensitive afferent neurons. *Curr Pharm Design* Vol.1, pp.133-144

Onodera, S.; Shibata, M.; Tanaka, M.; Inaba, N.; Arai, Y.; Aoyama, M.; Lee, B. & Yamaura, T. (1999b). Gastroprotective mechanism of lafutidine, a novel anti-ulcer drug with histamine H_2-receptor antagonistic activity. *Arzneimittelforschung* Vol.49, No.6, pp.519-526, ISSN 0004-4172

Onodera, S.; Tanaka, M.; Aoyama, M.; Arai, Y.; Inaba, N.; Suzuki, T.; Nishizawa, A.; Shibata, M. & Sekine, Y. (1999a). Antiulcer effect of lafutidine on indomethacin-induced gastric antral ulcers in refed rats. *Jpn J Pharmacol* Vol.80, No.3, pp.229-235, ISSN 0021-5198

Ota, H. & Katsuyama, T. (1992). Alternating laminated array of two types of mucin in the human gastric surface mucous layer. *Histochem J* Vol.24, No.2, pp.86-92, ISSN 0018-2214

Ota, H.; Katsuyama, T.; Ishii, K.; Nakayama, J.; Shiozawa, T. & Tsukahara, Y. (1991). A dual staining method for identifying mucins of different gastric epithelial mucous cells. *Histochem J* Vol.23, No.1, pp.22-28, ISSN 0018-2214

Robert, A. (1979). Cytoprotection by prostaglandins. *Gastroenterology* Vol.77, No.4, pp.761-767, ISSN 0016-5085

Rokutan, K.; Teshima, S.; Kawai, T.; Kawahara, T.; Kusumoro, K.; Mizushima, T. & Kishi, K. (2000). Geranylgeranylacetone stimulates mucin synthesis in cultured guinea pig gastric pit cells by inducing a neuronal nitric oxide synthase. *J Gastroenterol* Vol.35, No.9, pp.673-681, ISSN 0944-1174

Ruat, M.; Traiffort, E.; Bouthenet, M.L.; Schwartz, J.C.; Hirschfeld, J.; Buschauer, A. & Schunack, W. (1990). Reversible and irreversible labeling and autoradiographic localization of the cerebral histamine H2 receptor using [^{125}I]iodinated probes. *Proc Natl Acad Sci USA* Vol.87, No.5, pp.1658-1662, ISSN 0027-8424

Saegusa, Y.; Ichikawa, T.; Iwai, T.; Goso, Y.; Ikezawa, T.; Nakano, M.; Shikama, N.; Saigenji, K. & Ishihara, K. (2008). Effects of acid antisecretory drugs on mucus barrier of the rat against 5-fluorouracil-induced gastrointestinal mucositis. *Scand J Gastroenterol* Vol.43, No.5, pp.531-537, ISSN 1502-7708

Sato, H.; Kawashima, K.; Yuki, M.; Kazumori, H.; Rumi, M.A.; Ortega-Cava, C.F.; Ishihara, S. & Kinoshita, Y. (2003). Lafutidine, a novel histamine H_2-receptor antagonist, increases serum calcitonin gene-related peptide in rats after water immersion-restraint stress. *J Lab Clin Med* Vol.141, No.2, pp.102-105, ISSN 0022-2143

Sekine, Y.; Hirakawa, N.; Kashiwaba, N.; Matsumoto, H.; Kutsuma, T.; Yamaura, T. & Sekine, A. (1998). A novel histamine 2 (H_2) receptor antagonist with gastroprotective activity. I. Synthesis and pharmacological evaluation of N-phenoxypropylacetamide derivatives with thioether function. *Chem Pharm Bull (Tokyo)* Vol.46, No.4, pp.610-615, ISSN 0009-2363

Shimatani, T.; Inoue, M.; Kuroiwa, T.; Xu, J.; Nakamura, M.; Tazuma, S.; Ikawa, K. & Morikawa, N. (2006). Lafutidine, a newly developed antiulcer drug, elevates postprandial intragastric pH and increases plasma calcitonin gene-related peptide and somatostatin concentrations in humans: comparisons with famotidine. *Dig Dis Sci* Vol.51, No.1, pp.114-120, ISSN 0163-2116

Shiratsuchi, K.; Fuse, H.; Hagiwara, M.; Mikami, T.; Miyasaka, K. & Sakuma, H. (1988). Cytoprotective action of roxatidine acetate HCl. *Arch Int Pharmacodyn Ther* Vol.294, pp.295-304, ISSN 0301-4533

Sugiyama, T.; Hatanaka, Y.; Iwatani, Y.; Jin, X. & Kawasaki, H. (2008). Lafutidine facilitates calcitonin gene-related peptide (CGRP) nerve-mediated vasodilation via vanilloid-1 receptors in rat mesenteric resistance arteries. *J Pharmacol Sci* Vol.106, No.3, pp.505-511, ISSN 1347-8613

Szabo, S.; Trier, J.S. & Frankel, P.W. (1981). Sulfhydryl compounds may mediate gastric cytoprotection. *Science* Vol.214, No.4517, pp.200-202, ISSN 0036-8075

Tarnawski, A.; Hollander, D.; Gergely, H. & Stachura, J. (1985). Comparison of antacid, sucralfate, cimetidine, and ranitidine in protection of the gastric mucosa against ethanol injury. *Am J Med* Vol.79, No.2C, pp.19-23, ISSN 0002-9343

Tsubokawa, D.; Goso, Y.; Sawaguchi, A.; Kurihara, M.; Ichikawa, T.; Sato, N.; Suganuma, T.; Hotta, K. & Ishihara, K. (2007). A monoclonal antibody, PGM34, against 6-sulfated blood-group H type 2 antigen, on the carbohydrate moiety of mucin. *FEBS J* Vol.274, No.7, pp.1833-1848, ISSN 1742-464X

Tsubokawa, D.; Nakamura, T.; Goso, Y.; Takano, Y.; Kurihara, M. & Ishihara, K. (2009). Nippostrongylus brasiliensis: increase of sialomucins reacting with anti-mucin monoclonal antibody HCM31 in rat small intestinal mucosa with primary infection and reinfection. *Exp Parasitol* Vol.123, No.4, pp.319-325, ISSN 1090-2449

2

Approach to Role of Capsaicin - Sensitive Afferent Nerves in the Development and Healing in Patients with Chronic Gastritis

Gyula Mozsik[1], Imre L. Szabo[1] and Andras Dömötör[2]
[1]*First Department of Medicine, Medical and Health Centre, University of Pécs*
[2]*County Teaching Hospital, Veszprém*
Hungary

1. Indroduction

The intact gastrointestinal mucosa can be kept as good equilibrium between the aggressive and defensive factors. These factors have not been fully discovered, however the main aggressive factors are well defined. Gastritis is defined as a pathomorphological appearance of inflammation in the gastric mucosa. Gastritis may be caused by different factors such as *Helicobacter pylori* (*H. pylori*), bacterial overgrowth in a hypochlorohydric stomach, autoimmune mechanisms or chemical agents such as short and long-term nonsteroidal anti-inflammatory drug therapy.

The possible physiological, pathological and pharmacological role(s) of afferent nerves has (have) not been analyzed just recent studies search on its most important role(s) in GI physiology, pathology and pharmacology. Our attention has been focused on capsaicin-sensitive afferent nerves during the last decades.

The possible roles of the capsaicin-sensitive afferent nerves have been approached to gastrointestinal tract from the years of 1980 by our work-team in animal experiments, in healthy human subjects with histological intact and in patients with different disorders (Mózsik et al., 1997, 2001, 2005a, 2007). Capsaicin (given it in small doses) protected the gastrointestinal mucosal damage induced by different necrotizing agents (such as physical, chemical, drugs, etc.) in animal experiments and in human healthy subjects, in patients with different gastrointestinal disorders (Mózsik et al., 1997, 2005a, 2007, 2009). The functional state of some part of afferent nerves (capsaicin-sensitive afferent nerves) can be modified by application of capsaicin by a dose-dependent process (capsaicin, given in small doses stimulates, meanwhile given in higher dose produces reversible and irreversible inhibition or impairment) (Szolcsányi et al., 1984a; Mózsik et al., 2001).

1.1 Aims of observations

The aims of our observations were:

To study the distribution of capsaicin receptor (TRVP1), calcitonin gene-related peptide (CGRP) and substance P (SP) in the human gastric mucosa in histologically intact with functional dyspepsia, chronic gastritis (diagnosed histologically);

To evaluate the possible role of capsaicin-sensitive afferent nerves in the development of gastritis produced by *H. pylori*;
To analyse the role of capsaicin afferent nerves (e.g.immunhistochemical distribution of TRVP1, CGRP, SP) in the the gastric mucosa of the same patients with chronic gastritis produced by *H. pylori* before and after eradication treatment;
To approach the possible gastric mucosal defensive mechanisms of capsaicin-sensitive afferent nerves (immunhistochemical distribution of TRVP1, CGRP, SP) in the development of gastritis and its treatment;
To demonstrate a new pathway (namely the possible productions of new chemical compounds acting on the capsaicin-sensitive afferent nerves) to introduce (as one of the possibilities) in the treatment of chronic gastritis.

1.2 Patients and methods

The patients with symptoms suffering from functional complaints (n=40), chronic gastritis with *H. pylori* negative (gastric discomfort sensation, nausea, loss of appetite, vomiting) (n=30) and *H. pylori* positive (n=39) infection. The age of patients was between 39 to 68 years, and these patients were near to be equal to males and females.
Gastric biopsies were collected from the hyperaemic areas of the corpus and antrum of the stomach by oesophago-gastrosco-bulboscopy. The *H. pylori* infection was detected using the ^{14}C urea breath test (^{14}C UBT), the rapid urease test, and specific histological examinations. The gastric tissue samples were classified into the different groups of chronic gastritis to the updated Sydney system by an independent histopathologist (Dömötör et al., 2007, Lakner et al., 2010).
The immunhistochemical studies were carried out on formalin fixed, paraffin embedded tissue samples using anti-TRVP1 receptor, anti-SP and anti-CGRP antibodies.
18 patients with *H. pylori* positive chronic gastritis went over the same physical, laboratory, ultrasonographic, endoscopic and histological examinations (mentioned above) before and after eradication treatment.

1.3 Results

Distribution of TRVP1 positive (20%) and negative (80%), CRGP positive (30%) and negative (70%), SP weak (75) and strong (25%) in gastric mucosa of healthy human subjects. TRVP1 positive 82%, and negative 18%, CGRP positive 80% and negative 20%, SP weak 85% and strong 15% in patients with *H. pylori* positive chronic gastritis. TRVP1 positive 70% and negative 30%, CGRP positive 63% and negative 37%, SP weak 59% and strong 28% in patients with *H. pylori* negative chronic gastritis.
The eradication treatment for *H. pylori* infection was successful (in 16 from 18, 89%) and complaints (epigastrial pain, heart burn, abdominal expansion) also decreased. Histologically healthy gastric mucosa could be detected only in 22% (4 from 18) and appearance of gastric mucosa (just in moderate histological picture) was obtained.
TRVP1 positive 89% and negative 11%, CGRP positive 100%, SP positive 6% and negative 94% in patients with *H. pylori* positive gastritis, before eradication treatment. TRVP1 positive 72% and negative 18%, CGRP positive 100%, SP negative 100% in patients with *H. pylori* positive chronic gastritis after classical eradication treatment.

1.4 Main conclusions

H. pylori does not represent an exclusive factor for the development of chronic gastritis in patients. The many other compounds (physical, chemical agents) are able also to produce chronic gastritis in patients.

The expression of TRVP1 and increased CGRP participated in the development of chronic gastritis (without and with *H. pylori* infection), meanwhile the SP probably does not participate in this process. These results clearly indicate that the histological picture of chronic gastritis is independent from the presence of commonly emphasized role of *H. pylori* infection in patients, and much more complicated series of mechanisms are present in the development of human chronic gastritis (as we now suggest those at this time).

The classical eradication human therapy does not modify the immunhistological distribution of TRVP1, CGRP and SP in the human gastric mucosa with *H. pylori* infection. Many animal and human observations indicated that the stimulation of capsaicin-sensitive afferent nerves by application by small doses of capsaicin (or other compounds) produced defensive effects against the different physical, chemical, bacteriological, immunological agents.

The capsaicin-sensitive afferentation (s) has (have) a permanent defensive role(s) against gastric mucosal damage by different noxious agents, in the human gastric mucosa. The innovative pharmacological research may offer a new pathway to prevent the gastric mucosa induced by different agents (including the *H. pylori* infection).

2. Introduction

The principle role of efferent vagal nerves has been emphasized in the development of gastrointestinal mucosal damage and prevention, as well as in medical treatment involving anticholinergic agents, histamine H_2 receptor inhibitors, proton pump inhibitors during the last century. From the initial observation of capsaicin desensitation phenomenon, a long-lasting chemoanalgesia and impairment of thermoregulation in the 1970s, chain of new discoveries led to the discovery of the capsaicin receptor, a type of C-polymodal nociceptors (Szolcsányi, 2004b). The effects of capsaicin depend on the applied doses and duration of exposure (Mózsik et al., 2001; Szolcsányi, 2004a). These different effects of capsaicin are: (1) excitation; (2) sensory-blocking effect; (3) long-term selective neurotoxic impairment and (4) irreversible cell destruction.

Neurogenic inflammation is mediated by these C-afferents, which are supplied by the putative capsaicin receptor. These afferents are called capsaicin-sensitive chemoreceptive afferents. They opened new avenues of local peptidegic regulation in peripheral tissues. It has been suggested that, in contrast to classical axon theory, capsaicin-sensitive sensory system has a dual sensory-afferent function, whereby initiation of afferent signals and neuropeptide release are coupled at the same nerve endings. Furthermore, for instance in the skin at threshold stimuli which do not evoke sensation already maximum efferent response as enhanced microcirculation is elicited. Recently, the capsaicin receptor has been cloned and named as transient receptor potential vanilloid-1 (TRVP1) (Caterina et al., 1997). TRPV1 was detected in the area postrema and in the nucleus tractus solitarii where the afferent fibres of the vagal nerve come to an end. Studies with capsaicin receptor led to discovery of the first temperature-gated ion channel gated by noxious heat, protons, vanilloids and endogenous ligands as anadamide, N-oleodopamine and lypoxygenase products. Another recent achievement was the discovery of a novel neurohormonal regulatory mechanisms mediated by somatostatin. Somatostatin released from the TRVP1-expressing nerve endings reaches the circulation and elicits anti-inflammatory and analgetic sensory functions (Szolcsányi, 2004; Helyes et al., 2004).

The vagal nerve contains also only 10% efferent and 90% of afferent nerve fibres, and 9% of these afferent fibres are the capsaicin-sensitive afferent nerves (Gabellla & Pease, 1973;

Grijalva & Novin, 1990). Thus, the amount of the efferent nerves and the capsaicin-sensitive afferent nerves are roughly the same amount in the vagal nerve.

The possible role of afferent vagal nerve was studied in the last decades both in development of gastrointestinal mucosal damage and protection (Mózsik et al., 1997; 2004a; Holzer, 1999; Abdel-Salam et al., 1999). Recently, the gastroprotective effect of capsaicin against chemical agents (ethanol, indomethacin) has been proven in human healthy subjects (Mózsik et al., 2004b, 2005). The beneficial effect of capsaicin has also been shown in patients with functional gastrointestinal disorders (Bartolotti et al. 2002; Bhat & Bielefeldt, 2006).

The integrity of gastric mucosa is an equilibrium state between aggressive and defensive factors. The loss of this balance leads to the development of most gastric disorders, like gastric mucosal ulceration and most likely chronic gastritis.

One of the aggressive factors is *H. pylori* infection, which is a wide spread bacteria, one of the commonest pathogen bacillus in humans (Hocker & Hohenberger, 2003). At least half of the world's population could be infected with this organism (Logan & Walker, 2001). *H. pylori* - as a causative factor - increases the risk for development of human gastrointestinal disorders such as acute gastritis, chronic gastritis, gastric ulcer, gastric mucosa-associated lymphoid tissue (MALT) lymphoma, gastric adenocarcinoma, duodenal ulcer and it may be implicated in iron deficiency anemia and also in extra-gastrointestinal disorders (ischemic heart disease, ischemic cerebrovascular disease, atherosclerosis etc) (Parsonet, 1995; Peng et al., 1998; Pakodi et al., 2003; Mitani et al, 2004; Janulaityte-Gunther et al., 2005; Salih et al., 2005; Zhang et al., 2005a). The eradication of this organism has generally been associated with histological improvement of gastritis (Salih et al., 2005).

On the other hand, one of the defensive mechanisms is the capsaicin-sensitive afferentation. During administration of small doses of capsaicin (from ng/kg to µg/kg body weight) neurotransmitters such as substance-P (SP), calcitonin-gene related peptide (CGRP) and somatostatin (SS) are released from this nerve endings (Holzer, 1998, 1999; Szolcsányi, 2004). These mediators can increase mucosal blood flow by vasodilatation (Holzer et al., 1991), can activate mast cells and immunocells in the mucosa (Stead, 1992), and somatostatin can elicit systemic anti-inflammatory and analgetic "sensory functions". The immunodistribution of neuropeptides (SP, VIP, NPY, SOM, GAL, and TH) released from the sensory neurons and their neuroimmune function are known in *H. pylori* positive gastritis, but not have been examined in gastritis without *H. pylori* infection (Sipos et al., 2006).

The presence of this receptor and released neurotransmitters could be studied in the development of human gastrointestinal disorders including gastritis, peptic ulcer, polyp without and with dysplasia, tumour and inflammatory bowel diseases by immunhistological method (Kihara et al., 2003; Zhang et al., 2005b; Dömötör et al., 2005; Mózsik et al., 2007). In our further research significant changes were observed in the immunhistological distribution of TRPV1, CGRP and SP in patients with chronic *H. pylori* positive gastritis and in histological healthy subjects but no change could be detected between the patients suffered from chronic gastritis without or with *H. pylori* infection (Dömötör et al., 2006). The effect of omeprazole and omeprazole-like compounds could also be demonstrated in the gastric mucosa of rats by the changes of the TRPV1, CGRP and SP immunodistribution and by the reduction of number and severity of gastric mucosal lesions (Mózsik et al., 2005b).

3. Materials and methods

The symptoms of patients suffering from chronic gastritis with or without H. pylori infection (21 H. pylori positive, 30 *H. pylori* negative) were nonspecific (gastric discomfort

sensation, nausea, loss of appetite, vomiting). The patients underwent physical, laboratory, ultrasonographic, endoscopic and histological examinations at the First Department of Medicine, Medical and Health Centre, University of Pécs, Hungary (Table 1).
Twenty people with functional dyspepsia (all of them underwent the aforementioned medical, laboratory, iconographic, and histological examinations and all of these examinations indicated absolutely negative results) were taken as healthy controls. The age of patients was 39 to 68 years; there were 22 males and 29 females with chronic gastritis and 10 males and 10 females in the functional dyspepsia group (Table 1).

Patients:	127 patients, age: 21 – 84 years (68 males, 59 females) Preliminary study by *Dömötör et al, 2005*
Study 1:	51 patients with chronic gastritis age: 39 – 68 years (22 males, 29 females) 21 *H. pylori* positive, 30 *H. pylori* negative 20 persons with functional dyspepsia (controls) age: 41 – 67 years (mean: 52,1 years) (10 males, 10 females)
Study 2:	18 patients with *H. pylori* positive chronic gastritis (6 males, 12 females) age: 39 – 68 years (mean: 56.4 years) 20 with functional dyspepsia (controls) age: 41 – 67 years (mean: 52,1 years) (10 males, 10 females)

Table 1. Study design. The immunhistological studies for capsaicin-sensitive sensory nerves were carried out on biopsy specimens of gastric mucosa obtained from patients.

Eighteen patients with *H. pylori* positive chronic gastritis went over physical, laboratory, ultrasonographic, endoscopic and histological examinations at the Department of Medicine and Gastroenterology, Markusovszky Teaching Hospital, Szombathely (Hungary). The age of patients (6 males, 12 females) was 39 to 68 years (mean=56,4 yrs). The symptoms of the patients were measured with the same questionnaire. These patient received eradication therapy involving a seven days treatment with double dose proton-pump inhibitor (PPI; pantoprazole 2x40 mg/ day), amoxycillin (1000 mg twice daily) and clarithromycin (500 mg twice daily) according to the actual European guidelines (Malfertheiner et al., 2007). After the first week, the patients medicated normal dose of PPI for another week (Table 1). Six weeks after eradication therapy these patients underwent second gastroscopy with gastric biopsy.
Gastric biopsies were collected from hyperaemic areas of the corpus and antrum of the stomach by gastroscopy. H. pylori infection was detected using the ^{14}C UBT, the rapid urease test and specific histological examinations (Warthin-Starry silver staining). Gastric tissue samples were analyzed at the Department of Pathology and classified into different groups of chronic gastritis according to the updated Sydney system (Prince, 1991). The biopsies showed moderate and severe activity of inflammation. Gastric biopsies of patients with chronic gastritis and histologically healthy people were classified into groups by an independent pathologist.

Immunhistological studies were carried out on formalin-fixed, paraffin-embedded tissue samples using the peroxidase-labelled polymer method (Lab Vision Corp., USA). SP was detected by the NC1/34HL rat monoclonal antibody and TRPV1 receptor and CGRP were labelled using polyclonal rabbit antibody (all from Abcam Ltd., Cambridge, UK) (Table 2).

Antiserum	Abbreviation	Species	Dilution	Source
Transient receptor potential vanilliod 1	TRVP1	Rabbit	1:400	Abcam, Cambridge, UK
Calcitonin gene-realted peptide	CGRP	Rabbit	1:200	Abcam
Substance P	SP	Rat	1:200	Abcam

Table 2. Antibodies used as primary.

Immunhistochemical analysis was assessed by light microscopy (Olympus). TRPV1 and CGRP were detected as positive or negative, while the immunhistochemical distribution of SP was characterized using the "SP index." This index was calculated by counting immunopositive spots in at least five high-magnification fields. For fields without immunostaining, the score was 0; for fields containing only one positive spot, the score was 1; and for fields with two or more stained elements, the score was 2. The total score in one specimen was divided by the number of scanned fields to obtain the SP index. Based on these results, biopsies were classed into three categories: weak, medium, and strong (Table 3).

SP evaluation	SP index
Weak	<0.5
Medium	≥ 0.5 but < 1
Strong	≥ 1

Table 3. Semiquantitative quantitation of immunhistochemical SP staining in gastric mucosa of healthy subjects and patients with chronic gastitis

Observations were carried out according to Good Clinical Practice (GCP). Human examinations were carried out from 1997 to 2010 and were permitted by the Regional Ethical Committee of University of Pécs, Hungary. Written informed consent was obtained from all participants.
TRPV1 and CGRP were statistically evaluated by chi-square probe, while SP results were semi-quantitatively evaluated by Mann-Whitney's U test. The results were taken to be significant at P values of < 0.05.

4. Results

Results are presented as the typical pictures of the immunomorphological appearance of the studied receptor and mediators in the gastric mucosa in healthy human subjects and in patients with chronic gastritis with or without *H. pylori* infection (Figs. *1-4)*.

The immunhistochemical results are summarized in Table 4. showing the SP scores (mean ± SE) in healthy persons and in patients with *H. pylori* positive and negative chronic gastritis. In TRPVl-positive cases of chronic gastritis with or without *H. pylori* infection and in healthy subjects, immunostaining was detected as fine granular cytoplasmic immunosigns in epithelial cells in the gastric mucosa (Fig. 2). TRPVl-positive cases of chronic gastritis were significantly more frequent ($p<0.01$) than in controls, while no significant difference was detected in immunomorphology of TRPV1 between patients with H. pylori negative and those with H. pylori positive chronic gastritis.

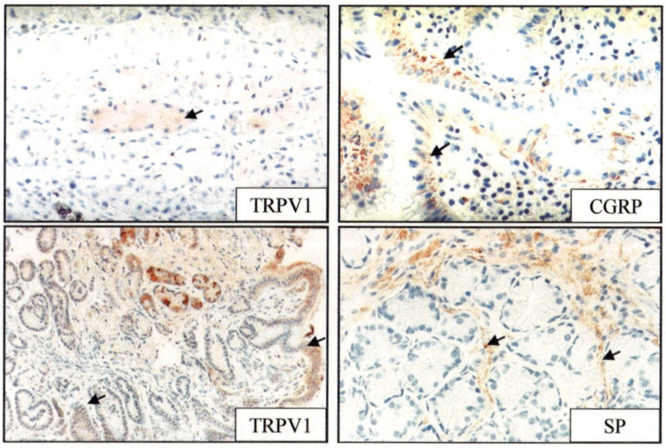

Fig. 1. Immunhistochemical distribution of TRPV1, CGRP and SP in mucosa of the stomach. Arrows show the immunosigns in the epithelial layer of the gastric mucosa (original magnification: 100x).

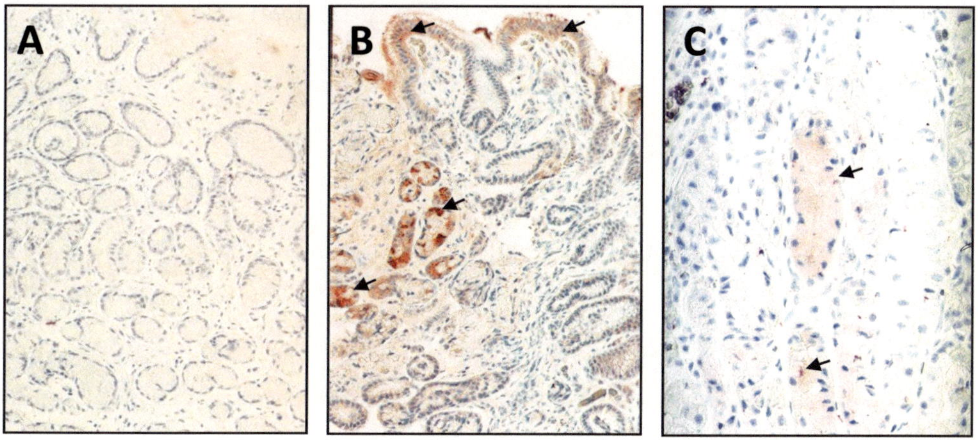

Fig. 2. Immunodistribution of TRPV1 in the gastric mucosa of a healthy subject (A) and of patient with *H. pylori* negative (B) and *H. pylori* positive (C) chronic gastritis. Arrows show the immunosigns in the epithelial layer of the gastric mucosa (original magnification: 100x).

The characteristic immunodistribution of CGRP was as a fine granular cytoplasmatic positivity in epithelial cells in the gastric mucosa of patients with chronic gastritis with or without *H. pylori* infection and in healthy persons (Fig. 3). Regarding the immunhistological distribution of CGRP, significant differences were observed between healthy controls and *H. pylori negative* chronic gastritis ($p<0.01$) and no significant difference was found between the two types (*H.* pylori negative and positive) of chronic gastritis. Although the number of the positive tissue samples increased in *H. pylori* positive gastritis, it did not reach a significantly different level compared to healthy controls.

Before *H. pylori* eradication, the symptoms of the patients with *H. pylori* positive chronic gastritis were unspecific, epigastrial pain (14/18; 77%), heart burn (13/18; 72%), nausea/vomiting (9/18; 50%) abdominal expansion (9/18; 50%), constipation (6/18; 38%). The gastric biopsies of patients with *H. pylori* positive chronic gastritis before eradication indicated moderate and severe activity of inflammation during the regular/common histopathological examinations. The *H. pylori* eradication therapy was successful in 16 from 18 patients (89%) (Figs. 5 and 6). The symptoms were moderated in seven patients (7/18; 39%) and 11 patients (11/18; 61%) had no complaints after eradication treatment.

The immunomorphology of SP was detected as small granular spot-like signals along the mucosal blood vessels in gastric mucosa of healthy subjects and of patients with chronic gastritis with or without the presence of *H. pylori* infection (Fig. 4). No significant difference was observed in the number of low and high SP scores between healthy subjects and patients with chronic gastritis, while medium SP immunhistological samples appeared in *H. pylori negative* and positive chronic gastritis.

The gastroscopy with gastric biopsy was carried out in all patients after *H. pylori* eradication. Histologically healthy gastric mucosa could be detected only in 4 (4/18; 22 %) of the control biopsies and in 14 (14/18; 78%) patients the appearance of chronic gastritis (just in moderate histological picture).

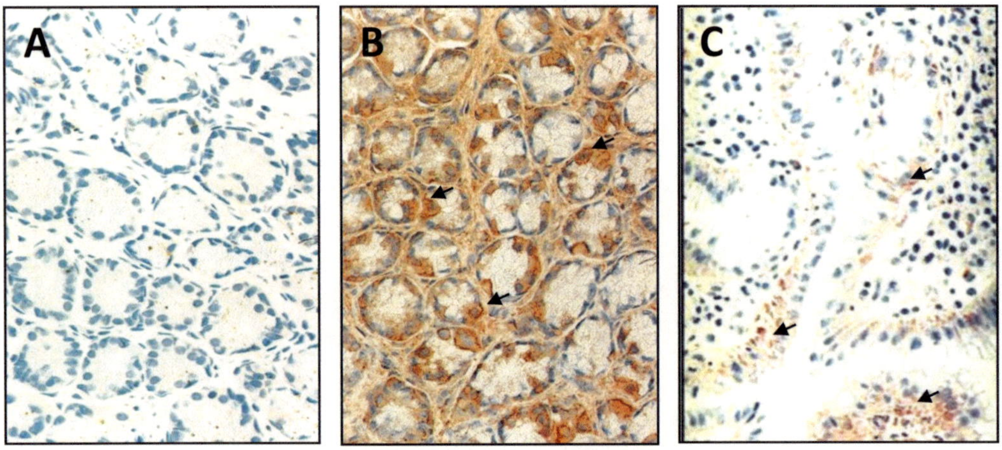

Fig. 3. Immunodistribution of CGRP in gastric mucosa of a healthy subject (A), of patient with *H. pylori* negative (B) and *H. pylori* positive (C) chronic gastritis. Arrows show the immunosigns in the epithelial layer of the gastric mucosa (original magnification: 100x).

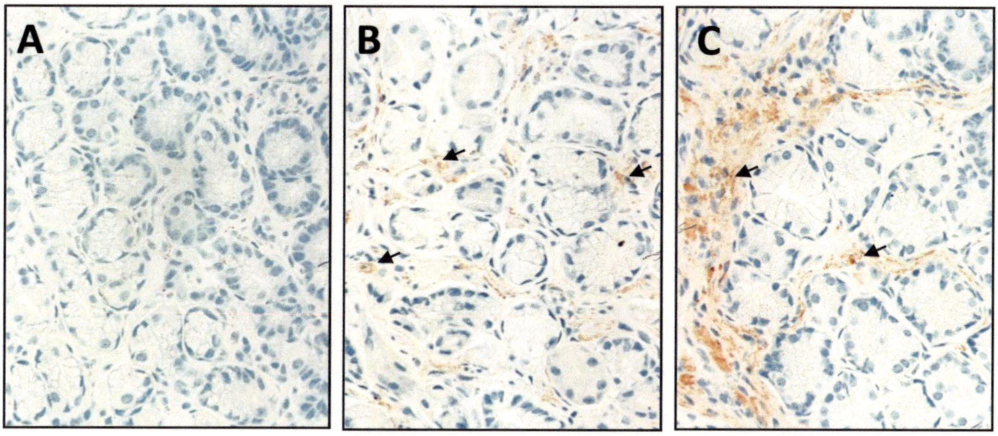

Fig. 4. Immunodistribution of SP in gastric mucosa of a healthy subject (A) and of patient with *H. pylori* negative (B) *H. pylori* positive (C) chronic gastritis (original magnification: 100x).

	TRVP1		CGRP		SP			
	+	–	+	–	–	Weak	Medium	Strong
Healthy (n=20)	20%	80%	30%	70%	0	75%	0	25%
H. pylori **positive (n=21)**	82%	18%	80%	20%	0	85%	0	15%
H. pylori **negative (n=30)**	70%	30%	73%	27%	0	70%	0	30%
H. pylori **positive before eradication (n=18)**	89%	11%	100%	0	94%	0	6%	0
H. pylori **positive after eradication (n=18)**	72%	18%	100%	0	100%	0	0	0

Table 4. Result of immunhistochemistry examinations for TRVP1, CGRP and SP in gastric mucosa of healthy subjects (n=40), patients with *H. pylori* negative chronic gastritis (n=30) and *H. pylori* positive chronic gastritis (n=18) before and after eradication therapy.

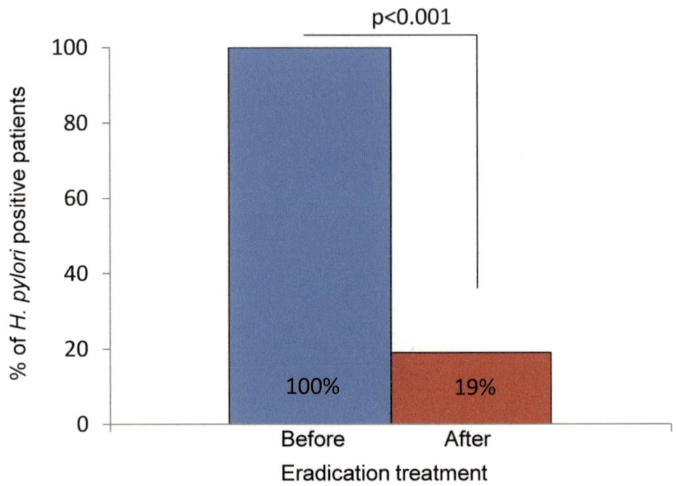

Fig. 5. The efficacy of the traditional *H. pylori* eradication treatment in patients with chronic gastritis (n=18) measured by urea breath test.

The TRPV1 was positive in 20% (5/20) in the healthy subjects, that value was 89 % (16/18; $p< 0.001$) before and 72% (13/18; $p< 0.03$) after eradication therapy in patients with chronic *H. pylori* positive patients.

Immunhistochemistry of CGRP was positive in 100% (18/18; $p<0.001$) of patients before and after eradication (18/18; $p< 0.001$). The SP immunostaing was positive in 25% of control persons (20/20), and in 5.5 % (1/18; $p> 0.05$) before and in 0% (0/18; $p>0.05$) after eradication. The results of the immunhistological examinations are characterized by the typical histological pictures of the TRPV1 receptor and the mediators (CGRP and SP) and are summarized in Tables 5 and 6.

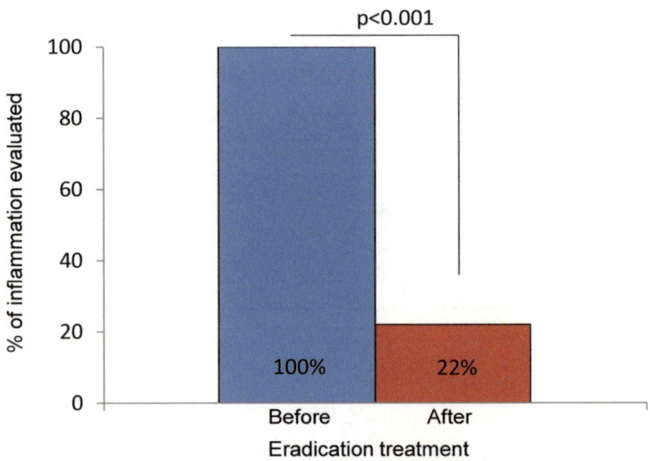

Fig. 6. Presence of histological inflammation in gastric mucosa of patients with chronic gastritis after classical *H. pylori* eradication therapy treatment (n=18).

TRVP1	Healthy subjects	vs.	*H.p.* - (+)	↑	p<0.0001	
		vs.	*H.p.* +	↑	p<0.0001	before eradication
		vs.	*H.p.* +	↑	p<0.0001	after eradication
CGRP	Healthy subjects	vs.	*H.p.* - (+)	↑	p<0.0001	
		vs.	*H.p.* +	↑	p<0.0001	before eradication
		vs.	*H.p.* +	↑	p<0.0001	after eradication
SP	Weak (strong)	vs.	*H.p.* - (+)		p>0.005	
		vs.	*H.p.* +	↑	p<0.0001	before eradication
		vs.	*H.p.* +	↑	p<0.0001	after eradication

p values were calculated between the identical results obtained in healthy subjects (n=40), in patients with *H. pylori* negative (n=30) and *H. pylori* positive chronic gastritis before (n=18) and after (n=18) eradication therapy.
↑ means increase.

Table 5. Summary of differences in result obtained in immunhistochemistry examinations for TRVP1, cGRP and SP in gastric mucosa of healthy subjects (n=40), patients with *H. pylori* negative chronic gastritis (n=30) and *H. pylori* positive chronic gastritis (n=18) before and after eradication therapy.

5. Discussion

The possible role(s) of the capsaicin-sensitive afferent vagal nerve has been studied by our work-team since the 1980s under physiological and different pathological conditions in animal experiments (Mózsik et al, 1997, 2001, 2004b; Abdel Salam et al., 1999), healthy subjects (Mózsik et al., 2004b, 2005a) and in patients with different gastrointestinal disorders (Dömötör et al., 2005, Mózsik et al., 2006, 2007).

The distribution of TRVP1, CGRP significantly increased in *H. pylori* positive chronic gastritis (in comparison with their distribution in gastric mucosa of healthy subjects), which data suggests that the TRPV1 and CGRP are involved in the development of human chronic gastritis (Tables 6 and 7). However, no significant changes were obtained before vs. after classical eradication treatment in patients with *H. pylori* positive chronic gastritis (Table 8). The SP decreased in patients with *H. pylori* chronic gastritis and its value unchanged before and after eradication treatment.

Histologically healthy gastric mucosa could be detected only 4 (4/18; 22%) *H. pylori* positive patients chronic gastritis at 6 weeks after classical eradication treatment. It was interesting to note, that the distribution of gastric mucosal TRPV1, CGRP and SP did not change in the *H. pylori* positive gastritis before and after classical eradication treatment.

How can we explain these unchanged immunodistribution in the gastric mucosa of *H. pylori* positive gastric chronic gastritis before and after eradication treatment?

We have to start from basic observed facts: 1. TRPV1, CGRP and SP can be immunhistologically detected in the rat and human gastric mucosa under healthy and different pathological circumstances; 2. the changes in expression of TRPV1, CGRP and SP are consequence of activation in the capsaicin-sensitive afferent nerves; 3. the *H. pylori* positivity was proven in all patients with chronic gastritis; 4. the eradication of *H. pylori* was successfully carried out, that associated with significant decrease of patients' complaints; 5. the gastric mucosa became to be negative (intact gastric mucosa) in 25%, and 75% of patients indicate moderate histological signs of gastritis after eradication treatment; 6. independently from that the exact proof, the chronic gastritis is in association with *H. pylori* positivity, the histological picture of gastric mucosa indicates only a moderate remission.

	TRVP1 positive		**TRVP1 negative**	
Healthy subjects (n=20)	20%		80%	
H. pylori neg/pos gastritis (n=51)	↑ (p<0.001)		↓ (p<0.001)	
H. pylori pos gastritis (n=18)				
Before eradication	↑ (p<0.001)	NS	↓ (p<0.001)	NS
After eradication	↑ (p<0.001)		↓ (p<0.001)	

↑ means increase. ↓ means decrease. NS means no significant difference. pos means postive. neg means negative.

Table 6. Summary of result obtained in immunhistochemistry examinations for TRVP1 in gastric mucosa of healthy subjects and patients with *H. pylori* negative chronic gastritis (n=30) and *H. pylori* positive chronic gastritis before and after eradication therapy (n=18).

	CGRP positive		**CGPR negative**	
Healthy subjects (n=20)	30%		70%	
H. pylori neg/pos gastritis (n=51)	↑ (p<0.001)		↓ (p<0.001)	
H. pylori pos gastritis (n=18)				
Before eradication	↑ (p<0.001)	NS	↓ (p<0.001)	NS
After eradication	↑ (p<0.001)		↓ (p<0.001)	

↑ means increase. ↓ means decrease. NS means no significant difference. pos means postive. neg means negative.

Table 7. Summary of result obtained in immunhistochemistry examinations for CGRP in gastric mucosa of healthy subjects and patients with *H. pylori* negative chronic gastritis (n=30) and *H. pylori* positive chronic gastritis before and after eradication therapy (n=18).

The TRVP1, CGRP expressions increased significantly in the gastric mucosa with *H. pylori* infection (in comparison with the immunodistribution of TRVP1 and CGRP obtained in the gastric mucosa with healthy subjects, and no significant changes were obtained in the distribution of SP.
In the second series of human observation, it was an unexpected result, that the distribution of TRVP1, CGRP and SP remained unchanged after the classical eradication treatment in patients, although the urea breath test showed high successful rate in bacterial eradication. The gastric mucosa did not become to be histologically negative after the eradication treatment. Interestingly the ratio between the TRVP1, CGRP positivity vs. negative remained the similar before and after eradication.
To understand the changes in histochemical distribution in the gastric mucosa, we performed acute animal experiment, when the rat gastric mucosa was exposed to endogenous (HCl) and exogenous (indomethacin) noxious agents. In these experiments presence of positive immunodistribution of TRPV1, CGRP and SP decreased acutely, that could be abolished by omeprazole (or omeprazole-like compounds) treatment (at 4 hour) (Mózsik et al., 2005b) (Figs. 7-10).

	SP negative	**SP positive**		
		weak	**medium**	**strong**
Healthy subjects (n=20)	0%	70%	5%	25%
			100%	
H. pylori pos gastritis (n=21)	0%	85%	5%	15%
H. pylori neg gastritis (n=30)	0%	70%	0	30%
			100%	
H. pylori pos gastritis (n=18)				
Before eradication	94%	0	6%	0
After eradication	100%	0	0%	0

↑ means increase. ↓ means decrease. pos means postive. neg means negative.

Table 8. Summary of result obtained in immunhistochemistry examinations for SP in gastric mucosa of healthy subjects and patients with *H. pylori* negative chronic gastritis (n=30) and *H. pylori* positive chronic gastritis before and after eradication therapy (n=18).

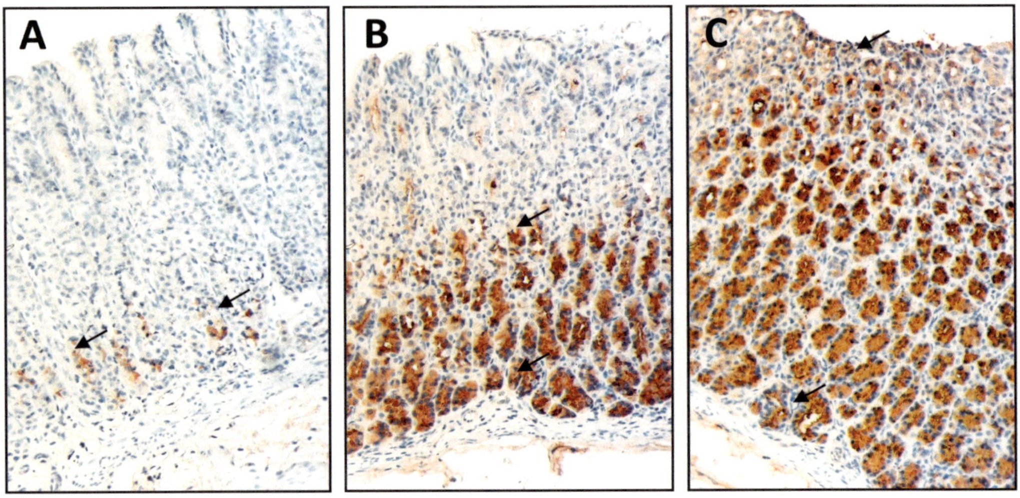

Fig. 7. Immunostaining for TVRP1 in rat gastric mucosa. Weak (A), medium (B) and strong (C) expression of TRVP1 by glandular cells. The weak antigen expression corresponds with immunostaining of some glands in the basal layer. In biopsies with medium expression, positive glands are found at the most in half of the mucosa, and in cases with strong TRVP1 positivity, almost all glands are stained (original magnification: 100x).

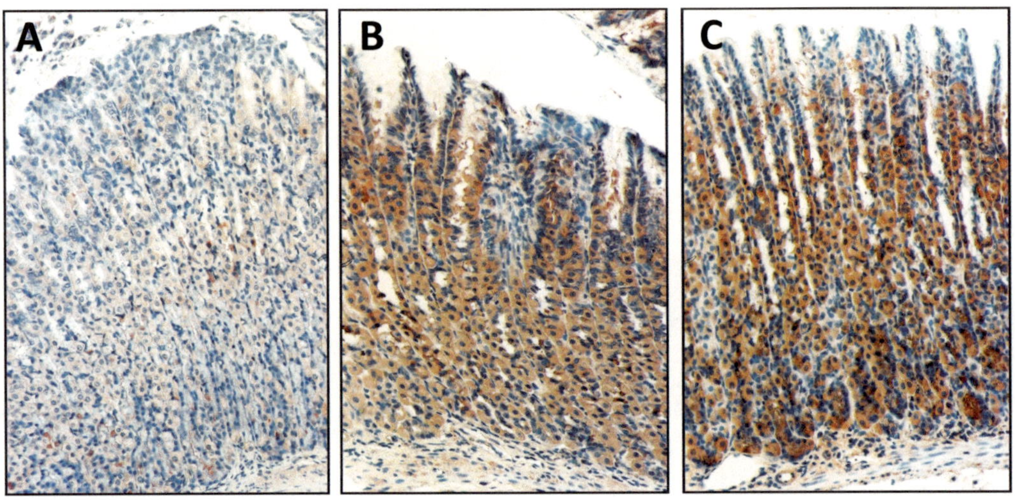

Fig. 8. Immunostaining for CGRP in rat gastric mucosa. Weak (A; only some glandular cells are positive in the mucosa), medium (B; fine granular cytoplasmic staining) and strong (C; predominantly in the basal zone, larger granular staining is observed with higher intensity) CGRP expression (original magnification: 100x).

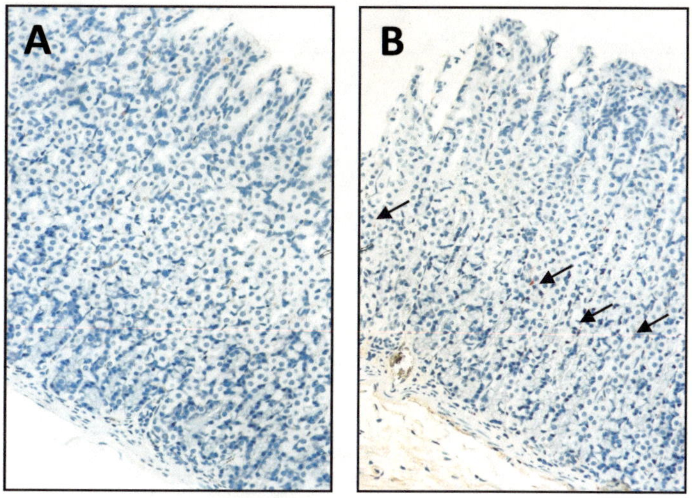

Fig. 9. Immunostaining for SP in rat gastric mucosa. The weakly stained mucosa (A) is almost negative, however, in positive cases; some fine granular immunostaining was observed (B), corresponding to perivascular neural elements (original magnification: 100x).

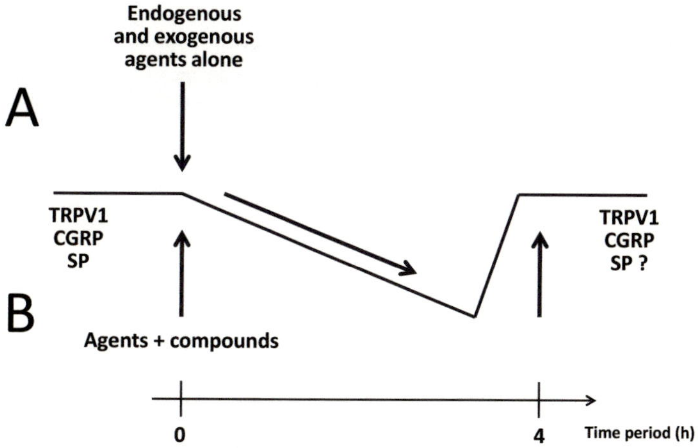

Fig. 10. Schematic presentation of hypothesis for the changes in immunhistochemically demonstrated changes of TRPV1 receptor, CGRP and SP in rat gastric mucosa after application of endogenous (HCl) and exogenous (indomethacin) chemical agents without (A) and with application of omeprazole and omeprazole like compounds (B) during 4-h experimental time period.

	Histochemical expression	Number of mucosal lesions	Severity of mucosal lesions
TRVP1 **Omeprazole** (n=5-10)	↑	↓	↓
TRVP1 ***Omeprazole like*** (n=5-10)	↑	↓	↓
CGRP ***Omeprazole*** (n=5-10)	Dose dependently ↑	↓	↓
CGRP ***Omeprazole like*** (n=5-10)	No significant change	↓	↓
SP ***Omeprazole*** (n=5-10)	No significant change	↓	↓
SP ***Omeprazole like*** (n=5-10)	No significant change	↓	↓

↑ means increase.
↓ means decrease.

Table 9. Correlation between the drug actions and histochemistry in indomethacin-treated rats (n=5-10).

	Histochemical expression	**HCl secretion**
TRVP1		
Omeprazole **(n=5-10)**	Dose dependent ↑	↓
Omeprazole like **(n=5-10)**	Dose dependent ↑	↓
CGRP		
Omeprazole **(n=5-10)**	Dose dependent ↑	↓
Omeprazole like **(n=5-10)**	Dose dependent ↑	↓
SP		
Omeprazole like **(n=5-10)**	No significant change	↓
Omeprazole like **(n=5-10)**	No significant change	↓

↑ means increase.
↓ means decrease.

Table 10. Correlation between the drug actions and immunhistochemistry in pylorus-ligated rats.

In this case the proton pump inhibitor acts at the level of efferent nerves. The classical eradication treatment does not link specifically to efferent or afferent nerves of the vagus.

There is no question that the 6-week time period after eradication therapy does not offer enough time for the histologically restoration of gastric mucosa in patients with chronic *H. pylori* positive gastritis.

Our explanation for the unchanged immunhistochemical distribution of TRPV1, CGP and SP of gastric *H. pylori* positive chronic gastritis before vs. after eradication treatment:

1. Six-week time period (including the time of eradication) is not enough time for the complete healing of chronic gastritis. Because of patients' complaints decreased (and the eradication treatment was mostly successful), however, the changes in gastrointestinal mucosal histology (and immunhistology) showed a lower infection, successful eradication treatment, traditional and specific immunhistological distribution of TVPV1, CGRP and SP differ from each other.
2. The six-week time period (after eradication) is probably not enough time for complete histologically recovery of chronic *H. pylori* in patients in term of histology and immunhistology.
3. The *H. pylori* bacteria as etiological factors might represent only one of the factors causing chronic gastritis (in term of histology).
4. The immunhistological distribution of TRVP1, CGRP and SP are independent on the chronic gastritis produced by different physical, chemical, bacteriological or immunological agents. It's true, that the gastric mucosa did not become histologically intact after eradication treatment. These changes in the histological picture in the gastric mucosa (before and after eradication treatment) suggest that the time period (6 weeks) was short for healing the chronic gastritis by eradication treatment. That fact is confirmed by the repeated histological examinations. Histologically healthy gastric mucosa could be studied only in 4 cases of the control biopsies. In 14 cases, the appearance of chronic gastritis became just moderated.
5. It can be suggested, that other *permanent factors* (stress, drugs) also *take also part in the development of chronic gastritis* which is in accordance with our further observations. The immunomorphology of TRVP1, CGRP and SP do not differ in chronic gastritis evoked by different factors (*H. pylori*, drugs, etc).
6. Low percentage of participants was refractory to the eradication therapy, so the persistent *H. pylori* infection before and after eradication could maintain the same immunhistochemical appearance, the same inflammatory answer.

We demonstrated that the immunodistribution of vanilloid receptor, CGRP and SP increased in patients with chronic gastritis, however, no differences were obtained in the immunhistochemical distribution of examined parameters in the gastric mucosa with *H. pylori* positive and *H. pylori* negative patients (Dömötör et al., 2006). Our presented results clearly indicate that the immunhistochemical distribution of vanilloid receptor, CGRP and SP after classical eradication treatment in patients with *H. pylori* positive chronic gastritis (by other words the capsaicin-sensitive afferent nerves) are independent from the eradication treatment.

The knowledge, that the capsaicin is able to reduce the indomethacin-induced gastric microbleeding in human healthy subjects and the involvement of TRVP1, CGRP and SP in different gastrointestinal disorders show the importance of continuation of such studies to reach a better understanding of gastric mucosal defensive mechanisms in humans (Mózsik et al., 2005a).

Similar conclusions were obtained from the results of animal experiments and human observations, when we co-applied drugs acting on efferent and afferent vagal nerve fibres (Mózsik et al., 1997, 2009) and received combined actions.

Recently, different molecular-pharmacological observations were carried out (and calculated, based on the dose-responses curves of drugs) with capsaicin, atropine, pirenzepine, cimetidine, ranitidine, famotidine, nizatidine, omeprazole, esomeprazole, PGI_2, vitamin A, β-carotene on the gastric basal acid output (BAO) in healthy human subjects (Mózsik et al., 2005), on changes of gastric transmucosal potential difference produced by ethanol (5 ml, 30 v/v% topically applied directly into the gastric mucosa by the way of endoscopic biopsy channel), on indomethacin-induced (3x25+25 mg orally) gastric microbleeding in healthy human subjects (Mózsik et al., 2007), and on gastric (basal and stimulated by betanechol, histamine and pentagastrin) acid secretion of pylorus-ligated rats (Mózsik et al., 2006) or on gastric mucosal damage produced by different chemicals (Indomethacin, HCl, ethanol, NaOH, concentrated NaCl solution) in rats (Mózsik et al., 2006).

The values of affinity (pD) and intrinsic activity (α) curves of these compounds were calculated according to standard procedures employed in molecular-pharmacology (Csáky, 1969). The values of the pD_2 (dose necessary to inhibit the gastric acid secretion and gastric mucosal damage by 50%) and pA_2 (dose necessary to produced 50% decrease in gastric acid secretion and in gastric mucosal damage) were calculated from the affinity and intrinsic activity curves. The intrinsic activity values obtained in relation to atropine ($\alpha_{atropine} = 1.00$) were taken as standard values.

The knowledge of affinity, intrinsic activity curves, values of pD_2 and pA_2 gives us an exact approach to understand the physiological and pharmacological roles of different compounds (Mózsik et al., 2006, 2007, 2009).

The following pD_2 values were obtained for the different drugs or substances inhibiting the gastric basal acid secretion (BAO): capsaicin, 5.88; atropine, 5.40; pirenzepine, 3.93; cimetidine, 2.23; ranitidine, 3.33; famotidine, 3.77; nizatidine, 3.23; omeprazole, 3.97 and esomeprazole, 3.97 (Mózsik et al., 2007). Similar results were obtained for these compounds inhibiting gastric mucosal damage produced by intragastric administration of ethanol or by orally applied indomethacin in healthy human subjects (Mózsik et al, 2005a).

The results of these observations led us to conclude that the capsaicin-sensitive afferent nerves have the most important physiological regulation of gastric basal acid secretion (BAO) and of chemicals-induced gastric mucosal damage in human healthy subjects (Mózsik et al, 2005a, 2007, 2009). Similar results obtained in animals experiments for regulation of gastric acid secretion and of gastric mucosal damage (Mózsik et al, 2006).

The unchanged functional state of capsaicin-sensitive afferentation, before and after classical eradication treatment in patients also offers to conclude an important regulatory function of gastric mucosa in patients with H. pylori chronic gastritis (in comparison the results obtained in patients with *H. pylori* positive gastritis vs. healthy persons) by TRVP1, CGRP and substance P during the eradication treatment.

The most important message of this work (study) is that the gastric capsaicin-sensitive afferentation has a permanent defensive role(s) in the gastric mucosal defence. Consequently the modification in the function of capsaicin-sensitive afferent nerves offer new possibilities in human medical therapy.

6. Acknowledgement

The authors express their thanks for the financial support of grant Baross (REG_DD_KFI_09, CAPSATAB, Hungary).

7. References

Abdel Salam, O. M. E., Debreceni, A. & Mózsik, Gy. (1999). Capsaicin-sensitive afferent sensory nerves in modulating gastric mucosal defense against noxious agents, Journal of Physiology, Vol.93, pp. 443-54

Bhat, Y.M. & Bielefeldt, K. (2006). Capsaicin receptor (TRVP1) and non-erosive reflux disease. *European Journal of Gastroenterology and Hepatology*, Vol.18, pp. 63-270

Bortolotti, M., Coccia, G., Grossi, G. & Miglioli, M. (2002). The treatment of functional dyspepsia with red pepper. *Alimentary Pharmacology and Therapeutic*, Vol.16, pp. 1075-82

Caterina, M.J., Chumacher, M.A., Tominaga, M., Rosen, T.A., Levine, J.D. & Julius, D. (1997). The capsaicin receptor: a heat-activated ion channel in the pain pathway, *Nature*, Vol.389, pp. 816-24

Csáky, T.Z. (1969). *Introduction to General Pharmacology*. Appleton Century- Craft Education Division, New York, Meredith Corporation, pp. 17-34

Dömötör, A., Peidl, Zs., Vincze, A., Hunyady, B., Szolcsányi, J., Kereskay, L., Szekeres, Gy. & Mózsik Gy. (2005). Immunhistochemical distribution of vanilloid receptor, calcium gene-related peptide and substance P in the gastrointestinal mucosa of patients with different gastrointestinal disorders. *Inflammopharmacology*, Vol.13, No.1-3, pp. 161-77

Dömötör, A., Kereskay, L., Szekeres, G., Hunyady, B., Szolcsányi, J. & Mózsik, G. (2006). Participation of capsaicin-sensitive afferent nerves in the gastric mucosa of patients with *Helicobacter pylori*-positive or-negative chronic gastritis. *Digestive Diseases and Sciences*, Vol.52, No.2, pp. 411-7

Gabella, G. & Pease, H. (1973). Number of axons in the abdominal vagus of the rat. *Brain Research*, Vol.58, pp. 465-69

Grijalva, C.V. & Novin, D. (1990). The role of hypothalamus and dorsal vagal complex in gastrointestinal function an pathophysiology. *Annals of New York Academy of Sciences*, Vol.597, pp 207-21

Helyes, Zs., Szabó, Á., Németh, J., Jakab, B., Pintér E., Bánvölgyi, Á., Kereskai, L. & Szocsányi, J. (2004). Anti-inflammatory and Analgesic Effects of Somatostatin Released From Capsaicin-Sensitive Sensory Nerve Terminals in a Freund's Adjuvant-Induced Chronic Arthritis Model in the Rat, *Arthritis & Rheumatism*, Vol.50, No.5, pp 1677–1685

Hocker, M. & Hohenberger P. (2003). *Helicobacter pylori* virulence factors – one part of a big picture. *Lancet*, Vol. 362: pp. 1231-3

Holzer, P., Livingston, E.H., Saria, A. & Guth, P.H. (1991). Sensory neurons mediate protective vasodilatation in rat gastric mucosa. *Americal Journal of Physiology*, Vol.260, pp. 363-70

Holzer, P. (1998). Neural emergency system in the stomach. *Gastroenterology*, Vol.114, pp. 823-83

Holzer, P. (1999). Capsaicin cellular targets, mechanisms of action and selectivity for thin sensory neurons. *Pharmacological Reviews*, Vol.43, pp. 143-201

Janulaityte-Gunther, D., Kucinskiene, R., Kupcinskas, L., Pavilonis, A., Labanauskas, L., Cizauskas, A., Schmidt, U., Wadstrom, T. & Andersen, L.P. (2005) Humoral immuneresponse to *Helicobacter pylori* infection in children with gastrointestinal symptoms. *FEMS Immunology and Medical Microbiology*, Vol.44, pp. 205-12

Kihara, N., de la Fuente, S.G., Fujino, K., Takahashi, T., Pappas, T.N. & Mantyh, C.R. (2003). Vanilloid receptor-1 containing primary sensory neurones mediate dextran sulphate sodium induced colitis in rats. *Gut*, Vol.52, No.5, pp. 713-9

Lakner, L., Dömötör, A., Tóth, Cs., Meczker, A., Hajós, R., Kereskai, L., Szekeres, Gy., Döbrönte, Z. & Mózsik, Gy. (2011). Immunhistochemical distribution of gastric mucosal TRVP1, CGRP and substance P in healthy subjects and in patients with *H.pylori* positive patients before and after eradication treatment. *World Journal of Gastrointestinal Pharmacology and Therapeutics*, (submitted for publication)

Logan, R.P.H. & Walker, M.M. (2001). Epidemiology and diagnosis of *Helicobacter pylori* infection 2001; *British Medical Journal*, Vol.323, pp. 920-2

Malfertheiner, P., Megraud, F., O'Morain, C., Bazzoli, F., El-Omar, E., Graham, D., Hunt, R., Rokkas, T., Vakil, N. & Kuipers, E.J. (2007). Current concepts in the management of *Helicobacter pylori* infection. The Maastricht III. Consensus Report, *Gut*, Vol.56, pp 772

Mózsik, Gy., Abdel-Salam, O.M.E. & Szolcsányi, J. (1997). *Capsaicin-Sensitive Afferent Nerves in Gastric Mucosal Damage and Protection.* Akadémiai Kiadó, Budapest, Hungary

Mózsik, Gy., Vincze, A. & Szolcsányi, J. (2001). Four response of capsaicin-sensitive primary neurones to capsaicin and its analogue. Gastric secretion , gastric mucosal damage and protection. *Journal of Gastroenterology and Hepatology*, Vol. 16, pp. 193-7

Mózsik, Gy., Pár, A., Pár, G, Juricskay, I., Figler, M. & Szolcsányi, J. (2004a). Insight into the molecular pharmacology to drugs acting on the afferent and efferent fibres of vagal nerve in the gastric mucosal protection, In: *Ulcer Research, Proceedings of the llth International Conference,* Sikiric, P., Seiwerth, R., Mózsik, Gy., Arakawa, T., Takeuchi, K. (Ed.), 163-8. Monduzzi, Bologna, Italy

Mózsik, Gy., Belágyi, J.,Szolcsányi, J., Pár, G., Pár, A., Rumi, Gy. & Rácz, I. (2004b). Capsaicin-sensitive afferent nerves and gastric mucosal protection in human healthy subjects. A critical overview. In: *Medicators in Gastrointestinal Protection and Repair, Takeuchi, K., Mózsik, Gy. (Ed.), 43-62.* Research Signpost, Kerala, India

Mózsik, Gy., Szolcsányi, J., Rácz, I. (2005a). Gastroprotection induced by capsaicin in healthy human subjects. *World Journal of Gastroenterology*, Vol.11, pp. 5180-4

Mózsik, Gy., Peidl, Zs., Szolcsányi, J., Dömötör, A., Hideg, K., Szekeres, Gy., Karádi, O. & Hunyady, B. (2005b). Participation of vanilloid/capsaicin receptors, calcitonin gene-related peptide and substance P in gastric protection of omeprazole and omeprazole-like compounds. *Inflammopharmacology*, Vol.13, pp. 139-59

Mózsik, Gy., Dömötör, A. & Abdel Salam, O.M.E. (2006). Molecular pharmacological approach to drug actions on the afferent and efferent fibres of vagal nerve in the gastric mucosal protection in rats. *Inflammopharmacology*, Vol.14, pp. 243-9

Mózsik, Gy., Szolcsányi, J. & Dömötör, A. (2007). Capsaicin research as a new tool to approach of the human gastrointestinal physiology, pathology and pharmacology. *Inflammopharmacology*, Vol.15, pp. 232-45

Mózsik, Gy., Dömötör, A., Past, T., Vas, V., Perjési, P., Kuzma, M., Blazsik, Gy. & Szolcsányi, J. (2009). *Capsaiconoids: from the Plant Cultivation to the Production of the Human Medical Therapy*. Akadémiai Kiadó, Budapest, Hungary

Mózsik Gy., Past T., Dömötör A., Kuzma M., Perjési P. (2010). Production of orally applicable new drug or drug combinations from natural origin capsaicinoids for human medical therapy. *Current Pharmaceutical Design*, Vol.16, No.10, pp. 1197-208

Mitani, K., Tatsuta, M., Iishi, H., Yano, H., Uedo, N., Iseki, K. & Narahara H. (2004). *Helicobacter pylori* infection as a risk factor for gastric ulceration. Hepato-Gastroenterology, Vol.51, pp. 309-12

Pakodi, F., Abdel-Salam, O.M., Debreceni, A. & Mózsik, G. (2003). Helicobacter pylori. One bacterium and a broad spectrum of human disease! An overview. *Journal of Physiology (Paris)*, Vol.94, pp. 139-52

Parsonet, J. (1995). The incidence of Helicobacter pylori infection. *Pharmacology & Therapeutics*, Vol.2, pp. 45-51

Peng, H., Ranaldi, R., Diss, T.C., Isaacson, P.G., Bearzi, I. & Pan, L. (1998). High frequency of CagA+ Helicobacter pylori infection in high-grade gastric MALT B-cell lymphomas. *Journal of Pathology*, Vol.185, pp. 409-12

Price, A.B. (1991). The Sydney System: histological division. *Journal of Gastroenterology and Hepatology*, Vol.6, pp. 209-22

Salih, B.A., Abasiyanik, M.F., Saribasak, H., Huten, O. & Sander, E. (2005). A follow-up study on the effect of Helicobacter pylori eradication on the severity of gastric histology. *Digestive Diseases and Sciences*, Vol.50, pp. 1517-22

Sipos, G., Altdorfer, K., Pongor, É., Chen, L.P. & Fehér, E. (2006). Neuroimmune-link in the mucosa of chronic gastritis with *Helicobacter pylori* infection. *Digestive Diseases and Sciences*, Vol.51, pp. 1810-7

Stead, R.H. (1992). Innervation of mucosal immune cells in the gastrointestinal tract. [Review] *Regional Immunology*, Vol.4, pp. 91-9

Szolcsányi J. (1984a). Capsaicin and neurogen inflammation: history and early findings. In: *Antidromic Vasodilatation and Nurogenic Inflammation*. Chahl, L.A., Szolcsányi, J. & Lembeck, F. (Ed.), 27-56, Akadémiai Kiadó, Budapest, Hungary

Szolcsányi, J. (1984b). Capsaicin sensitive chemoprotective neural system with dual sensory-afferent function, In: *Antidromic Vasodilatation and Neurogenic Inflammation*, Chalh L.A., Szolcsányi J., Lembeck F. (Ed.), 27-56, Akadémiai Kiadó, Budapest, Hungary

Szolcsányi, J. (2004). Forty years in capsaicin research for sensory pharmacology and physiology. *Neuropeptides*, Vol. 38, pp. 377-84

Zhang, C., Yamada, N., Wu, Y.L., Wen, M., Matsuhisa, T. & Matsukura, N. (2005a). Comparison of *Helicobacter pylori* infection and gastric mucosal histological features of gastric ulcer patients with chronic gastritis patients. *World Journal of Gastroenterology*, Vol.11, pp. 976-81

Zhang, C., Yamada, N., Wu, Y.L., Wen, M., Matsuhisa, T. & Matsukura, N. (2005b). *Helicobacter pylori* infection, glandular atrophy and intestinal metaplasia in superficial gastritis, gastric erosion, erosive gastritis, gastric ulcer and early gastric cancer. *World Journal of Gastroenterology*, Vol.11, pp. 791-6

3

Oxidative Stress Pathway Driven by Inflammation in Gastric Mucosa

Dovhanj Jasna[1] and Švagelj Dražen[2,3]
[1]*Medical School Osijek, Dept. of Clinical and Laboratory Diagnostics, Osijek*
[2]*Medical School Osijek, Dept. of Pathology, Osijek*
[3]*General Hospital Vinkovci, Dept. of Pathology and Cytology, Vinkovci*
Croatia

1. Introduction

Oxidative stress is a state in which toxic reactive oxygen species (ROS) overcomes the endogenous antioxidant defence of the host (Bulger & Helton, 1998). This state results in an excess of free radicals, which can react with cellular lipids, proteins, and nucleic acids, leading to cellular injury and eventual organ dysfunction. Gastric inflammation is a highly complex biochemical protective response to cellular/tissue injury. A large amount of evidence suggests that *Helicobacter pylori* (H. pylori) infection and nonsteroidal anti-inflammatory drug (NSAID) ingestion are major causative factors in the pathogenesis of gastric mucosal oxidative injury in humans. In response to *H. pylori* infection or NSAID, neutrophils are recruited to the site of inflammation and generate ROS and nitrogen reactive species (RNS) (Yoshikawa & Naito, 2000; Naito & Yoshikawa, 2002). The sources of radicals are mucosal xanthine oxidase and NADPH oxidase found in the resident leukocytes of the lamina propria (Otamiri & Sjodahl, 1991). However, recent results suggest that NOX family of NADPH oxidases might also be expressed in gastric epithelial cells. ROS mediates inflammation by activating redox-sensitive transcription factors such as NF-kappaB and activator protein (AP)-1 which upregulate a number of proinflammatory genes, resulting in the production of proinflammatory cytokines, adhesion molecules, receptors, etc. The generation of ROS and cytokines not only that is associated but also amplifies each other (positive feedback regulation). Not only is increased ROS formation a trigger of inflammation but inflammation itself again triggers ROS production (Glorie et al., 2006).

2. Free radicals and oxidative stress

Free radicals are atoms or atomic groups that contain unpaired electrons. Since electrons have a very strong tendency to exist in a paired rather than an unpaired state, free radicals indiscriminately pick up electrons from other atoms, converting those other atoms into secondary free radicals. Thus a chain reaction is triggered that can cause substantial biological damage. Reactive oxygen species are oxygen-derived small molecules, including oxygen radicals [superoxide ($O_2^{\cdot-}$), hydroxyl ($\cdot OH$), peroxyl ($RO_2^{\cdot}$), and alkoxyl ($RO^{\cdot}$)] and certain nonradicals that are either oxidizing agents and/or are easily converted into radicals, such as hypochlorous acid (HOCl), ozone (O_3), singlet oxygen ($^1O_2$), and hydrogen peroxide

(H_2O_2). RNS are nitrogen-containing oxidants, such as nitric oxide (Freitas et al. 2009,2010). The physiological generation of free radicals can occur as a byproduct of biological reactions in mitochondria, peroxisomes, cytochrome *P*-450. In a resting cell, superoxide anion is produced at 1–2% of total daily oxygen consumption during electron transfer and oxidative phosphorylation for ATP generation by mitochondria. Mitochondrial ROS are recognised as regulators of mitochondrial functions including electron transfer chain enzymes and mitochondrial membrane potential (Balaban et al., 2005, Finkel & Holbrook, 2005; Gottlieb, 2003). Overproduction of ROS, most frequently either by excessive stimulation of NADPH oxidase by cytokines, or by the mitochondrial electron transport chain and xanthine oxidase result in oxidative stress. Oxidative stress is a deleterious process that can be an important mediator of damage to cell structures and consequently various disease states and ageing (Jomova & Valko 2011; Valko, 2007).

During inflammation, phagocytic cells such as macrophages and neutrophils produce microbicidal oxidants whose formation is accompained by a transient episode of oxidative metabolism known as the respiratory burst. Reactive oxygen species, such as superoxide anion, hydrogen peroxide, the hydroxyl radical, and hypochlorous acid, together with microbicidal peptides and proteases, constitute their antimicrobial arsenal. The generation of microbicidal oxidants by neutrophils leads to the activation of a multiprotein enzyme complex known as the reduced nicotinamide adenine dinucleotide phosphate (NADPH) oxidase, which is responsible for transferring electrons from NADPH to O_2, resulting in the formation of superoxide anion. This multicomponent enzyme system is composed of cytosolic proteins (p47phox, p67phox, p40phox, and rac1/2) and membrane proteins (p22phox and gp91phox, which form cytochrome b558) which assemble at membrane sites upon cell activation. NADPH oxidase activation is tightly regulated because of potential damage of surrounding tissues (Babior, 1999; Bedard & Krause, 2007; El Benna et al., 2005; Krause& Bedard, 2008). ROS generation is generally a cascade of reactions that starts with the production of superoxide. Superoxide rapidly dismutates to hydrogen peroxide either spontaneously, particularly at low pH or catalyzed by superoxide dismutase. The cascade of ROS generation include the reaction of superoxide with nitric oxide to form peroxynitrite, the peroxidase-catalyzed formation of hypochlorous acid from hydrogen peroxide, and the iron-catalyzed Fenton reaction leading to the generation of hydroxyl radical (Klebanoff, 1980). Free radicals may act as direct or indirect damaging agents through their reaction with other chemical or structural components in cells. ROS and RNS also recruit other inflammatory cells with secondary amplification of the damage. An enzymatic and non-enzymatic antioxidant defence systems, including catalase (CAT), superoxide dismutase (SOD) and glutathione peroxidase (GPx) scavenge and regulate overall ROS levels to maintain physiological homeostasis. Lowering ROS levels below the homeostatic set point may interrupt the physiological role of oxidants in cellular proliferation and host defence. Under certain conditions, e.g., the presence of an elevated concentration of transition metal (Fe/Cu) ions, drug metabolism, or ischemia-reperfusion, ROS generation overwhelms cellular antioxidant defence resulting in oxidative stress. ROS may serve as cellular second messengers through the regulation of numerous signal transduction pathways at a concentration much below that required for formation of oxidative damage (Engelhardt et al., 2001). A rise in ROS levels may also constitute a stress signal that activates specific redox-sensitive signalling pathways. Once activated, these diverse signalling pathways may have either damaging or potentially protective functions (Finkel & Holbrook, 2000). Redox status has dual effects on upstream signaling system and downstream transcription factors.

Oxidants can stimulate many upstream kinases in signaling pathway cascades and yet inhibit transcription factors AP-1 and NF-kappaB activation (Kamata & Hirata, 1999). The signaling molecule, H_2O_2, mediates inflammation by activating NF kappaB and AP-1. Biological effects of NOX-derived O_2^- include: reaction with nitric oxide (NO) leading to NO degradation, peroxynitrite formation, protein tyrosine nitration, and the addition of glutathione (GSH) to thiols; reduction of iron centers within enzymes (e.g., aconitase) and alkalinization of intracellular organelles (Bedard & Krause, 2007). The current medical focus in this area has been directed toward the understanding of redox-driven physiological and pathophysiological processes in the cell.

3. Inflammation-induced oxidative stress in gastric mucosa

3.1 Ischemia- reperfusion injury-induced oxidative stress in gastric mucosa

Ischemia–reperfusion injury is important pathological process in gastric mucosal inflammation. Massive production of ROS during ischemia/reperfusion in turn lead to tissue injury. When production of ROS occurs in an uncontrolled manner, the result is excessive cellular/tissue damage that results with chronic inflammation and destruction of normal tissue (Yoshikawa & Naito, 2000; Sasaki & Joh, 2007). Neutrophils are the principal effector cells of reperfusion injury. Under the conditions of ischemia/ reperfusion, xanthine dehydrogenase is converted into xanthine oxidase which uses oxygen as a substrate. During ischemia, utilisation leads to a depletion of ATP and accumulation of the purine catabolites hypoxanthine and xanthine, which are metabolized by xanthine oxidase to produce enormous amounts of superoxide radical and hydrogen peroxide upon subsequent reperfusion and influx of oxygen (Granger et al., 2001).

In the extracellular space adenosine and ATP act as important endogenous signaling molecules in immunity and inflammation through activation of purinergic receptors (Swenen et al., 2005). Swennen et al. examined the ex vivo immunomodulatory effects of ATP in whole blood from healthy subjects. These data indicate that ATP is an anti-inflammatory agent with simultaneous TNF-alfa suppressing and IL-10 augmenting activity.In addition, ATP has been shown to contribute to the initiation of oxidative burst. It appears to prime neutrophils for functional responses to various inflammatory mediators, as indicated by increased production of ROS (Fredholm, 1997; Zhang et al., 1996). Endoscopic studies using reflectance spectrophotometry and laser Doppler flowmetry have reported a decrease in mucosal blood flow resulting in impairment of gastric mucosal energy metabolism. Adenine nucleotides in biopsy samples from human gastric mucosa were measured using high-performance liquid chromatography (HPLC).

Energy charge (EC) was assessed from ATP, adenosine diphosphate (ADP) and adenosine monophosphate (AMP) and calculated as EC=ATP + 1/2 ADP)/ATP + ADP + AMP. Energy charge of antrum was lower compared to corpus in the gastric mucosa. In elderly, the impaired energy metabolism in human gastric mucosa may weaken their defensive mechanism (Kawano et al., 1991). In vitro studies suggest that extracellular nucleotides and nucleosides may be important regulators of inflammatory and immune responses (Di Virgillio et al., 2001). Acute gastric erosions following hemorrhagic shock (stress ulceration) have been attributed to gastric hyperacidity, altered gastric secretion of mucus and an abnormal permeability of the gastric mucosa to H^+. An energy deficit severe enough to cause cellular necrosis is the event linking shock-induced gastric mucosal ischemia and stress ulceration (Menguy & Master 1974a, 1974b, 1974c, 1974d). This studies support the

value of ATP as a highly potent natural compound, which able to modulate inflammation and oxidative stress.
The conditions of chronic inflammation predispose susceptible cells to neoplastic transformation. ROS appear to be the key regulatory factors in molecular pathways linked to tumour development and tumour dissemination (Valko, 2007).
The longer the inflammation persists, the higher the risk of cancer gets. Inflammatory processes may induce DNA mutations in cells via oxidative/nitrosative stress. Inflammatory cells and cancer cells themselves produce free radicals and soluble mediators such as metabolites of arachidonic acid, cytokines and chemokines, which act by further producing reactive species. These, in turn, strongly recruit inflammatory cells in a vicious cycle. Reactive intermediates of oxygen and nitrogen may directly oxidize DNA, or may interfere with mechanisms of DNA repair. The main substances that link inflammation with cancer via oxidative/nitrosative stress are prostaglandins and cytokines. The effectors are represented by an imbalance between pro-oxidant and antioxidant enzyme activities (lipoxygenase, cyclooxygenase and phospholipid hydroperoxide glutathione-peroxidase), hydroperoxides and lipoperoxides, aldehydes and peroxinitrite (Federico et al., 2007).

3.2 *Helicobacter pylori*-induced oxidative stress

Helicobacter pylori, a pathogenic bacterium, is highly adapted to its ecologic niche, the human gastric mucosa. The pathogenesis of *H. pylori* relies on its persistence in surviving a harsh environment, including acidity, peristalsis, and oxidative burst by phagocyte cells (McGee & Mobley, 1999). *H. pylori* infection causes chronic inflammation, accumulation of ROS and oxidative DNA damage in the gastric mucosa.
During the process of colonizing the host, *H. pylori* induces a strong inflammatory response, generating large amounts of ROS. To evade oxidative killing *H. pylori* prevents NADPH oxidase assembly at the phagosome, with release of NADP+ and large amounts of superoxide anions into the extracellular milieu (Allen, 2007a; Allen, 2007b). *H. pylori* injects bacterial proteins into the cytosol of the gastric host cell *via* the type IV injection system and regulates the intracellular signal transduction. This mechanism provides a approach to resolving how *H. pylori* survives in the acidic environment of the human stomach. (Suzuki, 2006a, 2006b).
A number of studies have shown that *H. pylori* infection is associated with generation of free radicals, which leads to oxidative stress in the gastric mucosa (Fukuhara et al., 2008; Davies et al. 1994a, 1994b; McGee & Mobley 1999; Pignatelli et al., 2001; Li et al., 2001; Baik et al., 1996). Exposure of gastric epithelial cells to *H. pylori* resulted in an inflammatory reaction with production of ROS and nitric oxide (Nardone et al., 2004).The effects of bacterial eradication on mucosal oxidative stress were investigated by measuring the changes of the expression of inducible nitric oxide synthase (iNOS) and levels of nitrotyrosine and 8-hydroxy-2|[prime]|-deoxyguanosine in antral biopsies from patients with chronic atrophic gastritis and peptic ulcer disease before and after bacterial eradication. *Helicobacter pylori* eradication attenuates oxidative stress in human gastric mucosa (Pignatelli et al., 2001). The adding of prescribed doses of vitamins E and C to antimicrobial therapy is effective in eradicating *H. pylori* infection (Sezikli et al., 2009). Recent studies demonstrated that increased levels of ROS are generated in *H. pylori*- infected gastric epithelial cells and that this may be one mechanism leading to apoptosis associated with infection (Ding et al., 2007).
Host intracellular iron has been noticed as an important cofactor in induction of NADPH-dependent oxidative burst. The changed equilibrium of intracellular iron could influence the

course of infection to the enhancement of the pathogen with regard to oxidative stress (Dovhanj et al., 2009).

The expression of eight proteins (78 kDa glucose-regulated protein precursor, endoplasmin precursor, aldehyde dehydrogenase 2 and L-lactate dehydrogenase B chain, intracellular chloride channel protein 1, glutathione S-transferase, heat-shock protein 60 and cytokeratin 8) were altered in the *H. pylori*-infected tissues compared with the non-infected tissues. These proteins are related to cell proliferation, carcinogenesis, cytoskeletal function and cellular defence mechanism. *H. pylori*-induced alterations of protein expression of these proteins indicate the involvement of oxidative stress in the pathogenesis of *H. pylori*-induced gastric diseases, including inflammation, ulceration and carcinogenesis (Baek et al., 2004).

3.3 Role of glutathione and Mn-SOD in oxidative stress -induced gastric mucosal injury

The NADPH oxidase complex causes a strong stimulation of the pentose phosphate pathway (PPP), which primarily control the most important antioxidant of gastric mucosa, glutathione (Beil et al. 2000; Matthews & Butler, 2005).

Glutathione is a co-substrate of many enzymes involved in cellular detoxification and protection mechanisms (Townsend & Tew 2003). Maintaining optimal reduced glutathione/oxidized glutathione (GSH/GSSG) ratio in the cell is critical to survival and tight regulation of the system is imperative. A deficiency of GSH puts the cell at risk for oxidative damage (Townsend et al., 2003). *H. pylori* directly decrease cellular glutathione. Concerning GSH, their recycling is dependent on the maintenance of an pool of NADPH mainly via the pentose phosphate pathway, in which the reaction catalyzed by the glucose-6-phosphate dehidrogenase (G6-PDH) is the rate-limiting step. Mutations in *ZWF1*, the gene which encodes G6-PDH, make cells hypersensitive to oxidants such as H_2O_2 (Juhnke et al., 1996). During normal detoxification, H_2O_2 is converted to H_2O by reduced glutathione peroxidase and the oxidized glutathione is converted back to the reduced form by glutathione reductase and NADPH.

Glutathione (gamma-L-glutamyl-L-cysteinylglycine), the main non-protein thiol found in cells, is synthesized exclusively in the cytosol in two steps that require ATP. The first step is the unusual coupling of the gamma-carboxylic acid of glutamic acid to cysteine by the enzyme gamma-glutamylcysteine synthetase, followed by the formation of GSH by GSH synthetase, which uses ATP and gamma-glutamylcysteine and glycine as substrates. The formation of gamma-glutamylcysteine is the rate-limiting reaction in GSH synthesis and is a feedback inhibited by GSH itself, a mechanism responsible for the regulation of cellular GSH concentration.

Glutathione S-transferase plays a key role in the detoxification of carcinogenes, therapeutic drugs, and products of oxidative stress. This enzyme utilizes glutathione in reactions contributing to the transformation of such substances.

Studied association between glutathione S-transferases polymorphisms and immunoglobin G titer levels in serum against *Helicobacter pylori* in healthy subjects seropositive for *H. pylori* suggests that glutathione S-transferases activity is possibly involved in the protection against mucosal atrophy caused by *H. pylori* (Tatemichi et al., 2009). Another data showed that GSH plays a major role in cytoprotection against ulceration (Demir et al., 2003). This study has shown that gastric mucosal malondialdehide (MDA) levels were significantly higher, and gastric mucosal concentrations of GSH were significantly lower in peptic ulcer and gastritis patients compared to controls. These results suggest that the depletion of gastric mucosal glutathione in peptic ulcers and gastritis is caused by accumulation of free radicals. The findings of the study also confirm that ROS play important pathological role in gastric mucosa. Therefore, effective treatment and prevention of gastritis and peptic ulcers should be based on using the antioxidants in order to enhance gastric mucosal defence. Antioxidant enzymes, superoxide dismutase catalase, glutathione peroxidase, or peroxiredoxins are vital to the regulation of oxidative stress within cells. Significant changes in the activity and expression of several isoforms of superoxide dismutase were observed in the human gastric disease.

In eukaryotic cells, three isoforms of superoxide dismutase are present: extracellular copper/zinc-containing SOD (EC-SOD), mitochondrial manganese containing SOD (Mn-SOD), and cytoplasmic/nuclear copper/zinc-containing SOD (Cu,Zn-SOD), although the latter also localizes to the mitochondrial intermembrane space (Okado-Matsumoto & Fridovich, 2001). While the SOD isoenzymes catalyze the identical dismutation reaction involving the conversion of superoxide anion to oxygen and hydrogen peroxide , the function of each SOD isoform in cellular physiology appears to be very different, and often one SOD cannot compensate for another. Manganese superoxide dismutase induced by oxidative stress and by several physiological stimuli including inflammatory cytokines, bacterial proteins and growth factors. Gotz *et al.* first reported an increase of Mn- SOD in *H. pylori* -positive gastric mucosa. The study showed a significant correlation between the level of Mn-SOD protein with the degree of inflammation in the gastric mucosa (Noguchi *et al.*, 2002; Smoot et al., 2000). Recently, we have reviewed the important role of Mn-SOD in inflammation (Dovhanj et al., 2010). Manganese superoxide dismutase expression has been evaluated in gastric cancer, but little is known about the expression changes that occur in Mn-SOD in normal gastic mucosa from non-cancer patients with chronic gastritis. The evaluation of Mn-SOD activity during inflammation of gastric mucosa could clear out whether its assessment may be important to prevent the accumulation of gastric epithelial cell oxidative damage.

Given the risk of Mn-SOD overexpression and the role of Mn-SOD in the response to oxidative stress we hypothesized that patients with chronic gastritis would have increased mucosal Mn- SOD expression associated with chronic inflammation in the gastric mucosa. The inverse correlation between Mn-SOD activity and cell growth is a paradoxical phenomenon because Mn-SOD functions only as an antioxidant enzyme to protect a cell from oxidative stress caused by $O_2^{\cdot-}$ (Oberley, 2001). Proposed hypotheses regarding mechanisms by which Mn-SOD exerts growth inhibition often emphasize increased H_2O_2 production secondary to elevated Mn-SOD activity resulting in oxidative environments first in mitochondria and subsequently in the cytoplasm (Li et al., 2001; Li & Oberley, 1998; Rodriguez et al., 2000).

Reactive oxygen species and glutathione levels were measured in various phases of the cell cycle in both parental NIH/3T3 cells and NIH/3T3 cells overexpressing Mn-SOD, to determine whether their levels could have a possible regulatory role in cell cycle progression. This results suggest that oxidative stress exists in M phase of the cell cycle with total glutathione levels increased to decrease oxidative stress while analysis of Mn-SOD-overexpressing cell clones showed correlation of decreased cell growth with an ROS increase in S phase of the cell cycle and decrease of glutathione in mitosis. The data strongly suggest that specific levels of cell redox state are necessary for cells to successfully progress through the various phases of the cell cycle (Li & Oberley, 1998).

However, overexpression of Mn-SOD exceeding physiological conditions can lead to accumulation of ROS and oxidative stress, which may contribute to tumor metastasis and angiogenesis. It is known that intracellular content of Mn-SOD is altered in gastric neoplasms compared with normal tissue (Janssen et al., 2000; Hermann et al., 2005; Kruidenier et al., 2003, Hwang et al., 2005). Mn-SOD overexpression inhibits cell growth in both nonmalignant and malignant cells. The studies on Mn-SOD expression in cancer cells have been conducted on human tumours by comparing the specific cancer cell type with a relevant control cell type (colorectal cancer/ adjacent normal mucosa, oesophageal and gastric cancer /normal mucosa). According to these studies, Mn-SOD expression is variable but often high in human tumours compared to their normal counterparts. Understanding of the regulation of antiproliferative pathways by Mn-SOD and its control of tumor invasion might aid in the design of novel therapies targeting the respective molecular pathways (Valko, 2007).

4. Oxidative damage to DNA, lipids and proteins

The inflammation of gastric mucosa activates various oxidant-producing enzymes such as NADPH oxidase and inducible nitric oxide synthase. Reactive oxygen metabolites and nitrogen metabolites generated by these enzymes react with each other to generate new or more potent reactive species. The specific types of cellular damage resulting from reactive oxygen metabolites include lipid peroxidation, protein oxidation, and oxidative DNA damage. At high concentrations, ROS can be important mediators of damage to cell structures. Consequences of this stress include modification to cellular proteins, lipids and DNA (Valko et al., 2006). The hydroxyl radical is known to react with all components of the DNA molecule, damaging both the purine and pyrimidine bases and also the deoxyribose backbone (Halliwell & Gutteridge, 1999). The most extensively studied DNA lesion is the formation of 8-nitroguanine while carbonyl derivatives of proteins are the most widely studied oxidative stress-induced protein modifications (Valko et al., 2007). Carbonyl formation can occur through a variety of mechanisms including direct oxidation of certain amino-acid side chains and oxidation-induced peptide cleavage. Although all organs and all proteins can potentially be modified by oxidative stress, certain tissues and specific protein targets may be especially sensitive (Stadtman, 1992; Yan at al., 1997). The side chains of all amino acid residues of proteins, in particular cysteine and methionine residues of proteins are susceptible to oxidation by ROS/RNS (Stadtman, 2004). Oxidation of cysteine residues may lead to the reversible formation of mixed disulphides between protein thiol groups (-SH) and low molecular weight thiols, GSH (*S*-glutathiolation). The concentration of carbonyl groups, generated by many different mechanisms is a good measure of ROS-mediated protein oxidation. A number of highly sensitive methods have been developed for the assay of protein carbonyl groups (Dalle-Donne, 2005).

Nitric oxide contributes to oxidative lesions and alterations of gastric mucosa structure. Urinary 8-nitroguanine, a product of nitrative nucleic acid damage caused by reactive nitrogen species such as peroxynitrite and nitrogen dioxide. Immunoreactivity of the 8-nitroguanine has been found in the cytosol as well as in the nucleus of inflammatory cells and epithelial cells in inflamed tissues, but not in normal tissues. 8-nitroguanine in DNA is potentially mutagenic, yielding G:C to T:A transversion, possibly through its rapid depurination to form an apurinic site and/or miscoding with adenine. 8-nitroguanine in RNA may interfere with RNA functions and metabolism. Nitrated guanine nucleosides and nucleotides in the nucleotide pool may contribute to oxidative stress via production of superoxide mediated by various reductases and may disturb or modulate directly various important enzymes such as GTP-binding proteins and cGMP-dependent enzymes (Ohshima, et al. 2006).

Determination of NO metabolites concentrations in gastric juice of *Helicobacter pylori* positive patients has shown that the increase of NO metabolites is correlated with inflammatory lesions in gastric mucosa (Walecka-Kapica, E., 2008). *Helicobacter pylori* infection is associated with oxidatively damaged DNA in human leukocytes and decreased level of urinary 8-oxo-7,8-dihydroguanine. The levels of 8-oxo-7,8-dihydroguanine in DNA isolated from leukocytes of *H.pylori* infected patients and in the group with gastritis without *H.pylori* infection were significantly higher than in DNA isolated from the control group while level of urinary 8-oxo-7,8-dihydroguanine of children infected with *H.pylori* was significantly lower compared to group with gastritis without *H.pylori* infection. This increase of 8-oxo-7,8-dihydro-2'-deoxyguanosine level in leukocytes was interpreted as a response to inflammation itself, not just *H.pylori* infection. However, observed decrease in the level of modified base in urine seems to be specific for *H.pylori* infection and possibly linked with nitric oxide mediated inhibition of a key base excision repair enzyme (human 8-oxo-7, 8-dihydroguanine glycosylase) responsible for the repair of 8-oxo-7,8-dihydroguanine (Siomek, 2006).

Amelioration of oxidative stress with ensuing inflammation contributes to chemoprevention of *H. pylori*-associated gastric carcinogenesis (Park 2004). Gastric mucosa of patients infected by CagA-positive strains is characterized by a higher generation of ROS and by greater neutrophil counts than that observed in CagA-negative subjects (Danese, 2001). In addition, the oxygen-free radicals-mediated damage due to *H. pylori* cytotoxic strains, CagA+ strains, could be a driving force that leads from chronic gastritis to gastric carcinoma (Papa, 2002). A double immunofluorescence labeling study demonstrated that the level of 8-nitroguanine and 8-oxo-7,8-dihydro-2'-deoxyguanosine (8-oxodG) apparent in gastric gland epithelium was significantly higher in gastritis patients with *H. pylori* infection than in those without infection. This results suggest that 8-nitroguanine could be a promising biomarker of inflammation (Ma, 2004).

Kawanishi et al. examined the formation of 8-nitroguanine, a nitrative DNA lesion, in humans and animals under inflammatory conditions. An immunofluorescence labeling study demonstrated that 8-nitroguanine was strongly formed in gastric gland epithelial cells in gastritis patients with *H. pylori* infection, in hepatocytes in patients with hepatitis C, and in oral epithelium of patients with oral lichen planus. 8-nitroguanine was also formed in colonic epithelial cells of model mice of inflammatory bowel diseases and patients with ulcerative colitis. Interestingly, 8-nitroguanine was formed at the sites of carcinogenesis regardless of etiology. Therefore, 8-nitroguanine could be used to evaluate the risk of inflammation-related carcinogenesis.

Oxidative damage of the gastric mucosa in *H. pylori* positive chronic atrophic and nonatrophic gastritis, was evaluated by nitrotyrosine immunohistochemistry in the mucosa before and after eradication. Total nitrotyrosine levels appeared significantly higher in *H. pylori* positive than in negative patients. Oxidative damage of the gastric mucosa increases from *H. pylori* -chronic gastritis to *H. pylori* - chronic atrophic gastrits, involving the foveolae and intestinal metaplasia. *H. pylori* eradication induces a complete healing of foveolae but not of intestinal metaplasia, reducing the overall oxidative damage in the mucosa (Iacopini, F. et al. 2003). *Helicobacter pylori* eradication has differential effects on oxidative DNA damage at the gastroesophageal junction and at the gastric antrum. The levels of DNA adducts in the antral mucosa are not modified by *H. pylori* eradication; conversely, *H. pylori* eradication significantly increases the oxidative adducts at the gastroesophageal junction (Farinti, 2004).

Enhanced understanding of the mechanisms of gastroduodenal defense and injury provides new insight into potential therapeutic targets, contributing towards the development of better tolerated and more effective therapies (deFoneska 2010). Albayrak et al, 2010 suggested that urinary 8-OHdG levels could be investigated in every patient with chronic gastritis, since it is a simple and completely noninvasive procedure. In patients with high levels of urinary 8-OHdG, endoscopic procedures or even pathological investigation may then be carried out, with the consideration that there is a high risk of intestinal metaplasia.

4.1 Monitoring of oxidative damage of gastric mucosa

The determination of oxidative stress in inflammation of gastric mucosa may be important for a better understanding of its pathophysiology. ROS and RNS react with each other to generate new or more potent reactive species. Specific types of cellular damage resulting from reactive oxygen metabolites include lipid peroxidation, protein oxidation, and oxidative DNA damage. There are direct and indirect markers for monitoring of oxidative damage of gastric mucosa. Measurement of oxidation markers (direct) is helpful to assess oxidant activity and to monitor the effectiveness of the antioxidant system in normal cell affected by inflammation. The techniques range for detecting free radicals and reactive oxygen species or their byproducts include advanced methodologies using high-performance liquid chromatography, mass spectrometry, and electron paramagnetic resonance. The HPLC techniques are applied to the electrochemical measurement of protein oxidation products, particularly nitrotyrosine and dityrosine, and to the electrochemical detection of DNA oxidation products (Sawa, 2006). There are also mass spectrometry methods for measuring lipid oxidation products. Determination of biological markers of in vivo oxidative DNA damage, 8-hydroxy-2'-deoxyguanosine, and well-known lipid peroxidation markers, malondialdehyde (MDA) and 4-hydroxy-2-nonenal (HNE) are important for oxidative damage of gastric mucosa . HNE and MDA produce DNA adducts such as exocyclic etheno- and propano-DNA adducts, which are strong promutagenic DNA lesions causing point mutations.

The enzymatic and nonenzymatic antioxidants have been proposed as indirect markers. Among them, ascorbic acid, a-tocopherol, glutathione, enzymatic redox system of glutathione, glutathione-S-transferase and superoxide dismutase are related to gastric mucosal damage. Urinary hydrogen peroxide was postulated to be a biomarker of oxidative stress. (Baneerje, 2003). Recently, Lianzhen Yu et al. studied the low-molecular-weight 15 metabolites (including antioxidants) in blood plasma to characterize different stages from chronic superficial gastritis to chronic atrophic gastritis, intestinal metaplasia, gastric dysplasia and finally gastric cancer. They applied gas chromatography time-of-flight mass spectrometry to determine metabolites levels in plasma. The discriminatory metabolites characterizing progressive stages from chronic superficial gastritis to gastric cancer might be the potential markers to indicate the risk of gastric cancer. After a critical review of the literature data, we conclude that the balance between antioxidants and by-products of oxidative stress in the organism might be the best approach for the evaluation of oxidative stress in patients with gastric mucosal inflammation.

5. Conclusion

The severity of active inflammation of infected mucosa is directly correlated to the presence of high concentrations of free radicals. Increased oxidative stress in normal mucosa that had undergone changes in intensity of inflammatory infiltrates in the lamina propria are due to presence of inflammatory cells within the gastric mucosa. The inflammation has a key promoting role in oxidative stress. During the inflammation, inflammatory cells migrate to the injured site followed by a respiratory burst generating superoxide anion and other ROS. Oxidants, as mediators of cell damage, should be eliminated in normal cells. Antioxidative enzyme, Mn-SOD, is critically important in the maintenance of mitochondrial function in a cell. Thus, the mitochondrial Mn-SOD represents a major cellular defense against oxidative stress. A number of studies have suggested that altered cell redox state prove oxidative stress in gastric mucosa and further strengthen the idea of antioxidative defence up-regulation as protection of normal cells against inflammatory cells-derived ROS. The precise mechanisms of association between inflammation of gastric mucosa and mucosal oxidative damage need to be evaluated. Previous findings support the general idea that the evaluation of oxidative stress could be a useful factor for estimating the importance of the inflammation of gastric mucosa.

6. References

Allen, L. A. (2007). Phagocytosis and persistence of Helicobacter pylori. *Cell Microbiology,* Vol.9, No.4, (March 2010), pp.817-828, ISSN: 1462-5814.

Allen, L. A., & McCaffrey, R. L. (2007). To activate or not to activate: distinct strategies used by Helicobacter pylori and Francisella tularensis to modulate the NADPH oxidase and survive in human neutrophils. *Immunol Rev,* Vol.219, (September, 2007), pp.103-117, ISSN: 0105-289.

Albayrak, F., Uyanik, M. H., Dursun, H., Albayrak, Y., Altas, S., Uyanik, A., et al. (2010). Should increased levels of urinary 8-hydroxydeoxyguanosine in chronic gastritis imply intestinal metaplasia or gastric atrophy? *South Med J,* Vol.103, No.8, (July 2010), pp. 753-757, ISSN: 0006-2952.

Babior, B. M. (1999). NADPH oxidase: an update. *Blood,* Vol.*93, No.*5, (February 1999), pp. 1464-1476, ISSN: 0006-4971.

Baek, H. Y., Lim, J. W., Kim, H., Kim, J. M., Kim, J. S., Jung, H. C., et al. (2004). Oxidative-stress-related proteome changes in Helicobacter pylori-infected human gastric mucosa. *Biochem J, Vol.379, No.*2, (January 2001), pp. 291-299, ISSN: 1470-8728.

Baik, S. C., Youn, H. S., Chung, M. H., Lee, W. K., Cho, M. J., Ko, G. H., et al. (1996). Increased oxidative DNA damage in Helicobacter pylori-infected human gastric mucosa. *Cancer Res, Vol. 56,* No.6, (March 1996), pp. 1279-1282, ISSN: 0008-5472.

Balaban, R. S., Nemoto, S., & Finkel, T. (2005). Mitochondria, oxidants, and aging. *Cell,* Vol.120, No.4, (March 2005), pp. 483-495, ISSN: 0092-8674.

Banerjee, D., Madhusoodanan, U. K., Nayak, S., & Jacob, J. (2003). Urinary hydrogen peroxide: a probable marker of oxidative stress in malignancy. *Clin Chim Acta,*Vol.334, No.1-2, (July 2003), pp. 205-209, ISSN: 0009-8981.

Bedard, K., & Krause, K. H. (2007). The NOX family of ROS-generating NADPH oxidases: physiology and pathophysiology. *Physiol Rev, Vol.87,*No.1, (January 2007), pp. 245-313, ISSN: 0031-9333.

Beil, W., Obst, B., Sewing, K. F., & Wagner, S. (2000). Helicobacter pylori reduces intracellular glutathione in gastric epithelial cells. *Dig Dis Sci,* Vol.*45, No.*9, (October 2000), pp. 1769-1773, ISSN: 0163-2116.

Bulger, E. M., & Helton, W. S. (1998). Nutrient antioxidants in gastrointestinal diseases. *Gastroenterol Clin North Am, Vol.*27, No.2, (July 1998), pp. 403-419, ISSN: 0889-8553.

Davies, G. R., Banatvala, N., Collins, C. E., Sheaff, M. T., Abdi, Y., Clements, L., et al. (1994). Relationship between infective load of Helicobacter pylori and reactive oxygen metabolite production in antral mucosa. *Scand J Gastroenterol,* Vol.29, No.5, (May 1994), pp. 419-424, ISSN: 0889-8553.

Davies, G. R., Simmonds, N. J., Stevens, T. R., Sheaff, M. T., Banatvala, N., Laurenson, I. F., et al. (1994). Helicobacter pylori stimulates antral mucosal reactive oxygen metabolite production in vivo. *Gut,* Vol.35, No.2, (February 1994), pp. 179-185, ISSN: 0017-5749.

Danese, S., Cremonini, F., Armuzzi, A., Candelli, M., Papa, A., Ojetti, V., et al. (2001). Helicobacter pylori CagA-positive strains affect oxygen free radicals generation by gastric mucosa. *Scand J Gastroenterol,* Vol.36, No.3, (April 2001), pp. 247-250, ISSN: 0036-5521.

deFoneska, A., & Kaunitz, J. D. (2010). Gastroduodenal mucosal defense. *Curr Opin Gastroenterol,* Vol.26, No.6, (October 2010), pp. 604-610, ISSN: 1531-7056.

Demir, S., Yilmaz, M., Koseoglu, M., Akalin, N., Aslan, D., & Aydin, A. (2003). Role of free radicals in peptic ulcer and gastritis. *Turk J Gastroenterol,* Vol.14, No.1, (November 2003), pp. 39-43, ISSN: 1300-4948.

Di Virgilio, F., Chiozzi, P., Ferrari, D., Falzoni, S., Sanz, J. M., Morelli, A., et al. (2001). Nucleotide receptors: an emerging family of regulatory molecules in blood cells. *Blood,* Vol.97, No.3,(February 2001), pp. 587-600, ISSN: 0006-4971.

Ding, S. Z., Minohara, Y., Fan, X. J., Wang, J., Reyes, V. E., Patel, J., et al. (2007). Helicobacter pylori infection induces oxidative stress and programmed cell death in human gastric epithelial cells. *Infect Immun,* Vol.75, No.8, (June 2007), pp. 4030-4039, ISSN: 0019-9567.

Dovhanj, J., Kljaic, K., Dodig-Curkovic, K., Curkovic, M., Volarevic, M., & Marjanovic, K. (2009). Helicobacter pylori, zinc and iron in oxidative stress-induced injury of gastric mucosa. *Mini Rev Med Chem,* Vol.9, No.1, (January 2009), pp. 26-30, ISSN: 1389-5575.

Dovhanj, J., Kljaic, K., Smolic, M., & Svagelj, D. (2010). NADPH and iron may have an important role in attenuated mucosal defense in Helicobacter pylori infection? *Mini Rev Med Chem,* Vol.10, No.14, (December 2010), pp. 1309-1315, ISSN: 1875-5607.

El-Benna, J., Dang, P. M., Gougerot-Pocidalo, M. A., & Elbim, C. (2005). Phagocyte NADPH oxidase: a multicomponent enzyme essential for host defenses. *Arch Immunol Ther Exp (Warsz),* Vol.53, No.3, (July 2005), pp. 199-206, ISSN: 0004-069X.

Engelhardt, J. F., Sen, C. K., & Oberley, L. (2001). Redox-modulating gene therapies for human diseases. *Antioxid Redox Signal,* Vol.3, No.3, (August 2001), pp. 341-346, ISSN: 1523-0864.

Farinati, F., Cardin, R., Russo, V. M., Busatto, G., Franco, M., Falda, A., et al. (2004). Differential effects of Helicobacter pylori eradication on oxidative DNA damage at the gastroesophageal junction and at the gastric antrum. *Cancer Epidemiol Biomarkers Prev,* Vol.13, No.11, (November 2004), pp. 1722-1728, ISSN: 1055-9965.

Farinati, F., Cardin, R., Russo, V. M., Busatto, G., Franco, M., Falda, A., et al. (2004). Differential effects of Helicobacter pylori eradication on oxidative DNA damage at the gastroesophageal junction and at the gastric antrum. *Cancer Epidemiol Biomarkers Prev,* Vol.13, No.11, (November 2004), pp. 1722-1728, ISSN: 1055-9965.

Federico, A., Morgillo, F., Tuccillo, C., Ciardiello, F., & Loguercio, C. (2007). Chronic inflammation and oxidative stress in human carcinogenesis. *Int J Cancer,* Vol.121, No.11, (September 2007), pp. 2381-2386 ISSN: 1097-0215.

Finkel, T., & Holbrook, N. J. (2000). Oxidants, oxidative stress and the biology of ageing. *Nature,* Vol.408, No.6809, (November 2000), pp. 239-247, ISSN: 0028-0836.

Fredholm, B. B. (1997). Purines and neutrophil leukocytes. *Gen Pharmacol,* Vol.28, No.3, (March 1997), pp. 345-350, ISSN: 0306-3623.

Freitas, M., Lima, J. L., & Fernandes, E. (2009). Optical probes for detection and quantification of neutrophils' oxidative burst. A review. *Anal Chim Acta,* Vol.649, No.1, (August 2009), pp. 8-23, ISSN: 1873-4324.

Freitas, M., Porto, G., Lima, J. L., & Fernandes, E. (2010). Zinc activates neutrophils' oxidative burst. *Biometals,* Vol.23, No.1, (September 2009), pp. 31-41, ISSN: 1572-8773.

Fukuhara, K., Osugi, H., Takemura, M., Lee, S., Morimura, K., Kishida, S., et al. (2008). Helicobacter pylori induces gastritis and oxidative stress after distal gastrectomy. *Hepatogastroenterology,* Vol.55, No.85, (September 2008), pp. 1484-1486, ISSN: 0172-6390.

Gloire, G., Legrand-Poels, S., & Piette, J. (2006). NF-kappaB activation by reactive oxygen species: fifteen years later. *Biochem Pharmacol,* Vol.72, No.11, (May 2006), pp. 1493-1505, ISSN: 0006-2952.

Gottlieb, R. A. (2003). Cytochrome P450: major player in reperfusion injury. *Arch Biochem Biophys,* Vol.420, No.2, (December 2003), pp. 262-267, ISSN: 0003-9861.

Gotz, J. M., Veenendaal, R. A., Biemond, I., Muller, E. S., Veselic, M., & Lamers, C. B. (1995). Serum gastrin and mucosal somatostatin in Helicobacter pylori-associated gastritis. *Scand J Gastroenterol,* Vol.30, No.11, (November 1995), pp. 1064-1068, ISSN: 0036-5521.

Granger, J. P., Alexander, B. T., Llinas, M. T., Bennett, W. A., & Khalil, R. A. (2001). Pathophysiology of hypertension during preeclampsia linking placental ischemia with endothelial dysfunction. *Hypertension,* Vol.38, No.3, (September 2001), pp. 718-722, ISSN: 1524-4563.

Hermann, B., Li, Y., Ray, M. B., Wo, J. M., & Martin, R. C., 2nd. (2005). Association of manganese superoxide dismutase expression with progression of carcinogenesis in Barrett esophagus. *Arch Surg,* Vol.140, No.12, (December 2005), pp. 1204-1209, ISSN: 0004-0010.

Hwang, T. S., Choi, H. K., & Han, H. S. (2007). Differential expression of manganese superoxide dismutase, copper/zinc superoxide dismutase, and catalase in gastric adenocarcinoma and normal gastric mucosa. *Eur J Surg Oncol,* Vol.33, No.4, (November 2006), pp. 474-479, ISSN: 0748-7983.

Iacopini, F., Consolazio, A., Bosco, D., Marcheggiano, A., Bella, A., Pica, R., et al. (2003). Oxidative damage of the gastric mucosa in Helicobacter pylori positive chronic atrophic and nonatrophic gastritis, before and after eradication. *Helicobacter,* Vol.8, No.5, (October 2003), pp. 503-512, ISSN: 1083-4389.

Janssen, A. M., Bosman, C. B., van Duijn, W., Oostendorp-van de Ruit, M. M., Kubben, F. J., Griffioen, G., et al. (2000). Superoxide dismutases in gastric and esophageal cancer and the prognostic impact in gastric cancer. *Clin Cancer Res,* Vol.6, No.8, (August 2000), pp. 3183-3192, ISSN: 1078-0432.

Jomova, K., & Valko, M. (2011). Advances in metal-induced oxidative stress and human disease. *Toxicology,* Vol.283, No.2-3, (March 2011), pp. 65-87, ISSN: 1879-3185.

Juhnke, H., Krems, B., Kotter, P., & Entian, K. D. (1996). Mutants that show increased sensitivity to hydrogen peroxide reveal an important role for the pentose phosphate pathway in protection of yeast against oxidative stress. *Mol Gen Genet,* Vol.252, No.4, (September 1996), pp. 456-464, ISSN: 0026-8925.

Kamata, H., & Hirata, H. (1999). Redox regulation of cellular signalling. *Cell Signal,* Vol.11, No.1, (April 1999), pp. 1-14, ISSN: 0898-6568.

Kawano, S., Tanimura, H., Sato, N., Nagano, K., Tsuji, S., Takei, Y., et al. (1991). Age-related change in human gastric mucosal energy metabolism. *Scand J Gastroenterol,* Vol.26, No.7, (July 1991), pp. 701-706, ISSN: 0036-5521.

Kawanishi, S., & Hiraku, Y. (2006). Oxidative and nitrative DNA damage as biomarker for carcinogenesis with special reference to inflammation. *Antioxid Redox Signal,* Vol.8, No.5-6, (June 2006), pp. 1047-1058, ISSN: 1523-0864.

Klebanoff, S. J. (1980). Oxygen metabolism and the toxic properties of phagocytes. *Ann Intern Med,* Vol.93, No.3, (September1980), pp. 480-489, ISSN: 0003-4819.

Krause, K. H., & Bedard, K. (2008). NOX enzymes in immuno-inflammatory pathologies. *Semin Immunopathol,* Vol.30, No.3, (June 2008), pp. 193-194, ISSN: 1863-2297.

Kruidenier, L., Kuiper, I., van Duijn, W., Marklund, S. L., van Hogezand, R. A., Lamers, C. B., et al. (2003). Differential mucosal expression of three superoxide dismutase isoforms in inflammatory bowel disease. *J Pathol,* Vol.201, No.1, (September 2003), pp. 7-16, ISSN: 0022-3417.

Li, C. Q., Pignatelli, B., & Ohshima, H. (2001). Increased oxidative and nitrative stress in human stomach associated with cagA+ Helicobacter pylori infection and inflammation. *Dig Dis Sci,* Vol.46, No.4, (May 2001), pp. 836-844, ISSN: 0163-2116.

Li, N., & Oberley, T. D. (1998). Modulation of antioxidant enzymes, reactive oxygen species, and glutathione levels in manganese superoxide dismutase-overexpressing NIH/3T3 fibroblasts during the cell cycle. *J Cell Physiol,* Vol.177, No. 1, (September 1998), pp. 148-160, ISSN: 0021-9541.

Ma, N., Adachi, Y., Hiraku, Y., Horiki, N., Horiike, S., Imoto, I., et al. (2004). Accumulation of 8-nitroguanine in human gastric epithelium induced by Helicobacter pylori infection. *Biochem Biophys Res Commun,* Vol.319, No.2, (June 2004), pp. 506-510, ISSN: 0006-291X.

Matthews, G. M., & Butler, R. N. (2005). Cellular mucosal defense during Helicobacter pylori infection: a review of the role of glutathione and the oxidative pentose pathway. *Helicobacter,* Vol.10, No.4, (August 2005), pp. 298-306, ISSN: 1083-4389.

McGee, D. J., & Mobley, H. L. (1999). Mechanisms of Helicobacter pylori infection: bacterial factors. *Curr Top Microbiol Immunol,* Vol.241, (March 1999), pp. 155-180, ISSN: 0070-217X.

Menguy, R., & Masters, Y. F. (1974). Gastric mucosal energy metabolism and "stress ulceration". *Ann Surg,* Vol.180, No.4, (October 1974), pp. 538-548, ISSN: 0003-4932.

Menguy, R., & Masters, Y. F. (1974). Mechanism of stress ulcer. 3. Effects of hemorrhagic shock on energy metabolism in the mucosa of the antrum, corpus, and fundus of the rabbit stomach. *Gastroenterology,* Vol.66, No.6, (June 1974), pp. 1168-1176, ISSN: 0016-5085.

Menguy, R., & Masters, Y. F. (1974). Mechanism of stress ulcer. II. Differences between the antrum, corpus, and fundus with respect to the effects of complete ischemia on gastric mucosal energy metabolism. *Gastroenterology,* Vol.66, No.4, (June 1974), pp. 509-516, ISSN: 0016-5085.

Menguy, R., & Masters, Y. F. (1974). Mechanism of stress ulcer. IV. Influence of fasting on the tolerance of gastric mucosal energy metabolism to ischemia and on the incidence of stress ulceration. *Gastroenterology,* Vol.66, No.6, (April 1974), pp. 1177-1186, ISSN: 0016-5085.

Naito, Y., & Yoshikawa, T. (2002). Molecular and cellular mechanisms involved in Helicobacter pylori-induced inflammation and oxidative stress. *Free Radic Biol Med,* Vol.33, No.3, (July 2002), pp. 323-336, ISSN: 0891-5849.

Nardone, G., Rocco, A., & Malfertheiner, P. (2004). Review article: helicobacter pylori and molecular events in precancerous gastric lesions. *Aliment Pharmacol Ther,* Vol.20, No.3, (July 2004), pp. 261-270, ISSN: 0269-2813.

Noguchi, K., Kato, K., Moriya, T., Suzuki, T., Saito, M., Kikuchi, T., et al. (2002). Analysis of cell damage in Helicobacter pylori-associated gastritis. *Pathol Int,* Vol.52, No.2, (April 2002), pp. 110-118, ISSN: 1320-5463.

Oberley, L. W. (2001). Anticancer therapy by overexpression of superoxide dismutase. *Antioxid Redox Signal,* Vol.3, No.3, (August 2001), pp. 461-472, ISSN: 1523-0864.

Obst, B., Wagner, S., Sewing, K. F., & Beil, W. (2000). Helicobacter pylori causes DNA damage in gastric epithelial cells. *Carcinogenesis,* Vol.21, No.6, (June 2000), pp. 1111-1115, ISSN: 0143-3334.

Ohshima, H., Sawa, T., & Akaike, T. (2006). 8-nitroguanine, a product of nitrative DNA damage caused by reactive nitrogen species: formation, occurrence, and implications in inflammation and carcinogenesis. *Antioxid Redox Signal,* Vol.8, No.5-6, (June 2006), pp. 1033-1045, ISSN: 1523-0864.

Okado-Matsumoto, A., & Fridovich, I. (2001). Subcellular distribution of superoxide dismutases (SOD) in rat liver: Cu,Zn-SOD in mitochondria. *J Biol Chem,* Vol.276, No.42, (August 2001), pp. 38388-38393, ISSN: 0021-9258.

Otamiri, T., & Sjodahl, R. (1991). Oxygen radicals: their role in selected gastrointestinal disorders. *Dig Dis,* Vol.9, No.3, (January 1991), pp. 133-141, ISSN: 0257-2753.

Papa, A., Danese, S., Sgambato, A., Ardito, R., Zannoni, G., Rinelli, A., et al. (2002). Role of Helicobacter pylori CagA+ infection in determining oxidative DNA damage in gastric mucosa. *Scand J Gastroenterol,* Vol.37, No.4, (May 2002), pp. 409-413, ISSN: 0036-552.

Park, S., Kim, W. S., Choi, U. J., Han, S. U., Kim, Y. S., Kim, Y. B., et al. (2004). Amelioration of oxidative stress with ensuing inflammation contributes to chemoprevention of H. pylori-associated gastric carcinogenesis. *Antioxid Redox Signal,* Vol.6, No.3, (May 2004), pp. 549-560, ISSN: 1523-0864.

Pignatelli, B., Bancel, B., Plummer, M., Toyokuni, S., Patricot, L. M., & Ohshima, H. (2001). Helicobacter pylori eradication attenuates oxidative stress in human gastric mucosa. *Am J Gastroenterol,* Vol.96, No.06, (June 2001), pp. 1758-1766, ISSN: 0002-9270.

Rodriguez, A. M., Carrico, P. M., Mazurkiewicz, J. E., & Melendez, J. A. (2000). Mitochondrial or cytosolic catalase reverses the MnSOD-dependent inhibition of proliferation by enhancing respiratory chain activity, net ATP production, and decreasing the steady state levels of H(2)O(2). *Free Radic Biol Med,* Vol.29, No.9, (November 2000), pp. 801-813, ISSN: 0891-5849.

Sato, D., Yanaka, A., Shibahara, T., Matsui, H., Nakahara, A., Yanagawa, T., et al. (2008). Peroxiredoxin I protects gastric mucosa from oxidative injury induced by H. pylori infection. *J Gastroenterol Hepatol,* Vol.23, No.4, (November 2007), pp. 652-659, ISSN: 1440-1746.

Sawa, T., Tatemichi, M., Akaike, T., Barbin, A., & Ohshima, H. (2006). Analysis of urinary 8-nitroguanine, a marker of nitrative nucleic acid damage, by high-performance liquid chromatography-electrochemical detection coupled with immunoaffinity purification: association with cigarette smoking. *Free Radic Biol Med,* Vol.40, No.4, (February 2006), pp. 711-720, ISSN: 0891-5849.

Siomek, A., Rytarowska, A., Szaflarska-Poplawska, A., Gackowski, D., Rozalski, R., Dziaman, T., et al. (2006). Helicobacter pylori infection is associated with oxidatively damaged DNA in human leukocytes and decreased level of urinary 8-oxo-7,8-dihydroguanine. *Carcinogenesis,* Vol.27, No.3, (October 2005), pp. 405-408, ISSN: 0143-3334.

Sasaki, M., & Joh, T. (2007). Oxidative stress and ischemia-reperfusion injury in gastrointestinal tract and antioxidant, protective agents. *J Clin Biochem Nutr,* Vol.40, No.1, (April 2008), pp. 1-12, ISSN: 0912-0009.

Sezikli, M., Cetinkaya, Z. A., Sezikli, H., Guzelbulut, F., Tiftikci, A., Ince, A. T., et al. (2009). Oxidative stress in Helicobacter pylori infection: does supplementation with vitamins C and E increase the eradication rate? *Helicobacter,* Vol.14, No.4, (August 2009), pp. 280-285, ISSN: 1523-5378.

Smoot, D. T., Elliott, T. B., Verspaget, H. W., Jones, D., Allen, C. R., Vernon, K. G., et al. (2000). Influence of Helicobacter pylori on reactive oxygen-induced gastric epithelial cell injury. *Carcinogenesis,* Vol.21, No.11, (November 2000), pp. 2091-2095, ISSN: 0143-3334.

Suzuki, H., Marshall, B. J., & Hibi, T. (2006). Overview: Helicobacter pylori and extragastric disease. *Int J Hematol,* Vol.84, No.4, (November 2006), pp. 291-300, ISSN: 0925-5710.

Suzuki, T., Matsuo, K., Sawaki, A., Ito, H., Hirose, K., Wakai, K., et al. (2006). Systematic review and meta-analysis: importance of CagA status for successful eradication of Helicobacter pylori infection. *Aliment Pharmacol Ther,* Vol.24, No.2, (July 2006), pp. 273-280, ISSN: 0269-2813.

Swennen, E. L., Bast, A., & Dagnelie, P. C. (2005). Immunoregulatory effects of adenosine 5'-triphosphate on cytokine release from stimulated whole blood. *Eur J Immunol,* Vol,35. No.3, (February 2005), pp. 852-858, ISSN: 0014-2980.

Tatemichi, M., Iwasaki, M., Sasazuki, S., & Tsugane, S. (2009). Association between polymorphisms in glutathione S-transferase Mu3 and IgG titer levels in serum against Helicobacter pylori. *J Hum Genet,* Vol.54, No.10, (August 2009), pp. 557-563, ISSN: 1435-232X.

Townsend, D. M., & Tew, K. D. (2003). The role of glutathione-S-transferase in anti-cancer drug resistance. *Oncogene,* Vol.22, No.47, (October 2003), pp. 7369-7375, ISSN: 0950-9232.

Townsend, D. M., Tew, K. D., & Tapiero, H. (2003). The importance of glutathione in human disease. *Biomed Pharmacother,* Vol.57, No.3-4, (June 2003), pp. 145-155, ISSN: 0753-3322.

Valko, M., Leibfritz, D., Moncol, J., Cronin, M. T., Mazur, M., & Telser, J. (2007). Free radicals and antioxidants in normal physiological functions and human disease. *Int J Biochem Cell Biol,* Vol.39, No.1, (September 2006), pp. 44-84, ISSN: 1357-2725.

Yoshikawa, T., & Naito, Y. (2000). The role of neutrophils and inflammation in gastric mucosal injury. *Free Radic Res,* Vol.33, No.6, (March 2001), pp. 785-794, ISSN: 1071-5762.

Walecka-Kapica, E., Knopik-Dabrowicz, A., Klupinska, G., & Chojnacki, J. (2008). [The assessment of nitric oxide metabolites in gastric juice in Helicobacter pylori infected subjects in compliance with grade of inflammatory lesions in gastric mucosa]. *Pol Merkur Lekarski,* Vol.24, No.140, (July 2008), pp. 95-100, ISSN: 1426-9686.

Yu, L., A, J., Sun, M., Qian, S., Cheng, L., Yang, S., et al. (2011). Metabolomic phenotype of gastric cancer and precancerous stages based on gas chromatography time-of-flight mass spectrometry. *J Gastroenterol Hepatol.*

Zhang, Y., Palmblad, J., & Fredholm, B. B. (1996). Biphasic effect of ATP on neutrophil functions mediated by P2U and adenosine A2A receptors. *Biochem Pharmacol,* Vol.51, No.7, (April 1996), pp. 957-965, ISSN: 0006-2952.

4

Oxidative Stress Involved Autophagy and Apoptosis in *Helicobacter pylori* Related Gastritis

Jyh-Chin Yang[1] and Chiang-Ting Chien[2,3]
Departments of [1]Internal Medicine
[2]Medical Research
[3]Graduate Institute of Clinical Medicine, Hospital and College of Medicine, National Taiwan University, Taipei
Taiwan

1. Introduction

Gastritis, inflammation of gastric mucosa, is a very common condition in the world wide. There is no universally accepted classification of gastritis. Early classification was based mainly on the morphology, but recently pathogenic mechanisms have also been incorporated. The Sydney system, a classification of gastritis introduced in 1990, and updated in 1995, has included both an endoscopic and histologic divisions and is designed for an unambiguous uniform reporting system. (Dixon, Genta et al. 1996)

The histologic changes of acute gastritis include hyperemia, edema, and infiltration of polymorphonuclear cells, together with variable loss of epithelium. Endoscopically, these changes can be observed as edema, petechial or submucosal hemorrhage, erosions or ulcers. A lot of factors including nonsteroidal anti-inflammatory drugs (NSAIDs) and various noxious substances may result in these acute abnormalities. Excess production of reactive oxygen species evokes oxidative stress, which can induce apoptosis and autophagy in the damaged tissue or cells. Oxidative stress induced by the NSAIDs and various noxious substances may contribute to the pathophysiologic and histopathologic alterations including autophagy and apoptosis, leading to gastritis.

The discovery of *Helicobacter pylori* has markedly improved our understanding about the nature of chronic gastritis and other important gastroduodenal diseases. (Marshall 1983; Warren 1983) *H. pylori* have been accepted as the most common cause of chronic gastritis. (Suerbaum and Michetti 2002) Colonization of gastric mucosa by *H. pylori* is always associated with persistent inflammation. Several virulence factor derived from *H. pylori* may promote these inflammatory mucosal changes. *H. pylori*-associated chronic gastritis usually accompanies with polymorphonuclear infiltration and architectural change of the gastric mucosa. There are marked mucosal cellular and systemic humoral immunologic responses. The mucosal damage seen in patients with *H. pylori* may result from both the effect of immunologic response and the bacterial toxin. Apoptosis and autophagy may contribute to cell homeostasis in gastric epithelial cells subjected to *H. pylori* infection. The combination of antioxidant and anti-adhesion materials can be attenuated the severity of gastritis.

2. Epidemiology

More than 50% of population in the world is infected with this bacterium. The prevalence of infection is increased with age and thought to be a cohort effect.

Epidemiologic studies show this infection is generally acquired during childhood and the majority of *H. pylori* transmission is through close person-to-person contact. The oral-oral, gastro-oral, or fecal-oral exposure seems the most probable explanation for infection. (Brown 2000; Amieva, El-Omar et al. 2008)

3. Pathogenesis

Bacterial factor and colonization

H. pylori infection is closely associated with chronic active type B gastritis, peptic ulcers, gastric cancer and gastric MALT lymphoma. The pre-neoplastic lesions, such as glandular atrophy and intestinal metaplasia, may consequently result from persistent chronic gastritis in some patients. The outcome of *H. pylori* infection depends on the combination of bacterial and host factors in addition to less well-defined environmental conditions.

H. pylori are one of few organisms capable of colonizing the harsh environment of the human stomach. The initial step in *H. pylori* infection is the penetration and adherence of the bacterium to mucin and epithelial cells. *H. pylori* generate large amounts of cytosolic and cell surface-associated urease. The urease helps the organism to avoid the bactericidal activity of gastric acid. *H. pylori* can use its polar flagella to migrate rapidly to a more favorable environment below the mucus layer very close to the surface of the epithelium where the pH is near neutral.

After *H. pylori* migrate to the gastric epithelium, the bacteria adhere to the surface of host cells and may damage them in order to obtain nutrients and establish persistent colonization. Several different adhesion molecules have been identified and classified as adhesins. (Boren, Falk et al. 1993) The best studied *H. pylori* adhesins are outer membrane proteins that bind carbohydrate modifications in the glycoproteins of epithelial cells. The specific bacterial gene product, BabA, act as the ligand for the fucosylated blood group antigen Lewis b receptor. (Ilver, Arnqvist et al. 1998) The SabA protein adheres to sialated glycoproteins, specifically to sialyl-Lewis-X. (Mahdavi, Sonden et al. 2002)

A segment of bacterial DNA, known as the cag pathogenicity iland (cag PAI), direct the key interaction between *H. pylori* and the host cells. Many of the genes adjacent to *cagA* encode proteins that provide a type IV secretion system (TFSS) that allows the transfer of bacterial products from pathogenic bacteria into the host cell. (Censini, Lange et al. 1996; Christie, Atmakuri et al. 2005) cag PAI plays an important role in the pathogenesis of gastritis. Patients infected with *cagA* positive strain of *H. pylori* are generally associated with increase interleukin-8 (IL-8) expression and inflammation in their gastric mucosa. (Blaser and Atherton 2004) CagA protein translocates into the cytoplasm of epithelial cell where it is tyrosine phosphorylated by host Src kinases and subsequently results in the change of cell morphology and cell function. (Higashi, Tsutsumi et al. 2002; Higashi, Tsutsumi et al. 2002)

The response of epithelial cell to *H. pylori* infection is complex and a summary of interaction with several influencing variables, such as bacterial virulence factors, the signaling linked to specific receptors, reaction of immune and hormones.

The *vacA* gene is present in all strains of this organism. However, only more than half of *H. pylori* strains are able to express the vacuolating cytotoxin (VacA). The association of the structure and function of VacA with the severity of disease has been demonstrated. (Cover 1996; Van Doorn, Figueiredo et al. 1999; Blaser and Atherton 2004). Specific *vacA* alleles (s1 and m1) can result in more severe disease and epithelial cell apoptosis. (Atherton, Cao et al. 1995; Cover, Krishna et al. 2003)

H. pylori strains that express outer inflammatory protein A (OipA) are also associated with increased expression of IL-8, neutrophil infiltration, and more severe clinical outcomes. (Yamaoka, Kikuchi et al. 2002)

Host response

The host response to *H. pylori* infection plays a very important role in the pathogenesis of this organism related gastrointestinal disease. The IL-1 is known as a strong inhibitor of gastric acid secretion. The genetic polymophisms of IL-1β have been demonstrated to be associated with an increased incidence of hypochlorhydria, atrophic gastritis and gastric cancer. (El-Omar, Carrington et al. 2000; Furuta, El-Omar et al. 2002) The development of gastric cancer can be related to increase IL-1 expression, more severe gastritis and greater colonization of *H. pylori*.

H. pylori infection can result in changes in epithelial cell morphology, disruption of the tight junction, production of cytokines, increased epithelial cell proliferation, and increased rates of epithelial cell death via apoptosis. (Amieva, Vogelmann et al. 2003; Naumann and Crabtree 2004; Ernst, Peura et al. 2006)

The induction and expression of genes in epithelial cells responding to *H. pylori* stimulation is regulated by several transcription factors which are controlled by a series of signaling mechanisms. The nuclear factor-kappa B (NF-$_k$B) seems to be the most studied molecule in these transcription factors. NF-$_k$B activity in *H. pylori* infected epithelium is markedly enhanced, correlating with increased secretion of IL-8 protein and infiltration of inflammatory cell. (Naumann and Crabtree 2004) The changes of cell functions, including cell profiferation, inflammation, and survival in response to *H. pylori* infection are mostly regulated by mitogen-activated protein (MAP) kinase cascades. (Keates, Keates et al. 1999)

The acid secretion is a major function of gastric epithelial cells. The net effect of *H. pylori* infection on acid secretion is related to the duration and distribution of infection and the presence of mucosal atrophy. The epithelial barrier function is altered as a consequence of both direct effects of *H. pylori* and its accompanying inflammatory response. Humans infected by *H. pylori* develop a unique inflammatory response in which infection persists despite the recruitment and activation of lymphocytes, phagocytic cells, and other immune cell populations. (Ernst, Peura et al. 2006)

It is known that *H. pylori* can induce an infiltration with T lymphocytes, plasma cells, mononuclear phagocytes and neutrophils. Furthermore, expression of cytokines such as tumor necrosis factor (TNF), IL-1, IL-6 and IL-8 is also enhanced by the infection. However, it is not well known how the immune response and the mechanisms behind it related to disease outcome. The immunoregulatory and proinflammatory cytokines induced by *H. pylori* may influence the nature of the local T cell response. It is thought that helper T (Th) cells can be divided into two subsets, Th1, and Th2. The Th1 subset promotes cell-mediated immunity by producing mainly IL-2, TNF-α, and interferon-gamma (IFN-γ), and the Th2 subset, which is important for antibody response produces IL-4, IL-5 and IL-10. Evidences in recent research have strongly suggested that T cell mediated immune response may play an important role in induction of disease in *H. pylori* infection. (Crowe, Alvarez et al. 1995; D'Elios, Manghetti et al. 1997; Mohammadi, Nedrud et al. 1997) It is still not clear whether different outcome of the disease is modulated by the different type of T cell immune response, although some studies suggested that Th1 type dominant cellular response may be involved in the *Helicobacter* disease. (Haeberle, Kubin et al. 1997) Little is known about whether Th2 response can be protective or whether modulation of these responses can change the outcome of infection.

Apoptosis and autophagy

Some bacterial components may reach the lamina propria where it can activate underlying phagocytosis through the damaged epithelial barrier. One of these bacterial factors is the *H. pylori* neutrophil-activating protein (Hp-NAP). This protein can promote the adhesion of neutrophil to the endothelial cells and stimulate chemotaxis of monocytes and neutrophils and production of reactive oxygen intermediates. (Satin, Del Giudice et al. 2000) Recruitment and activation of neutrophils and macrophages result in the release of various inflammatory mediators.

H. pylori urease has been shown to bind to class II major histocompatibility complex (MHC) molecules on the surfaces of gastric epithelial cells and induce apoptosis. (Fan, Gunasena et al. 2000) *H. pylori* VacA can be inserted into mitochondrial membranes where it induces cytochrome c release and activates the caspase-3-dependent cell-death signaling cascade. (Galmiche, Rassow et al. 2000) Also, Th1 cytokines induced by *H. pylori* can stimulate apoptosis through a Fas-mediate pathway by inducing expression of the cell-surface receptor Fas and Fas ligand. (Wagner, Beil et al. 1997; Jones, Day et al. 1999; Smythies, Waites et al. 2000)

The expression of inducible nitric oxide synthase (iNOS) is increased in *H. pylori* infected gastric mucosa. Nitric oxide (NO) and Superoxide (O_2^-) may be produced by infiltrating neutrophils. These reactive oxygen species (ROS) can react to form peroxynitrite which is a potent oxidant and reducing agent. Apurinic–apyrimidinic endonuclease-1 (redox factor-1) plays an important role in the regulation of redox-sensitive signaling and is expressed in epithelial cell during infection with *H. pylori*. (Ding, O'Hara et al. 2004; O'Hara, Bhattacharyya et al. 2006) The increased oxidative DNA damage by ROS is thought to play a causal role in malignant transformation. The cells which undergo apoptosis are removed by phagocytes. This engulfment of *H. pylori* infected epithelial cells by phagocytes plays an important role in the cytokine induction and the activation of host adaptive response.

An increase of chronic inflammatory cells in the gastric mucosa indicates the presence of a chronic gastritis that may result from the increased oxidative stress. Apoptosis and autophagy are two types of programmed cell death that play a critical role in tissue homeostasis and disease development. Exacerbated production of ROS in the inflamed tissue results in substantial type I programmed cell death, apoptosis, including increases in Bax/Bcl-2 ratio, caspase-3 activity, DNA fragmentation and apoptotic cell formation in the damaged tissue. (Baik, Youn et al. 1996; Smoot, Elliott et al. 2000; Chien, Lee et al. 2001; Yu, Chien et al. 2004; Yu, Lin et al. 2005)

Autophagy is type II programmed cell death and is a major lysosomal catabolic pathway for cytoplasmic macromolecules and organelles. Autophagy could be mediated by Beclin-1, a novel Bcl-2-interacting protein, to promote autophagocytosis and a cell-survival response. (Blommaart, Luiken et al. 1997; Liang, Jackson et al. 1999) Previous studies have indicated that *H. pylori*-induced gastric epithelial cell damage by increased Bax/Bcl-2-related proapoptotic cell death and decreased autophagy survival and/or repair. (Catrenich and Chestnut 1992; Lee, Yeo et al. 2004)

4. Clinical and therapeutic application

How to prevent and cure *H. pylori* infection associated with gastritis is an important issue. Nowadays the first-choice of therapy for *H. pylori* infection is one-week combination of a proton pump inhibitor and antibiotics. Following failure of the first-line treatment, second-line therapies, including alternative triple and quadruple regimens, have frequently been applied to the patients. (Chey, Wong et al. 2007; Malfertheiner, Megraud et al. 2007) Although, the current antibiotic-based therapies are generally effective, it may still fail because of the rising trend of antibiotic resistance or the low compliance. (Megraud 2004; Vakil, Megraud et al. 2007) To find out an alternative agent or mixture with preventive and therapeutic potential on *H. pylori* infection is therefore urgently required.

Some strains of *Lactobacillus* and *Bifidobacterium* can inhibit *H. pylori* growth. However, probiotics do not eradicate *H. pylori* but maintain a lower level of this pathogen in the stomach.(Gotteland, Brunser et al. 2006) A vaccine can be used either propbylactically or therapeutically for *H. pylori* infection. In the mice, vaccination can result in significantly reduced *H. pylori* colonization but it cannot achieve satisfactory eradication or prevention of *H. pylori* infection. (Del Giudice, Covacci et al. 2001)

A successful *H. pylori* infection requires the penetration and adherence of the bacterium to mucin and gastric epithelial cells. *H. pylori* that adheres to gastric mucosa subsequently causes gastric epithelial cell damage and atrophy via oxidative stress and the type I apoptotic or type II autophagic programmed cell death-related pathway. Sialylated glycoconjugates are responsible for the adherence of *H. pylori* to gastric epithelium. Cumulated studies have shown that anti-adhesive therapy using 3'-sialyllactose can prevent the binding of *H. pylori* to human gastrointestinal epithelial cells and decrease *H. pylori* colonization in rhesus monkeys without side-effects. (Simon, Goode et al. 1997; Mysore, Wigginton et al. 1999)

Catechins, known as one kind of antioxidants, have been shown to possess anti-oxidative, anti-inflammatory, anti-apoptotic and cancer prevention activity. (Katiyar and Mukhtar 1996; Lin and Lin 1997; Yu, Lin et al. 2005) Besides, catechins including their major active component, epigallocatechin-3-gallate (EGCG), have antibacterial effect against *H. pylori* by inhibiting the activity of urease and VacA of this organism. (Mabe, Yamada et al. 1999; Matsubara, Shibata et al. 2003; Ruggiero, Tombola et al. 2006)

Although catechins or 3'-sialyllactose have an inhibitory effect on *H. pylori* infection in vitro, these two compounds fail to effectively control infection in animal model in vivo when each is used alone. (Mabe, Yamada et al. 1999; Mysore, Wigginton et al. 1999; Matsubara, Shibata et al. 2003) However, effective prevention and treatment of *H. pylori* infection using a combination of catechins and sialic acid in AGS cells and BALB/c mice have been shown in a recent study. (Yang, Shun et al. 2008) The combination of catechins and sialic acid showed synergistic or additive anti-*H. pylori* activity and significantly reduced iNOS expression and Bax/BCl-2-mediated apoptosis but enhanced Becline-1 mediated autophage. Pretreatment with catechins/sialic acid completely prevented *H. pylori* infection and resulted in normal histology. Post-treatment with catechins/sialic acid decreased the bacterial load and gastritis score and eradicated up to 60% of *H. pylori* infectious in a dose-dependent manner.

The rationale of this treatment model which can effectively control *H. pylori* infection includes several points. (Yang and Chien 2009) First, by reviewing the literature, we can find that monotherapy using a single drug such as PPI, bismuth salt, or antibiotics always fail to eradicate *H. pylori* in humans, although each of these drugs can work in vitro. (Bamba,

Kondo et al. 1997) Thus, dual therapy, then triple therapy, and even quadruple therapy have been recommended step by step. Second, catechins have antioxidant and anti-microbial effects (Lin and Lin 1997; Mabe, Yamada et al. 1999), whereas sialic acid has anti-adhesive and antioxidant effects. (Simon, Goode et al. 1997; Teneberg, Jurstrand et al. 2000) Together, they may have additive or synergistic effect against *H. pylori*. Third, both catechins and sialic acid can exist in the foodstuff are wildly accepted to be very safe to humans.

5. Conclusions

It is now clear that both bacterial factors and host response play a role in the pathogenesis of *H. pylori* related gastroduodenal disease. *H. pylori* infection can cause gastric mucosal injury, including oxidative stress, inflammation, and apoptosis formation but inhibit the autophagic survival response in gastric epithelial cell as indicated in **Figure 1**. A new strategy for control of *H. pylori* infection is to interfere with the interaction between the bacteria and target cells and to eradicate bacteria but not target cells at the same time. The combination of compounds with anti-adhesive, antioxidant, and anti-microbial activities may protect gastric mucosa from infection by *H. pylori* and treat its related gastritis via downregulation of apoptosis and upregulation of autophagy.

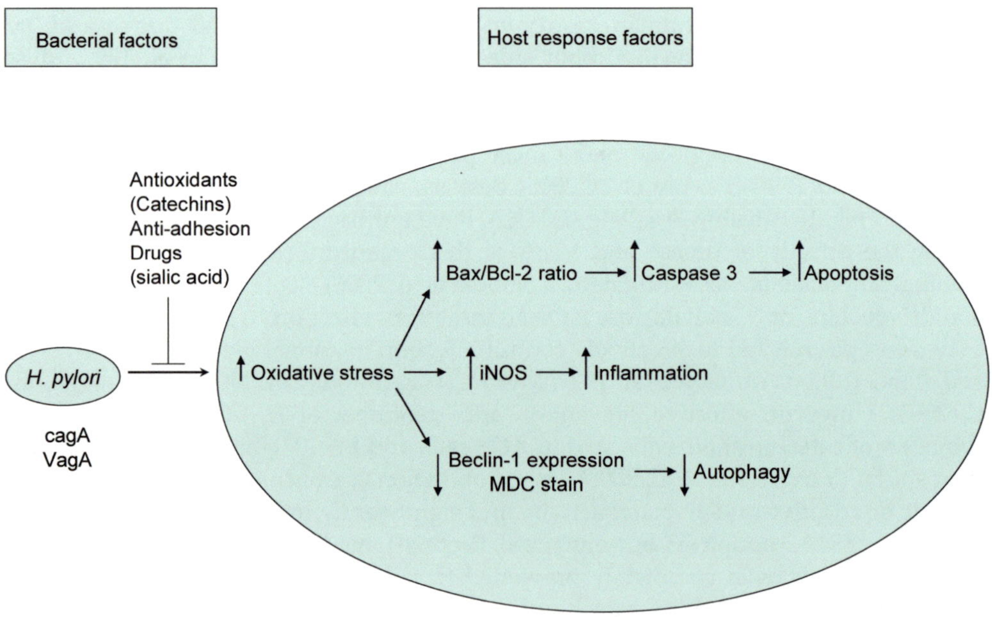

Fig. 1. Possible pathways of *H. pylori* invade gastric epithelium via a upregulation in oxidative stress, inflammation and apoptosis and a downregulation in autophagy. The combination of antioxidants and anti-adhesion drug may reduce *H. pylori*-induced gastritis.

6. References

Amieva, M. R., E. M. El-Omar, et al. (2008). "Host-bacterial interactions in Helicobacter pylori infection." Gastroenterology 134(1): 306-323.

Amieva, M. R., R. Vogelmann, et al. (2003). "Disruption of the epithelial apical-junctional complex by Helicobacter pylori CagA.[see comment]." Science 300(5624): 1430-1434.

Atherton, J. C., P. Cao, et al. (1995). "Mosaicism in vacuolating cytotoxin alleles of Helicobacter pylori. Association of specific vacA types with cytotoxin production and peptic ulceration." Journal of Biological Chemistry 270(30): 17771-17777.

Baik, S. C., H. S. Youn, et al. (1996). "Increased oxidative DNA damage in Helicobacter pylori-infected human gastric mucosa." Cancer Research 56(6): 1279-1282.

Bamba, H., Y. Kondo, et al. (1997). "Minimum inhibitory concentration of various single agents and the effect of their combinations against Helicobacter pylori, as estimated by a fast and simple in vitro assay method." American Journal of Gastroenterology 92(4): 659-662.

Blaser, M. J. and J. C. Atherton (2004). "Helicobacter pylori persistence: biology and disease." Journal of Clinical Investigation 113(3): 321-333.

Blommaart, E. F., J. J. Luiken, et al. (1997). "Autophagic proteolysis: control and specificity." Histochemical Journal 29(5): 365-385.

Boren, T., P. Falk, et al. (1993). "Attachment of Helicobacter pylori to human gastric epithelium mediated by blood group antigens.[see comment]." Science 262(5141): 1892-1895.

Brown, L. M. (2000). "Helicobacter pylori: epidemiology and routes of transmission." Epidemiologic Reviews 22(2): 283-297.

Catrenich, C. E. and M. H. Chestnut (1992). "Character and origin of vacuoles induced in mammalian cells by the cytotoxin of Helicobacter pylori." Journal of Medical Microbiology 37(6): 389-395.

Censini, S., C. Lange, et al. (1996). "cag, a pathogenicity island of Helicobacter pylori, encodes type I-specific and disease-associated virulence factors." Proceedings of the National Academy of Sciences of the United States of America 93(25): 14648-14653.

Chey, W. D., B. C. Wong, et al. (2007). "American College of Gastroenterology guideline on the management of Helicobacter pylori infection." American Journal of Gastroenterology 102(8): 1808-1825.

Chien, C. T., P. H. Lee, et al. (2001). "De novo demonstration and co-localization of free-radical production and apoptosis formation in rat kidney subjected to ischemia/reperfusion." Journal of the American Society of Nephrology 12(5): 973-982.

Christie, P. J., K. Atmakuri, et al. (2005). "Biogenesis, architecture, and function of bacterial type IV secretion systems." Annual Review of Microbiology 59: 451-485.

Cover, T. L. (1996). "The vacuolating cytotoxin of Helicobacter pylori." Molecular Microbiology 20(2): 241-246.

Cover, T. L., U. S. Krishna, et al. (2003). "Induction of gastric epithelial cell apoptosis by Helicobacter pylori vacuolating cytotoxin." Cancer Research 63(5): 951-957.

Crowe, S. E., L. Alvarez, et al. (1995). "Expression of interleukin 8 and CD54 by human gastric epithelium after Helicobacter pylori infection in vitro." Gastroenterology 108(1): 65-74.

D'Elios, M. M., M. Manghetti, et al. (1997). "T helper 1 effector cells specific for Helicobacter pylori in the gastric antrum of patients with peptic ulcer disease." Journal of Immunology 158(2): 962-967.

Del Giudice, G., A. Covacci, et al. (2001). "The design of vaccines against Helicobacter pylori and their development." Annual Review of Immunology 19: 523-563.

Ding, S.-Z., A. M. O'Hara, et al. (2004). "Helicobacter pylori and H2O2 increase AP endonuclease-1/redox factor-1 expression in human gastric epithelial cells." Gastroenterology 127(3): 845-858.

Dixon, M. F., R. M. Genta, et al. (1996). "Classification and grading of gastritis. The updated Sydney System. International Workshop on the Histopathology of Gastritis, Houston 1994." American Journal of Surgical Pathology 20(10): 1161-1181.

El-Omar, E. M., M. Carrington, et al. (2000). "Interleukin-1 polymorphisms associated with increased risk of gastric cancer.[erratum appears in Nature 2001 Jul 5;412(6842):99]." Nature 404(6776): 398-402.

Ernst, P. B., D. A. Peura, et al. (2006). "The translation of Helicobacter pylori basic research to patient care." Gastroenterology 130(1): 188-206; quiz 212-183.

Fan, X., H. Gunasena, et al. (2000). "Helicobacter pylori urease binds to class II MHC on gastric epithelial cells and induces their apoptosis." Journal of Immunology 165(4): 1918-1924.

Furuta, T., E. M. El-Omar, et al. (2002). "Interleukin 1beta polymorphisms increase risk of hypochlorhydria and atrophic gastritis and reduce risk of duodenal ulcer recurrence in Japan.[erratum appears in Gastroenterology 2002 Sep;123(3):957 Note: Sugimurra Haruhiko [corrected to Sugimura Haruhiko]]." Gastroenterology 123(1): 92-105.

Galmiche, A., J. Rassow, et al. (2000). "The N-terminal 34 kDa fragment of Helicobacter pylori vacuolating cytotoxin targets mitochondria and induces cytochrome c release." EMBO Journal 19(23): 6361-6370.

Gotteland, M., O. Brunser, et al. (2006). "Systematic review: are probiotics useful in controlling gastric colonization by Helicobacter pylori?" Alimentary Pharmacology & Therapeutics 23(8): 1077-1086.

Haeberle, H. A., M. Kubin, et al. (1997). "Differential stimulation of interleukin-12 (IL-12) and IL-10 by live and killed Helicobacter pylori in vitro and association of IL-12 production with gamma interferon-producing T cells in the human gastric mucosa." Infection & Immunity 65(10): 4229-4235.

Higashi, H., R. Tsutsumi, et al. (2002). "Biological activity of the Helicobacter pylori virulence factor CagA is determined by variation in the tyrosine phosphorylation sites." Proceedings of the National Academy of Sciences of the United States of America 99(22): 14428-14433.

Higashi, H., R. Tsutsumi, et al. (2002). "SHP-2 tyrosine phosphatase as an intracellular target of Helicobacter pylori CagA protein." Science 295(5555): 683-686.

Ilver, D., A. Arnqvist, et al. (1998). "Helicobacter pylori adhesin binding fucosylated histo-blood group antigens revealed by retagging." Science 279(5349): 373-377.

Jones, N. L., A. S. Day, et al. (1999). "Helicobacter pylori induces gastric epithelial cell apoptosis in association with increased Fas receptor expression." Infection & Immunity 67(8): 4237-4242.

Katiyar, S. K. and H. Mukhtar (1996). "Tea consumption and cancer." World Review of Nutrition & Dietetics 79: 154-184.

Keates, S., A. C. Keates, et al. (1999). "Differential activation of mitogen-activated protein kinases in AGS gastric epithelial cells by cag+ and cag- Helicobacter pylori." Journal of Immunology 163(10): 5552-5559.

Lee, K.-M., M. Yeo, et al. (2004). "Protective mechanism of epigallocatechin-3-gallate against Helicobacter pylori-induced gastric epithelial cytotoxicity via the blockage of TLR-4 signaling." Helicobacter 9(6): 632-642.

Liang, X. H., S. Jackson, et al. (1999). "Induction of autophagy and inhibition of tumorigenesis by beclin 1." Nature 402(6762): 672-676.

Lin, Y. L. and J. K. Lin (1997). "(-)-Epigallocatechin-3-gallate blocks the induction of nitric oxide synthase by down-regulating lipopolysaccharide-induced activity of transcription factor nuclear factor-kappaB." Molecular Pharmacology 52(3): 465-472.

Mabe, K., M. Yamada, et al. (1999). "In vitro and in vivo activities of tea catechins against Helicobacter pylori." Antimicrobial Agents & Chemotherapy 43(7): 1788-1791.

Mahdavi, J., B. Sonden, et al. (2002). "Helicobacter pylori SabA adhesin in persistent infection and chronic inflammation." Science 297(5581): 573-578.

Malfertheiner, P., F. Megraud, et al. (2007). "Current concepts in the management of Helicobacter pylori infection: the Maastricht III Consensus Report." Gut 56(6): 772-781.

Marshall, B. J. (1983). "Unidentified curved bacilli on gastric epithelium in active chronic gastritis." Lancet i: 1273-1275.

Matsubara, S., H. Shibata, et al. (2003). "Suppression of Helicobacter pylori-induced gastritis by green tea extract in Mongolian gerbils." Biochemical & Biophysical Research Communications 310(3): 715-719.

Megraud, F. (2004). "H pylori antibiotic resistance: prevalence, importance, and advances in testing." Gut 53(9): 1374-1384.

Mohammadi, M., J. Nedrud, et al. (1997). "Murine CD4 T-cell response to Helicobacter infection: TH1 cells enhance gastritis and TH2 cells reduce bacterial load." Gastroenterology 113(6): 1848-1857.

Mysore, J. V., T. Wigginton, et al. (1999). "Treatment of Helicobacter pylori infection in rhesus monkeys using a novel antiadhesion compound.[see comment]." Gastroenterology 117(6): 1316-1325.

Naumann, M. and J. E. Crabtree (2004). "Helicobacter pylori-induced epithelial cell signalling in gastric carcinogenesis." Trends in Microbiology 12(1): 29-36.

O'Hara, A. M., A. Bhattacharyya, et al. (2006). "Interleukin-8 induction by Helicobacter pylori in gastric epithelial cells is dependent on apurinic/apyrimidinic endonuclease-1/redox factor-1." Journal of Immunology 177(11): 7990-7999.

Ruggiero, P., F. Tombola, et al. (2006). "Polyphenols reduce gastritis induced by Helicobacter pylori infection or VacA toxin administration in mice." Antimicrobial Agents & Chemotherapy 50(7): 2550-2552.

Satin, B., G. Del Giudice, et al. (2000). "The neutrophil-activating protein (HP-NAP) of Helicobacter pylori is a protective antigen and a major virulence factor.[see comment]." Journal of Experimental Medicine 191(9): 1467-1476.

Simon, P. M., P. L. Goode, et al. (1997). "Inhibition of Helicobacter pylori binding to gastrointestinal epithelial cells by sialic acid-containing oligosaccharides." Infection & Immunity 65(2): 750-757.

Smoot, D. T., T. B. Elliott, et al. (2000). "Influence of Helicobacter pylori on reactive oxygen-induced gastric epithelial cell injury." Carcinogenesis 21(11): 2091-2095.

Smythies, L. E., K. B. Waites, et al. (2000). "Helicobacter pylori-induced mucosal inflammation is Th1 mediated and exacerbated in IL-4, but not IFN-gamma, gene-deficient mice." Journal of Immunology 165(2): 1022-1029.

Suerbaum, S. and P. Michetti (2002). "Helicobacter pylori infection.[see comment]." New England Journal of Medicine 347(15): 1175-1186.

Teneberg, S., M. Jurstrand, et al. (2000). "Inhibition of nonopsonic Helicobacter pylori-induced activation of human neutrophils by sialylated oligosaccharides." Glycobiology 10(11): 1171-1181.

Vakil, N., F. Megraud, et al. (2007). "Eradication therapy for Helicobacter pylori." Gastroenterology 133(3): 985-1001.

Van Doorn, L. J., C. Figueiredo, et al. (1999). "Geographic distribution of vacA allelic types of Helicobacter pylori." Gastroenterology 116(4): 823-830.

Wagner, S., W. Beil, et al. (1997). "Regulation of gastric epithelial cell growth by Helicobacter pylori: offdence for a major role of apoptosis." Gastroenterology 113(6): 1836-1847.

Warren, J. R. (1983). "Unidentified curved bacilli on gastric epithelium in active chronic gastritis." Lancet i: 1273.

Yamaoka, Y., S. Kikuchi, et al. (2002). "Importance of Helicobacter pylori oipA in clinical presentation, gastric inflammation, and mucosal interleukin 8 production." Gastroenterology 123(2): 414-424.

Yang, J.-C. and C.-T. Chien (2009). "A new approach for the prevention and treatment of Helicobacter pylori infection via upregulation of autophagy and downregulation of apoptosis." Autophagy 5(3): 413-414.

Yang, J. C., C. T. Shun, et al. (2008). "Effective prevention and treatment of Helicobacter pylori infection using a combination of catechins and sialic acid in AGS cells and BALB/c mice." Journal of Nutrition 138(11): 2084-2090.

Yu, H. J., C. T. Chien, et al. (2004). "Hypoxia preconditioning attenuates bladder overdistension-induced oxidative injury by up-regulation of Bcl-2 in the rat." Journal of Physiology 554(Pt 3): 815-828.

Yu, H. J., B. R. Lin, et al. (2005). "Sympathetic vesicovascular reflex induced by acute urinary retention evokes proinflammatory and proapoptotic injury in rat liver." American Journal of Physiology - Renal Physiology 288(5): F1005-1014.

Part 2

Molecular Pathogenesis and Treatment of Chronic Gastritis

5

Chronic Gastritis

Wojciech Kozlowski[1], Cezary Jochymski[1] and Tomasz Markiewicz[1,2]
[1]*Military Institute of Medicine / Pathology Department,*
[2]*Warsaw University of Technology,*
Poland

1. Introduction

Proper definition, recognition and classification of chronic gastritis are fundamental for its successful therapy. Gastric inflammation based on clinical/endoscopic classification is not a pathomorphologically homogenous diagnostic group. From histopathological point of view, it seems most likely that chronic gastritis is characterized by morphological indices of chronic inflammatory changes in different parts of gastric mucosa. Chronic superficial gastritis is associated with lymphocyte and plasma cells infiltrate of the foveolar part of gastric mucosa. Chronic gastritis is associated with the inflammatory cell infiltrate predominantly consisting of lymphocyte and plasma cells in total gastric mucosa. Current classification of chronic gastritis and the worldwide accepted knowledge of the natural history of gastritis are combined in the 1994 Houston-updated Sydney System. Helicobacter pylori is by far the most important etiologic factor in chronic gastritis. Helicobacter pylori infection accompanies chronic (or chronic active) and/or superficial (or atrophic) gastritis in about 90% and the process of development of the lesions usually lasts from 20 to 40 years. Chronic gastritis, especially caused by Helicobacter pylori, is accompanied by disturbances in secretion of HCL, pepsinogen as well as gastrin and somatostatin. It has been reported that Helicobacter pylori induces increased apoptosis and hyperproliferation of gastric epithelial cells. These changes (increased apoptosis, hyperproliferation and secretion disturbances) are reduced after Helicobacter pylori eradication. It is worth mentioning that regenerative abilities of gastric mucosa glandular epithelium cells are the main mechanism determining their right functions concerning both integrity of the mucosa and normal function of its all epithelial cellular elements. In chronic atrophic gastritis, a significantly higher percentage of cells in mitotic phase is found as compared to both normal condition and chronic superficial gastritis. Moreover the proliferative activity of glandular epithelial cells is directly proportional to the increasing degree of gastric mucosa atrophy. An increase in proliferative activity of glandular epithelium in gastric mucosa was also observed in chronic, particularly atrophic, gastritis, independently of its etiology. There is strong evidence on possible progression of changes from chronic atrophic gastritis to intestinal metaplasia, dysplasia and finally adenocarcinoma. It is worth mentioning that not much attention has been drawn to the importance of the examination of regenerative activity of the gastric mucosa epithelium, neuroendocrine and immune cells for the study of chronic gastritis pathogenesis.

2. Evaluation of the morphological criteria used so far for diagnosis of superficial and atrophic chronic gastritis

Gastritis is a disorder generally acknowledged by both clinicians and pathomorphologists. At the same time it is the most frequently overused diagnosis mostly by clinicians and less commonly by pathomorphologists. On one hand, gastritis is considerably frequently diagnosed even in seemingly trivial complaints such as acid indigestion or dyspepsia. On the other hand, is should be taken into consideration that differently advanced histological indices of gastritis are diagnosed in about 40% of people with normal endoscopic picture of gaster and no digestive track complaints (Sipponen, 1992). It is worth noticing that according to population prognosis, about 50% of people would develop gastritis within their lives, mainly in occupational period. Therefore, the problem involves not only overuse of this type of diagnosis but also its omission in evaluating healthy people's condition. Based on the said assumption, it can be concluded that the fundament for diagnosing and classifying gastritis should be exclusively endoscopy with collection of samples and the final evaluations of the sample in histopathological test.

From pathomorphological standpoint gastritis could be defined as a syndrome caused by heterogenic group of pathogenic factors which lead to damage to gastric mucous membrane manifested by acute, chronic or mixed inflammatory reaction (Strickland, 1990). Scandinavian authors claim that chronic gastritis (CHG) is an age-independent progressing disease whose onset has a form of a superficial inflammatory infiltrate (gastritis chronica superficialis), through gradual loss of gastric proper glands (gastritis chronica atrophica), to complete atrophy of these glands inclusively (atrophia mucosae ventriculi; severe atrophic gastritis). Development of morphology studies on CHG was inseparably connected with progress within endoscopic techniques as well as methodics of pathomorpholgical tests. The following events had significant influence on gastropathomorphology process: introduction of endoscopic examination (beginning of 50s of the previous century), immunological tests (end of 50s of the previous century), improvement of endoscopic techniques (beginnings of 70s) , "rediscovery" of Helicobacter pylori in gastric mucous membrane and correlation of its presence with gastric lesions (beginning of 80s) (Strickland, 1990) as well as development of immunohistological techniques (beginning of 80s) and current development of molecular biology methods and molecular cytogenetics, especially the use of this type of examination techniques in pathomorphology.

The term "gastritis" (quote by Misiewicz et al., 1990) was first introduced in 1728 by Stahl who probably did not expect that in further years it would become the most commonly made diagnosis and at the same time one of the least clear ones. As it was mentioned above, classification of inflammation in gastric mucous membrane, especially chronic one, should be based only on morphological indices of its damage while the majority of current classifications of gastritis is to a great extent based on a pathomorphological diagnosis which is a combination the following criteria: etiologic, topographic and, according to some people, also immunological and histopathological (Correa, 1988; Dixon et al., 1996; Misiewicz et al., 1990; Owen, 1996; Price, 1991, 1999; Strickland, 1990; Tytgat, 1991). Therefore, this point of view lacks clear division into functional changes and morphological changes. In other words, the difference between the cause and the effect, morphological in this case, is blurred.

The first gastritis classification based on histopathological examination of samples collected by the so called blind biopsy and samples collected during surgical procedures was created by Schindler in 1947. Due to inability to define anatomotopography of the collected gastric mucous membrane sample Schindler first divided inflammation into superficial and atrophic and next distinguished the group of hypertrophic inflammations. Moreover, he was the first to use the term *gastritis chronica* with full awareness in its today's meaning (quote by Misiewicz et al., 1990).

The best recognition was given to the gastritis classification created by Whitehead in 1972 (Whitehead et al., 1972). It is based only on classic pathomorphological criteria and involves separate diagnosis for region of pylorus, corpus, cardia and gastric mucous membrane welding area. Similarly to Schindler's classification, Whitehead divided gastritis into superficial and atrophic. However, Whitehead distinguished two forms for each of them: active form with presence of granulocyte infilters in epithelium and/or interstitium and a non-active form with inflammatory infiltration from lymphoidal and plasmatic cells located in lamina propria. Atrophy of mucous membrane proper glands was evaluated in a three-level scale (mild, moderate and sever) as well as, in justified cases, the presence of intestinal and pseudopyloric metaplasia was noted.

One year later Strickland and McKay modified CHG classifications by combining etiologic and immunologic data with pathomorphological and anatomotopographic indices and by distinguishing type A and B gastritis (Strickland & Mackay, 1973). Type A gastritis referred only to gastric corpus and was accompanied by pernicious anaemia, while in the case of type B gastritis the lesions were localized in antral regions. In the same year (Glass & Pitchumoni, 1975) Glass and Pitchumoni completed the first classification by adding AB type gastritis which included types of extensive involvement of mucous membrane of the corpus and prepyloric regions. The cases of concurrent presence of antibodies of oxyntic cell were defined as AB-plus CHG.

In 1980 (Correa, 1980) Correa introduced etiopathogenetic element into histopathological diagnosis by dividing CHG into: autoimmunization CHG with pernicious anaemia; hypersecretion CHG connected with duodenal ulceration and environmental CHG dependent mainly on the diet but also on geographic localization. In 1988 (Correa, 1988) the same author modified his previous classification by dividing CHG into: diffuse antral gastritis, diffuse corporal gastritis and multifocal atrophic gastritis. Next, in 1992 along with Yardley (Correa & Yardley, 1992) in continuation of completing and developing the previous versions of his classification of CHG he divided the inflammation into: gastritis with and without atrophy of gastric proper glands. In the group of non-atrophic gastritis he distinguished superficial CHG as initial condition and/or stationary as well as diffuse CHG connected with prepyloric region. As regards diffuse inflammation of prepyloric regions, it might be accompanied by duodenal and pyloric ulcer. Moreover, in this case Helicobacter pylori is the first cause and the following are not observed: gland atrophy, intestinal metaplasia or carcinogenesis. Among the types of atrophic gastritis he distinguished the following: diffuse CHG connected with the corpus, autoimmunization CHG accompanied by pernicious anaemia and multifocal CHG usually affecting mucous membrane in lower regions of gastric lesser curvature. Multifocal CHG can be accompanied by duodenal ulcer and is frequently followed by occurrence of intestinal metaplasia of mucous membrane. Moreover, cases of atrophic multifocal CHG are accompanied by increased risk of neoplasm development.

The study by Marshall from 1983 (Marshall, 1983) on Helicobacter pylori revolutionized the view on CHG etiology, which, among others, contributed to creation of a new CHG classification finally accepted in Sydney in 1990 (Misiewicz et al., 1990; Price, 1991).

Basically, this classification included all the previous CHG divisions, yet an etiology factor was added as a permanent element of pathomorphological diagnosis. In this classification the previous CHG morphological quantifications were exchanged with evaluation of morphological change advancement level according to a four-level scale. One of the most important practical conclusions in the Sydney classification is a necessity of routine collection of a particular number of samples (four; two from the corpus and two from the antrum, from both anterior and posterior walls) and what is equally important - fixation of those samples in properly labeled separate containers. Moreover, it was clearly stated that any other lesion confirmed by endoscopic examination requires collection of additional samples from the *muscularis mucosae* depth.

It should be noted that chronic gastritis is not characterized by a specific clinical or endoscopic picture. This also refers to particular most common etiologic factors whose action is not characterized by a defined syndrome complex. Moreover, it is worth adding that there is no correlation between endoscopic picture of gastric mucous memrane and histopathological examination, especially in the case of mild changes. The most significant issue as regards this aspect of CHG diagnostics is the fact that even in 40% of CHG cases no endoscopic changes or presence of CHG microscopic indices of various level of advancement are observed. These dependencies lead to the issue called routine collection of samples in every endoscopy as well as relevant problems, not only connected with high cost.

From histopathological standpoint, the Sydney system distinguishes three basic types of inflammation: acute, chronic and special. Acute inflammation is usually characterized by subclinical course, which is rarely used as an indication to perform stomach endoscopy. Special forms of gastritis are not frequently examined by taking biopsy as this type of disorder is extremely rare. Therefore, routine gastrologic biopsy material is most frequently connected with cases of non-specific CHG of considerably repeatable picture of pathomorphological changes due to the fact that immunological mechanisms of reaction to different pathogens in gastric mucous membrane are generally not various. Therefore, the Sydney system included all the microscopic indices of gastric mucous membrane changes that are present in CHG and were described before 1990. Some of the indices are as follows: inflammatory infiltrate (consisting of lymphoid and plasmatic cells), atrophy of gastric proper glands, active inflammatory process (measured by the number of neutrophils and eosinophils), intestinal metaplasia and intensity of Helicobacter pylori colonization in gastric mucous membrane evaluated in a 4-level- scale (none, mild, moderate and severe). Other CHG microscopic changes, such as mucus content in cells, degenerative changes of epithelial cells, hyperplasia of foveolar layer glands, stroma oedema, erosions, fibrosis and dilation of vascular lumen are evaluated only in terms of quality.

According to the Sydney System, the following sites of sample collection in topographic part of pathomorphological diagnosis can be determined: antrum, corpus or the whole gaster (pangastritis, antrum predominant, corpus predominant). Therefore, in the case of collecting samples from only one anatomotopographic region the diagnosis based on the Sydney system is not possible (incomplete examination). The etiologic part, which is to a possible extent defined by a clinician, includes: Helicobacter pylori (currently the most common cause), autoimmunization, drug-induced disorder as well as infectious etiology (bacterial, viral, parasite, fungal). In the case of no evident cause (etiology) CHG is defined as idiopathic inflammation.

The assumptions described above suggest, among others, that the Sydney system replaced classic histopathological diagnosis which involves diagnosis based on miscroscopic indices of changes only by means of quantitative evaluation of the advancement level of inflammatory miscroscopic indices. This interpretation of changes allows for quantitative consideration of morphological changes in CHG (necessary for e.g. scientific works). However, it does not allow for making an accurate histopathological diagnosis which would allow the clinician to draw prognostic and therapeutic conclusions.

This approach towards pathomorphological phenomena in the Sydney system was a probable reason for excluding generic diagnosis - gastritis chronica superficialis (CHSG) which, according to opinion of both this work's and other authors, was very significant. Superficial chronic gastritis is characterized by presence of inflammatory infiltrate built up of lymphoid and plasmatic cells localized in 1/3 of the upper part of gastric mucous membrane, namely on foveolar layer. This inflammation usually affects also the layer of stem glands. Comparing to CHSG of antral and pyloric parts, corpus of the gaster is a site of a more common CHSG development. A key diagnostic element of CHSG is evaluation of inflammatory infiltrate localization which is analyzed in terms of strictly defined histotopographic structures of gastric mucous membranes. Therefore, it is a very accurate criterion which does not require additional examination tools and/or other supporting classifications/scales. It is worth mentioning that this type of diagnosis occurred in all the CHG classifications compiled before 1900 (Correa, 1980, 1988; Correa & Yardley 1992; Whitehead, 1972). Most authors consider CHSG as the initial part of CHG. As regards the difference between the two disorders, in the case of CHG the inflammatory infiltrate of similar cellular composition affects also deeper parts of gastric mucous membrane and reaches muscularis mucosa. In the presence of granulocytes (neutrophils and/or eosynophils) in the inflammatory infiltrate composition, active inflammation - CHSG activa and CHG activa - is diagnosed.

One of the most significant advantages of the Sydney classification is that it obliges clinicians and pathomorphologist to cooperate in the process of diagnosis gastritis from the very beginning and it makes the clinicians responsible for the etiologic and anatomotopographic part of the diagnosis. Clinicians frequently have justified doubts as regards etiology of the observed gastric lesion. However, establishment of topography of the collected oligobiopoints as well as their fixation in separate containers can in no way be problematic. Following its compilation, the Sydney classification was not fully accepted, especially by American authors (Correa & Yardley, 1992). This was, among others, the reason for its revision which was finally performed in Houston in 1994 (Dixon et al., 1996). The most significant element of the revision was giving a suitable role to classic histopathological nomenclature in making CHG diagnosis, especially regarding non-atrophic CHG, particularly for *gastritis chronica superficialis* which was "forgotten" in the Sydney classification (Correa & Yardley, 1992). Visual analogue scale was added to the quantitative evaluation of histopathological changes. Also, the following rule of routine collection of samples from gastric mucous membrane, slightly different from the Sydney classification, was suggested in Houston:

- two antrum samples; 2-3cm, from pylorus from lesser and greater curvature,
- two corpus samples; 8cm, from cardia from lesser and greater curvature,
- one sample from the region of angular incisure
- five samples from angular incisure for comparable evaluation of intestinal metaplasia and/or dysplasia level.

The authors also recommend HE and PAS with Alcjan Blue as a routine staining next to Helicobacter pylori identification (Giemsa's method).
This vast work from Houston, apart from the revision of the Sydney system, contains a number of detailed and valuable information on a wide range of aspects connected with cooperation between endocsopist and pathomorphologist and thus, it is suggested as a fundamental educational material for both parties. The modified Sydney classification causes different reactions among pathomorphologists –full acceptation (Chen et al., 1999; Wyatt, 1995) and a certain reserve (Guarner et al., 1999), especially with respect to implementation of the classification in pediatric gastropathology (Cohen et al., 2000). However, the authors supporting the concept of Sydney classification claim that this conceptual direction of CHG classification will be maintained. They are awaiting for the nearest non-histopathological criterion, namely dependencies arising from potential effects of using vaccination against Helicobacter pylori (Price, 1999).
One of the latest complete divisions of gastritis was published by Appelman in 1994 (Appelman, 1994). Traditional division into acute and chronic disease was maintained. The following were distinguished from chronic gastritis: inflammation connected with Helicobacter pylori and atrophy gastritis, lymphocitar gastritis - also called "chemical" and focal gastritis. Helicobacter pylori related gastritis, the most common one, is defined variously by different authors (Axon, 1992; Borchard, 2001; Correa, 1980, 1988; Glass & Pitchumoni, 1975; Green & Graham, 1990; Sipponen, 1989, 1992; Strickland & Mackay, 1973; Whitehead et al., 1972). Commonly used synonyms are as follows: gastritis chronica diffusa antralis, gastritis chronica typus B, gastritis chronica activa antralis, gastritis chronica non specifica and gastritis typus hypersecretions. Many publications (Arkkila et al., 2006; Axon, 1992; Correa & Yardley, 1992; Green & Graham, 1990; Marshall, 1983; Sipponen, 1992; Zhang et al., 2005a, 2005b) clearly confirmed that Helicobacter pylori causes chronic gastritis by affecting mainly prepyloric part of the stomach. It can lead to atrophy of gastric proper glands, cancer and less frequently to lymphoma. It usually accompanies duodenal ulcer. Its morphological indices are inflammatory infiltrates of neutrophils localized on the foveolar layer stroma of gastric mucous membrane in the case of acute gastritis. Chronic gastritis is characterized by an infiltrate of lymphoid cells, plasmatic cells and acidophilic granulocytes. Moreover, it is accompanied by lymphadenoplasia foci and the infiltrate affects the whole gastric mucous membrane (Appelman, 1994; Axon, 1992; Correa, 1988; Marshall, 1983; Misiewicz et al., 1990; Price, 1991; Sipponen, 1992; Strickland, 1990; Wyatt, 1995).
As regards autoimmunization inflammation, it is frequently defined as gastritis autoimmunogenes, gastritis chronica atrophica typus A, gastritis chronica typus A and gastritis chronica diffusa corporis. It is most frequently observed in Scandinavia and in northern areas of Europe. This inflammation affects gastric corpus and can be accompanied by: pernicious anaemia, autoimmunization Hashimoto thyroiditis, diabetes, adrenal insufficiency and thyroid function disorders. Common complications are stomach cancer and carcinoid. However, it is assumed that enterohormonal disorders (hypergastrinemia) which accompany carcinoid development are initiated by achlorhydria in the course of inflammation (Appelman, 1994; Strickland, 1990).
Interestingly, focal atrophic gastritis is more frequently observed in the USA and Japan. Its most common synonyms are: gastritis chronica atrophica typus B or environmental gastritis. In terms of frequency of occurrence it affects lesser curvature, prepyloric region and gastric corpus. The most serious complication is cancer, mainly intestinal (Correa, 1980, 1988; Correa & Yardley, 1992).

Lymphocitar gastritis can be divided into the previously distinguished types of inflammation: gastritis chronica superficialis, gastritis chronica erosiva, gastritis varioliformis and morbus Menetrier. Basic morphological index of the lesions is an infiltrate which consists mainly of lymphocytes localized within superficial epithelium of gastric mucous membrane foveolar layer. This group comprises lesions of gastric mucous membrane which accompany among others celiac disease (Appelman, 1994; Price, 1991; Wyatt, 1995).

The so called chemical gastritis is by some authors also referred to as: "chemica" gastropathy, gastritis refluxiva, gastritis biliaris, gastritis postmedicamentosa. Basic morphological indices of this inflammation are: proliferation of foveolar layer , decreased mucous secretion, stroma oedema with low inflammatory reaction (Appelman, 1994; Borchard, 2001; Strickland, 1990; Wyatt, 1995). According to both the authors as well as other authors (Borchard, 2001; Dixon et al., 1996), the number of mixed CHG cases, in which some of the most significant components are microscopic indices of chemical gastritis, is increasing (or they are more frequently diagnosed).

According to pathomorphological standpoint, the authors of this work, following prior mental, substantial and emotional acknowledgement of potential addresses, assume and suggest implementation of CHG classification based almost exclusively on pathomorphological criteria acknowledged also by other authors. Histopathological diagnoses used in this classification contain data on severity and distribution of inflammatory infiltrate, its activity and condition of potential atrophy of gastric proper glands (*gastritis chronica superficialis activa et nonactiva; gastritis chronica activa et nonactiva, gastritis chronica atrophica et atrophia mucosae ventriculi*) as well as they take into consideration also histotopographical data on the examined samples (*CHG antralis, corporis, fundi, cardiae, pylori*). In every justified case, dysplasia level is evaluated as well as the presence of : glandular *hyperplasia of foveolar layer, intestinal and pseudopyloric metaplasia*. Focal gastritis is a kind of systemic disease which causes among others lesion in the gaster and in characterized by specific morphological indices of diagnosis CHG type. The suggested classification also comprises other CHG types enumerated by Appelman: lymphocitar, the so called chemical CHG, and gastritis chronica erosiva. According to the Sydney classification system, identification of Helicobacter pylori is obligatorily taken into consideration in histological evaluation along with the assessment of this microorganism. However, etiopathogenetic standpoint is a supplementary element found in additional comment to the basic histopathological diagnosis.

A number of factors, such as different classifications, the increasing number of reports on the Sydney classification analysis, both initial and updated version, and the opinions of cooperating clinician groups, lead to a conclusion similar to Appelman's view: the best CHG classification is the one that both provides the best possible and the clearest contact between clinician and pathologist and most of all facilitates effective diagnostic and therapeutic management.

3. Analysis of the proliferative activity of gastric mucosa glandular epithelium in relation to the chronic gastritis type

Regenerative abilities of glandular epithelium cells of gastric mucosa constitute the main mechanism determining their correct functions concerning both integrity of the mucosa and normal function of all its epithelial cell elements (Goodlad & Wright, 1995). One of more important cell elements in this process are mucous cells of the cervical part of gastric glands (Goodlad & Wright, 1995; Hellander, 1981) and also isthmus cells, as stressed by other authors (Goodlad & Wright, 1987). Mucous cells of the cervical part of gastric glands are present singly and/or in cellular clusters in the epithelium of the cervical region of gastric glands (Goodlad & Wright, 1995) and are usually invisible after routine H-E staining. These cells, besides purely secretory function, are the pool of cells that are the source for regenerating cells of the glandular epithelium, among which the presence of primary alimentary tract cells for gastric mucosal epithelium (so called stem cells) can be observed (Goodlad & Wright, 1995; Solcia et al., 1979).

One of more frequently used immunocytochemical markers for cells in proliferation phase is proliferating cell nuclear antigen (PCNA) (Goodlad & Wright, 1995). It is a protein of 36 kDa mass, co-factor for DNA delta-polymerase and it participates in DNA synthesis (S-phase of cell cycle) and DNA repair (Keleman, 1997; Waseem & Lane, 1990). PCNA usually undergoes overexpression in conditions connected with activity of growth factors (Hall et al., 1990). PCNA expression is genetically regulated, and mRNA PCNA is present in both proliferating cells and those in resting phase (Hall et al., 1990).

The control of glandular epithelium regeneration centres in the alimentary tract, including the stomach is multidirectional, starting from simple negative feedback with damaged superficial epithelial cells, finishing on the effect of intragastric environment (Goodlad & Wright, 1995). The main point of this regulation includes hormonal, neuropeptide, peptide and genetic actions with simultaneous influence of immune-nervous factors and mesenchymal components on the stroma (Goodlad & Wright, 1995). Apart from the group of factors associated with enteroglucagon, a particular role in the stimulation of regenerative processes regulation in gastric mucosa is played by gastrin (Goodlad & Wright, 1995; Walsh, 1990). It should be stressed that drugs influencing gastrin level also exert indirect influence on glandular epithelium proliferation in gastric mucosa (Havu, 1986). Prostaglandins, in their broad spectrum of activity, have the ability to stimulate proliferation of glandular epithelial cells of gastric mucosa, including also acceleration of these cells' migration (Goodlad et al., 1989). As regards the growth factors, epidermal growth factor (EGF) plays the main role in the regulation of regeneration processes in gastric mucosa (Weaver & Walker, 1988).

Most of the regenerating cells of glandular epithelium migrate along the wall of foveolar layer glands to the surface of gastric mucosa during about seven days (Lee, 1985). This migration far less frequently occurs deep into gastric glands and takes longer time, i.e. about 200 days (Hattori, 1976). As it is commonly known, cell division includes four phases, making up jointly the so called cell cycle (cell cycle phases: G1, S, G2 and M), and the duration of this cycle depends mainly on the duration of the G1 phase (Goodlad & Wright, 1995; Preston-Martin et al., 1990). A cell may go out of the cell cycle to enter G0 resting state or may pass to maturation phase. It has been disclosed, however, that in the case of alimentary tract mucosal cells, the resting state is practically not observed, perhaps with the exception of the large bowel (Goodlad & Wright, 1995).

Apoptotic regulations of these cells, and, in the first place, genetically determined regulations, play, besides regenerative abilities of the epithelium, an important role in the homeostatic process of gastric mucosa (Goodlad & Wright, 1995; Oren, 1992; Yanagihara & Tsumuraya, 1992). Growth factors and other factors, for example c-myc, bcl-2, p53, TGF-beta, TNF and other cytokines participate in the apoptotic process (Oren, 1992; Yanagihara & Tsumuraya, 1992).

Proliferative activity of the glandular epithelium of stomach corpus and fundus mucosa is normally located in the cervical part of gastric glands, while in the prepyloric part it occupies the middle 1/3 part of the mucosa where also G cells are present (Ito et al., 1986). In this part an intensive expression of chromogranin-A-positive cells can also be observed. In own studies it has been demonstrated that these regions are the place where the most intensive PCNA expression is observed. Most authors think that proliferative activity of glandular epithelial cells in gastric mucosa increases with *Helicobacter pylori* colonization (Bechi et al., 1996; Jang & Kim, 2000; Lynch & Axon, 1995; Panella et al., 1996), which is particularly visible in the corpus (Bechi et al., 1996). On the other hand, after eradication, the proliferative activity returns to normal (Lynch & Axon, 1995). According to other authors, bile participates in the increase of gastric glandular epithelial activity in the course of *H.pylori* colonization (Lynch & Axon, 1995), while the markers of this activity are observed mainly within the epithelial zone of foveolar layer glands (Bechi et al., 1996). It is worth mentioning that other authors (Ito et al., 1986) found a deepening of proliferative zone within gastric glands in the same gastric mucosal inflammatory conditions, with accompanying significant reduction of EC cell number. According to some authors, increased proliferative activity of gastric mucosal glandular epithelium, particularly that measured by PCNA expression, in the course of chronic inflammatory conditions and *H.pylori* colonization may be even the marker of risk of malignancy development (Irazusta et al., 1998; Panella et al., 1996). Other authors (Diebold et al., 1998), however, demonstrated that during *H.pylori* colonization a decrease in the number of argyrophilic cells occurs along with simultaneous reduction of their proliferative potential. This seems to be in concordance with the studies in which an inhibitory effect of VacA on the proliferation of epithelial cells of gastric mucosal glands through impairment of their migration ability was demonstrated (Ricci et al., 1996). The same authors also proved that another antigen, CagA, exerts no effect on the proliferative potential of gastric mucosal glandular epithelium. The results of these studies may be, in a certain way, compared with own studies according to which no significant influence of *H.pylori* colonization on proliferative activity of gastric mucosal glandular epithelium was demonstrated. An increase in proliferative activity of glandular epithelium in gastric mucosa was also observed in chronic gastritis, independently of its etiology (Bechi et al., 1996; Deschner et al., 1972; Irazusta et al., 1998; Panella et al., 1996). It was usually accompanied by a decrease in G cell count, including adrenomodulin-containing cells (Kitani et al., 1999), particularly frequently when the gastritis was associated with atrophic lesions. According to the studies by other authors (Bielicki et al., 1993; Guerci et al., 1992), a significantly higher percentage of cells in division phase is found in chronic atrophic gastritis as compared to both normal condition and to chronic superficial gastritis, and the proliferative activity of glandular epithelial cells is directly proportional to the increasing degree of atrophy. Other authors (Ito et al., 1986) noted that, together with intensification of inflammatory processes in gastric mucosa, the zone of increased proliferation of glandular epithelial cells involves also deeper layers of the lamina propria of gastric mucosa, and also. the number of ECn cells is reduced. It should be added that in hypergastrinaemia, the expression of neuroendocrine cells and their proliferative abilities increase but such changes were not observed during antisecretory treatment. No such hypergastrinaemia inducing effect was observed during activation of gastric mucosal inflammatory processes or in biomorphotic process. In the course of *Helicobacter pylori* colonization other authors (Jang & Kim, 2000) found intensification of both apoptosis and proliferative activity of neuroendocrine cells, mainly G and D, correlated with gastritis activity and with the degree of *H.pylori* colonization.

Own studies are partially in concordance with the observations described above since they demonstrated that proliferative zone of mucosal epithelial cells becomes deeper with intensification of inflammatory lesions but only in the case of stomach corpus. At this point, however, it should be noted that this applies only to males who have higher proliferative activity in this zone of mucosa as compared with females. Regardless of that, in own studies a significantly higher proliferative activity was found, but only in superficial gastritis, in relation to deep gastritis, which had not been described by other authors. Apart from this, it was demonstrated that changes of proliferative activity of gastric mucosal epithelium were independent of age, location (prepyloric part - corpus), and also *Helicobacter pylori* colonization in gastric mucosa.

3.1 Conclusions (own studies)

1. Chronic superficial gastritis coexists with significantly higher proliferative activity of gastric mucosal glandular epithelium, particularly in relation to the prepyloric part.
2. Changes of proliferative activity of gastric mucosal glandular epithelium are independent of age, histotopography and *H.pylori* colonization.

4. Assessment of the current status of neuroendocrine and immune cells for the study of pathogenesis of chronic gastritis

Gastric mucosal neuroendocrine cells are usually located in the epithelial layer of the gastric glands in the corpus and prepyloric part, sometimes in their cervical zone, but they are never found in the superficial epithelium of the foveolar layer glands of gastric mucosa (Dayal, 1992; Kozlowski et al., 1993, 1995; Portela-Gomes & Grimelius, 1986). Modern classifications of gastric mucosal neuroendocrine cells tend to divide them according to anatomic-topographic location in the stomach (Bordi et al., 2000; Dayal, 1992; Tzaneva, 2001). The following neuroendocrine cells are present in the mucosa of gastric corpus and fundus: ECL (enterochromaffin-like), D (somatostatin), ECn (enterochromaffin), X/A, D1, and P cells. ECL cells occur almost exclusively in gastric fundus mucosa. However, the prepyloric part of the stomach contains G (gastrin), D, and ECn cells. D cells produce somatostatin and are present almost in the whole alimentary tract and also in the pancreas (Canese & Bussolati, 1977). In course of their long cytoplasmic processes they exert paracrine effect on other neighbouring gastric mucosal cells (Larsson et al., 1984). At least 20% of D cells have axon processes through which they are in contact with G cells in the prepyloric part and parietal cells in gastric corpus mucosa (Larsson et al., 1984), inhibiting their secretory function. Moreover, D cells in the prepyloric part have specialised tubules through which they are in contact with gastric lumen (autoregulation with intragastric environment). D cells in gastric fundus mucosa have no such contact with stomach lumen (Fenoglio-Preiser, 1999). As far as now, no publications on correlations between gastric mucosa neuroendocrine and degree of chronic gastritis can be found in scientific literature.

The applied own method of studying gastric mucosal neuroendocrine cells allowed for assessment of their count and rate of changes in the course of non-specific gastritis of various progression in a repeatable way. It is worth mentioning that on the basis of examination of one cross-section type it is possible to assess the most probable total count of a definite type of gastric mucosal neuroendocrine cells in a highly correlated way (about

95% confidence level). This type of histological quantitative examinations is very practical in routine histopathological diagnosis.

Contrary to the results reported by other authors (Coupe et al., 1990; Tzaneva & Julianov, 1999), changes concerning D cells and CgA cells located in the stomach corpus mucosa were found in own studies. The latter, however, demonstrated a significant decrease of D cell count in the oxyntic mucosa with simultaneous increase of CgA cell count in the prepyloric mucosa. It should be mentioned that the latter changes were observed only in patients with *Helicobacter pylori* colonization in gastric mucosa, which was in agreement with the results obtained by other authors (Chamouard et al., 1997; Graham et al., 1993; Kozlowski et al., 1993, 1995; Tzaneva & Julianov, 1999).

According to literature data, the most numerous neuroendocrine cells of gastric mucosa include the following cells: ECL, G, and D, since together they account for over 75% of all mucosal endocrine cells in the prepyloric part and corpus of the stomach (Dayal, 1992; Fenoglio-Preiser, 1999; Solcia et al., 1975). It can be assumed that the increasing number of CgA cells in the prepyloric mucosa means simultaneous increase of G cell count. Therefore, the results obtained in own studies may be regarded as a confirmation of the fact already known from papers by other authors (Chamouard et al., 1997; Graham et al., 1993; Kozlowski et al., 1993, 1995; Tzaneva & Julianov, 1999) and also obtained empirically (Lee et al., 1992) which point to participation of disturbances of interrelations between D and G cells in the pathomechanism of hypergastrinaemia that accompanies *Helicobacter pylori* colonization of gastric mucosa. It should be stressed that due to other causes, e.g. chronic atrophic gastritis in the corpus, the numbers of ECL as well as D cells in hypergastrinaemia increase (Borch et al., 1987; Bordi et al., 1987; Carney et al., 1983; Cattan et al., 1989; Hodges et al., 1981; Iacangelo et al., 1988), which is accompanied by characteristic vacuolar lesions observed under electron microscope in ECL cells (D'Adda et al., 1990; Rubin, 1972).

Chromogranin A, used, as mentioned above, for identification of neuroendocrine cells, is an acid protein of 49 kDa mass located in secretory granules of APUD system cells (Lloyd et al., 1984; Wiedemann & Huttner, 1989) which belongs to the family of proteins called granins/secretogranins. The most important members of this protein family include: chromogranin A, B, and secretogranin II (Lloyd et al., 1984). Chromogranin A is present in both endocrine and neuroendocrine cells (Cetin, 1992; Iacangelo et al., 1988). It is also present in most neuroendocrine tumours and, therefore, is serves as a commonly used marker for their identification (Wiedemann et al., 1989). At the same time, it participates in the biosynthesis of pancreatostatin (Iacangelo et al., 1988) which inhibits insulin and hydrochloric acid secretion. It is worth mentioning that Chromogranin A also binds intracellular calcium and catecholamines, significantly regulating intracellular homeostasis along this pathway (Iacangelo et al., 1988). It is distributed in neuroendocrine cell granules in rather close association with serotonin which is simultaneously connected with both its synthesis and accumulation (Tzaneva, 2001).Chromogranin A expression in a significant per cent of neuroendocrine cells agrees with argyrophilic reaction e.g. according to Grimelius (Cetin, 1992).

From the standpoint of methodological principles of indentifying individual neuroendocrine cell types in humans, an extremely important and frequently forgotten fact is that D cells (secreting somatostatin) give no positive argyrophilic reaction according to Grimelius, and show no Chromogranin A expression in immunohistochemical reaction (Cetin, 1992; Tzaneva, 2001). However, in neuroendocrine aminergic cells the both above mentioned colour reactions gave positive results (Cetin, 1992). It is worth mentioning that

even purely mathematical calculation of G cell number among CgA cells is more precise than analogous mode of ECL cell calculation since only G, D and ECn cells are present in the prepyloric part (Bordi et al., 2000; Dayal, 1992; Tzaneva, 2001).
Decreased D cell count was found in duodenal ulcer with *Helicobacter pylori* colonization of gastric mucosa and in cases of hypergastrinaemia, yet sometimes also in conditions without hypergastrinaemia (Zverkov et al., 1996). Many authors are convinced that hypergastrinaemia, observed in cases of *H.pylori* colonization of gastric mucosa, is just caused by reduction of D cell count (Haruma et al., 1995; Kozlowski et al., 1993; Kozlowski et al., 1995). No such hypergastrinaemia-inducing effect was observed during activation of gastric mucosal inflammatory processes or in biomorphotic process. As regards the course of *Helicobacter pylori* colonization, other authors (Jang & Kim, 2000) found intensification of both apoptosis and proliferative activity of endocrine cells, mainly G and D, correlated with gastritis activity and with the degree of *H.pylori* colonization. Not all authors (Tzaneva & Julianov, 1999) found lesions in CgA and D cells of gastric corpus mucosa with *H.pylori* colonization. At the same time, these authors stressed that D cells did not participate in the pathomechanism of hypergastrinaemia observed in this case.
Experimental pathology demonstrates that together with deepening biomorphosis, the expression of G cells decreases while D and ECn cells are more numerous (Sandstrom et al., 1999). However, these relations are not so easy to explain, what has been already reported by the authors cited above, due to e.g. the fact that it is not certain whether pathogenic factors other than biomorphosis leading to the above described lesions in G, D and ECn cells, can be excluded. The own study confirmed lack of changes in the neuroendocrine cells status in the gastric mucosa depending on the biomorphosis.
Studies of endocrine cells in gastric mucosa and gastrointestinal tract mucosa in general, require extensive continuation. However, in order to provide significant progress in medical knowldege, it is necessary to standardise, in the first place, the method of quantitative assessment of these cells and also to establish a generally accepted strictly histopathological classification of chronic gastritis.

5. Presented results and conclusions

Helicobacter pylori presence in about 50% of healthy population without any clinical symptoms, and in 30% also without any morphological changes in gastric mucosa, requires further evaluations, both clinical and pathological. Endoscopic biopsy evaluations have firmly indicated that there is a poor correlation between the gastric mucosal appearance and histological indices of superficial and atrophic chronic gastritis. The Sydney System and its updated 1994 Houston status of the gastritis classification remains incompletely accepted. Many pathological reports on gastritis have individual, non-standard styles, which poorly correlates with both clinical symptoms and endoscopic lesions. As chronic gastritis is both overdiagnosed and underdiagnosed, a cooperation between clinicians and pathologists in diagnostics of a particular type of chronic gastritis is a necessity. Finally, in order to provide significant progress in medical knowledge, it is necessary to standardize, in the first place, the clinic-pathological cooperation and the method of quantitative or semi-quantitative assessment of the inflammatory and epithelial (histoarchitectural structure) cells of the gastric mucosa and also to establish a generally accepted strictly histopathological classification of chronic gastritis.

6. References

Appelman H.D. (1994). Gastritis: terminology, etiology, and clinicopathological correlations: another biased view. *Hum Pathol*, Vol.25, No.10, (October 1994), pp.1006-1019, ISSN 0046-8177

Arkkila P.E., Seppala K., Farkkila M.A., et al. (2006). Helicobacter pylori eradication in the healing of atrophic gastritis: a one-year prospective study. *Scand J Gastroenterol*, Vol.41, No.7, (July 2006), pp.782-90, ISSN 0036-5521

Axon A.T.R. (1992). Clinical and histological consequences of Helicobacter pylori suppresion/eradication. *J Gastroenterol Hepatol*, Vol.4, Suppl.2, (1992), pp.49-52, ISSN 1440-1746

Bechi P., Balzi M., Becciolini A., et al. (1996). Helicobacter pylori and cell proliferation of the gastric mucosa: possible implications for gastric carcinogenesis. *Am J Gastroenterol*, Vol.91, No.2, (February 1996), pp.271-276, ISSN 0002-9270

Bielicki D., Markiewicz M., Marlicz K., et al. (1993). PCNA/cyclin defined proliferative activity of epithelial cells in normal gastric mucosa in chronic gastritis. *Polish J Pathol*, Vol.44, (1993), pp.75, ISSN 1233-9687

Borch K., Renvall H., Kullman E., et al. (1987). Gastric carcinoid associated with syndrome of hypergastrinemic atrophic gastritis: A prospective analysis of 11 cases. *Am J Surg Pathol*, Vol.11, No.,(1987), pp.435-444, ISSN 0147-5185

Borchard F. (2001). Chemical-reactive gastritis. *Pathologe*, Vol.22, No.1, (January 2001), pp.44-55, ISSN 0172-8113

Bordi C., D'Adda T., Azzoni C., et al. (2000). Classification of gastric endocrine cells at light and electron microscopical levels. *Microsc Res Tech*, Vol.48, No.5, (March 2000), pp. 258–271, ISSN 1097-0029

Bordi C., Ferrari C., D'Adda T., et al. (1986) Ultrastructural characterization of fundic endocrine cell hyperplasia associated with atrophic gastritis and hypergastrinemia. *Virchows Arch*, Vol.404, No., (1986), pp.335-347 , ISSN 0945-6317

Canese M.G., Bussolati G. (1977). Immuno-Electron-Cytochemical Localization of the Somatostatin Cells In The Human Antral Mucosa. *J Histochem Cytochem*, Vol.25, No., (1977), pp. 1111-1118, ISSN 0022-1554

Carney A., Go V., Fairbanks V., et al. (1983). The syndrome of gastric argyrophil carcinoid tumours and nonantral gastric atrophy. *Ann Intern Med*, Vol.99, No.6, (December 1983), pp.761-766, ISSN 0003-4819

Cetin Y. (1992). Chromogranin A immunoreactivity and Grimelius' argyrophilia. A correlative study in mammalian endocrine cells. *Anat Embryol*, Vol.185, No.3, (September 1992), pp.207-15, ISSN 0340-2061

Chamouard P., Walter P., Wittersheim C., et al. (1997). Antral and fundic D-cell numbers in Helicobacter pylori infection. *Eur J Gastroenterol Hepatol*, Vol.9, No.4, (April 1997), pp.361-365, ISSN 0954-691X

Chen X.Y., Van der Hulst R.W., Bruno M.J., et al. (1999). Interobserver variation in the histopathological scoring of Helicobacter pylori related gastritis. *J Clin Pathol*, Vol.52, No.8, (August 1999), pp.612-615, ISSN 0021-9746

Cohen M.C., Cueto-Rua E., Balcarce N., et al. (2000). Assessment of the Sydney System in Helicobacter pylori-associated gastritis in children. *Acta Gastroenterol Latinoam*, Vol.30, No.1, (January 2000), pp.35-40, ISSN 0300-9033

Correa P., Yardley J.H. (1992). Grading and classification of chronic gastritis: one american response to the Sydney System. *Gastroenterology,* Vol.102, No.1, (January 1992), pp.355-359, ISSN 0016-5085

Correa P. (1988). Chronic gastritis: a clinico-pathologic classifications. *Am J Gastroenterol,* Vol.83, No.5, (May 1988),pp.504-509, ISSN 0002-9270

Correa P. (1980). The epidemiology and pathogenesis of chronic gastritis. Three etiologic entities. *Front Gastroenterol Res,* Vol.6, (1980), pp.98-108, ISSN 0302-0665

Coupe M., Rees H., Springer C.J., et al. (1990). Gastric enterochromaffin-like (ECL) cells in hypergastrinaemic duodenal ulcer disease. *Gut,* Vol.31, No.2, (February 1990), pp.144-147, ISSN 0017-5749

D'Adda T., Corleto V., Pilato F.P., et al. (1990). Quantitative ultrastructure of endocrine cells of oxyntic mucosa in Zollinger-Ellison syndrome. *Gastroenterology,* Vol.99, No.1, (July 1990), pp.17-26, ISSN 0016-5085

Dayal Y. (1992). Hyperplastic proliferations of the ECL cells. *Yale J Biol Med,* Vol.65, No.6, (Nov-Dec 1992), pp.805-825, ISSN 0044-0086

Deschner E.E., Winawer S.J., Lipkin M. (1972). Patterns of nucleic acid and protein synthesis in normal human gastric mucosa and atrophic gastritis. *J Nat Cancer Inst,* Vol.48, No.6, (June 1972), pp.1567-1574, ISSN 0027-8874

Diebold MD, Richardson S, Duchateau A, et al (1998) Factors influencing corpus argyrophil cell density and hyperplasia in reflux esophagitis patients treated with antisecretory drugs and controls. *Dig Dis Sci,* Vol.43, No.8, (August 1998), pp.1629-1635, ISSN 0163-2116

Dixon M.F., Genta R.M., Yardley J.H., Correa P., et al., (1996), Classification and grading of gastritis. The updated Sydney System. *Am J Surg Pathol,* Vol.20, No.10,(October 1996), pp.1161-1181, ISSN 0147-5185

Fenoglio-Preiser CH (ed.). (1999). *Gastrointestinal Pathology.* Lippincott-Raven, ISBN 9780397516407, Philadelphia New York

Glass G.B.J., Pitchumoni C.S. (1975). Structural and ultrastructural alterations, exfoliative cytology and enzyme cytochemistry and histochemistry, proliferation kinetics, immunological derangements and other causes, and clinical associations and sequallae. *Hum Pathol,* Vol.6, No.2, (March 1975), pp.219-250, ISSN 0046-8177

Goodlad R.A., Madgwick A.J.A., Moffatt M.R., et al. (1989). Prostaglandins and the gastric epithelium: Effects of misoprostol on gastric epithelial cell proliferation in the dog. *Gut,* Vol.30, No.3, (March 1989), pp.316-21, ISSN 0017-5749

Goodlad R.A., Wright N.A. (1987). Peptides and epithelial growth regulation. *Experientia,* Vol.43, No.7, (July 1987), pp.780-784, ISSN 0014-475

Goodlad R.A., Wright N.A. (1995). Epithelial kineticks; control and consequences of alteration in disease. In: *Gastrointestinal and oesophageal pathology (2nd ed),* Whitehead R. (Ed.) , pp.97-115, Churchill Livingstone, ISBN 9780443047640, New York

Graham D.Y., Lew G.M., Lechago J. (1993). Antral G-cell and D-cell numbers in Helicobacter pylori infections effect of H. Pylori eradication. *Gastroenterology,* Vol.104, No.6, (June 1993), pp.1655-1660, ISSN 0016-5085

Green L.K., Graham D.Y. (1990). Gastritis in the elderly. *Clinics North Am,* Vol.19, No.2, (June 1990), pp.273-292, ISSN 0889-8553

Guarner J., Herrera-Goepfert R., Mohar A., et al. (1999). Interobserver variability in application of the revised Sydney classification for gastritis. *Hum Pathol*, Vol.30, No.12, (December 1999), pp.1431-1434, ISSN 0046-8177

Guerci A., Chambre J.F., Franck P., et al. (1992). Flow cytometric analysis of the cell cycle in chronic gastritis. *Anal Cell Pathol*, Vol.4, No.5, (September 1992), pp.381-338, ISSN 0921-8912

Hall P.A., Levison D.A., Woods A.L., et al. (1990). Proliferating cell nuclear antigen (PCNA) immunolocalization in paraffin sections: an index of cell proliferation with evidence of deregulated expression in some neoplasm. *J Pathol*, Vol.162, No.4, (December 1990), pp.285-294 , ISSN 1096-9896

Haruma K., Sumii K., Okamoto S., et al. (1995). Helicobacter pylori infection associated with low antral somatostatin content in young adults. Implication for the pathogenesis of hypergastrinemia. *Scandinavian J Gastroenterol*, Vol.30, No.6, (June 1995), pp.550-553, ISSN 0036-5521

Hattori T. (1976). Tritiated thymidine autoradigraphic study on cellular migration in the gastric gland of the golden hamster. *Cell Tiss Res*, Vol.172, No.2, (September 1976), pp.171-184, ISSN 0302-766X

Havu N. (1986). Enterochromaffin-like cell carcinoids of gastric mucosa in rats after life-long inhibition of gastric secretion. *Digestion*, Vol.35, Suppl.1, (1986), pp.42-55, ISSN 0012-2823

Hellander H.E. (1981). The cells of the gastric mucosa. *Int Rev Cytol*, Vol.70, (1981), pp.217-82, ISSN 0074-7696

Hodges J., Isacsson P., Wright R. (1981). Diffuse enterochromaffin-like (ECL) cell hyperplasia and multiple gastric carcinoids; complication of pernicious anemia. *Gut*, Vol.22, No.3, (March 1981), pp.237-241, ISSN 0017-5749

Iacangelo A., Fischer-Colbrie R., Koller K.J., et al. (1988). The sequence of porcine chromogranin A can serve precursor for the biologically active hormone, pancreastatin. *Endocrinology*, Vol.122, No.5, (May 1988), pp.2339-2341, ISSN 0013-7227

Irazusta S.P., Vassallo J., Magna L.A., et al. (1998). The value of PCNA and AgNOR staining in endoscopic biopsies of gastric mucosa. *Pathol Res Pract*, Vol.194, No.1, (1998), pp.33-39, ISSN 0344-0338

Ito H., Yokozaki H., Tokumo K., et al. (1986). Serotonin containing E cells in normal human gastric mucosa and in gastritis. Immunohistochemical, electron microscopic and autoradiographic studies. *Virchows Arch A*, Vol.409, No.3, (1986), pp.313-323, ISSN 0174-7398

Jang T.J., Kim J.R. (2000). Proliferation and apoptosis in gastric antral epithelial cells of patients infected with Helicobacter pylori. *J Gastroenterol*, Vol.35, No.4, (April 2000), pp.312-314, ISSN 0944-1174

Keleman Z. (1997). PCNA: Structure, Function and Interactions. *Oncogene*, Vol.14, No.6, (February 1997), pp.629-640, ISSN 0950-9232

Kimura N., Sassano N., Yamada R., et al. (1988). Immunohistochemical study of chromogranin in 100 cases of pheochromocytoma, carotid body tumor, medullary thyroid carcinoma and carcinoid tumour. *Virchows Arch*, Vol.413, No.1, (1988), pp.33-38, ISSN 0945-6317

Kitani M., Asada Y., Sakata J., et al. (1999). Cell density of adrenomedullin-immunoreactive cells in the gastric endocrine cells decreases in antral atrophic gastritis. *Histopathology*, Vol.34, No.2, (February 1999), pp.134-139, ISSN 0309-0167

Konecki D.S., Benedum U.M., Gerdes H.H., et al. (1987). The primary structure of human chromogranin A and pancreastatin. *J Biol Chem*, Vol.262, No.35, (December 1987), pp.17026-17030, ISSN 0021-9258

Kozlowski W., Kulig A., Czkwianianc E., et al. (1995). Morphological and immunohistochemical examinations of the dynamic changes of gastric mucosa associated with the treatment of Helicobacter pylori infection in children. *An Ac. Med Bial*,Vol.40, No.3, (1995), pp. 678-684, ISSN 1427-941X

Kozlowski W., Kulig A., Czkwianianc E., et al. (1993). Histochemical and immunohistoenzymatical evaluations of the gastric endocrine cells (ECL, EC, G and D) with Helicobacter pylori infection in children. *Przegl Pediatr*, Vol.XXIII, Suppl.1, (1993), pp.249-254, ISSN 0137-723X, (In polisch),

Larsson L., Rehfeld J., Stockbrugger R., et al. (1978). Mixed endocrine tumours associated with hypergastrinemia of antral origin. *Am J Pathol*, Vol.93, No.1, (October 1978), pp.53-68, ISSN 0002-9440

Larsson L.I. (1984). Evidence for anterograde transport of secretory granules in processes of gastric paracrine (somatostatin) cells. *Histochemistry*, Vol.80, No.8, (1984), pp.323-326, ISSN 0301-5564

Lee E.R. (1985). Dynamic histology of the antral epithelium in the mouse stomach. III. Ultrastructure and renewal of pit cells. *Am J Anat*, Vol.172, No.3, (March 1985), pp.225-240, ISSN 0002-9106

Lee H., Hakanson R., Karlsson A., et al. (1992). Lansoprazole and Omeprazole Have Similar Effect on Plasma Gastrin Levels, Enterochromaffin-Like Cells, Gastrin Cells and Somatostatin Cells in the Rat Stomach. *Digestion*, Vol.51, No.3, (1992), pp.125-132, ISSN 0012-2823

Lloyd R.V., Mervak T., Schmidt K., et al. (1984). Immunohistochemical detection of chromogranin and neuron-specific enolase in pancreatic endocrine neoplasms. *Am J Surg Pathol*, Vol.8, No.8,(August 1984), pp.607-614, ISSN 0147-5185

Lynch D.A., Axon A.T. (1995). Helicobacter pylori, gastric cancer and gastric epithelial kinetics: a review. *Europ J Gastroenterol Hepatol*, Vol.7, Suppl.1, (August 1995), pp.S17-23, ISSN 0954-691X

Warren J.R., Marshall B. (1983). Unidentified curved bacilli on gastric epithelium in active chronic gastritis. *Lancet*, Vol.321, No.8336, (June 1983), pp.1273-1274, ISSN 0140-6736

Mathews M.B., Bernstein R.M., Franza B.R., et al. (1984). Identity of the proliferating cell nuclear antigen and cyclin. *Nature*, Vol.309, No.5966, (May 1984), pp.374-376, ISSN 0028-0836

Misiewicz J.J., Tytgat G.N.J., Goodwin C.S., et al. (1990). The Sydney System: a new classification of gastritis. *World Congresses of Gastroenterology*; 1990 August 26–31. Sydney, pp.1-10

Murray S.S., Deaven L.L., Burton D.W., et al. (1987). The gene for human chromogranin A (CgA) is located on chromosome 14. *Biochem Biophys Res Commun*, Vol.142, No.1, (January 1987), pp.141-146, ISSN 0006-291X

Oren M. (1992) The involvement of oncogenes and tumour suppresor genes in the control of apoptosis. *Cancer and Metastatic Review*, Vol.11, No.2, (September 1992), pp.141-148, ISSN 0167-7659

Owen D.A., (1996) The Morphology of Gastritis. *Yale J Biol Med*, Vol.69, (1996), pp.51-60, ISSN 0044-0086

Panella C., Ierardi E., Polimeno L., et al. (1996). Proliferative activity of gastric epithelium in progressive stages of Helicobacter pylori infection. *Dig Dis Sci*, Vol.41, No.6, (June 1996), pp.1132-1138 ISSN 0163-2116

Portela-Gomes G.M., Grimelius L. (1986). Identification and characterisation of enterochromaffin cells with different staining techniques. *Acta Histochem*, Vol.79, (1986), pp.161-174, ISSN 0065-1281

Preston-Martin S., Pike M.C., Ross R.K., et al. (1990). Increased cell division as a cause for human cancer. *Cancer Research*, Vol.50, No.23, (December 1990), pp.415-421, ISSN 0008-5472

Price A.B. (1999). Classification of gastritis: yesterdey, today and tomorrow. *Verh Dtsch Ges Pathol*, Vol.83, (1999), pp.52-55, ISSN 0070-4113

Price A.B. (1991). The Sydney System: Histological division. *J Gastoenterol Hepatol*, Vol.6, No.3, (May-June 1991), pp.209-222, ISSN 1440-1746

Ricci V., Ciacci C., Zarrilli R., et al. (1996). Effect of Helicobacter pylori on gastric epithelial cell migration and proliferation in vivtro: role of VacA and CagA. *Infection Immunity*, Vol.64, No.7, (July 1996), pp.2829-2833, ISSN 0019-9567

Rosa P., Hille A., Lee R.W.H., et al. (1985). Secretogranins I and II: two tyrosinesulfated secretory proteins common to a variety of cells secreting peptides by the regulated pathway. *J Cell Biol*, Vo.101, No.5 Pt 1, (November 1985), pp.1999-2011, ISSN 0021-9525

Rubin W. (1972). Endocrine cells in the normal human stomach. A fine structural study. *Gastroenterology*, Vol.63, No.1, (November 1972), pp.784-800, ISSN 0016-5085

Sandstrom O., Mahdavi J., el-Salhy M. (1999). Age-related changes in antral endocrine cells in mice. *Histol Histopathol*, Vol.14, No.1, (January 1999), pp.31-36, ISSN 0213-3911

Sipponen P. (1989). Atrophic gastritis as a premalignant condition. *Ann Med*, Vol.21, No.4, (August 1989), pp.287-290, ISSN 0785-3890

Sipponen P. (1992). Long-term consequences of gastroduodenal inflammation. *J Gastroenterol Hepatol*, 1992, Vo.4, Suppl.2, (1992), pp.25, ISSN 1440-1746

Solcia E., Capella C., Buffa R., et al. (1979). Endocrine cells of the gastrointestinal tract and related tumors. *Pathobiol Ann*, Vol.9, (1979), pp.163-204, ISSN 0362-3025

Solcia E., Capella C., Vassallo G. (1975). Endocrine cells of the gastric mucosa. *Int Rev Cytol*, Vol.42, (1975), pp.223-286, ISSN 0074-7696

Strickland R.G., Mackay I.R. (1973). A reappraisal of the nature and significance of chronic gastritis. *Am J Dig Dis*, Vol.18, No.5, (May 1973), pp.426-440, ISSN 0002-9211

Strickland R.G. (1990). Gastritis. *Springer Seminars in immunopathology* 1990, Vol.12, No.2-3, (1990), pp.203-217, ISSN 0344-4325

Tytgat G.N.J. (1991). The Sydney System: Endoscopic division. Endoscopic appearance in gastritis/duodenitis. *J Gastroenterol Hepatol*, Vol.6, No.3, (May-June 1991), pp.223-234, ISSN 1440-1746

Tzaneva M. (2001). Electron microscopic immunohistochemical investigation of chromogranin A in endocrine cells in human oxyntic gastric mucosa. *Acta Histochem*, Vol.103, No.2, (April 2001), pp.179-194, ISSN 0065-1281

Tzaneva M., Julianov A. (1999). Chromogranin A-, somatostatin- and serotonin-containing endocrine cells in the corporal gastric mucosa of patients with Helicobacter pylori associated gastritis. *Endocr Regul*, Vol.33, No.2, (June 1999), pp.79-82, ISSN 1210-0668

Walsh J.H. (1990). Role of gastrin as a trophic hormone. *Digestion*, Vol.47, Suppl.1, (1990), pp.11-16, ISSN 0012-2823

Waseem N.H., Lane D.P. (1990). Monoclonal antibody analysis of the proliferating cell nuclear antigen (PCNA). Structural conservation and the detection of a nucleolar form. *J Cell Sci*, Vol.96, Pt.1, (May 1990), pp.212-219, ISSN 0021-9533

Weaver L.T., Walker W.A. (1988). Epidermal growth factor and the developing human gut. *Gastroenterology*, Vol.94, No.3, (March 1988), pp.845-847, ISSN 0016-5085

Whitehead R., Truelove S.C., Gear M.W.L. (1972). The histological diagnosis of chronic gastritis in fibreoptic gastroscope biopsy specimens. *J Clin Pathol*, 1972, Vol.25, No.1, (January 1972), pp.1-11, ISSN 0021-9746

Wiedemann B., Huttner W.B. (1989). Synaptophysin and chromogranin/secretogranins widespread constituents of distinct types of neuroendocrine vesicles and new tools in tumor diagnosis. *Virchows Arch B*, Vol.58, No.2, (1989), pp.95-121, ISSN 0340-6075

Wilson B.S., Lloyd R.V. (1984). Detection of chromogranin in neuroendocrine cells with a monoclonal antibody. *Am J Pathol*, Vol.115, No.3, (June 1984), pp.458-468, ISSN 0002-9440

Wyatt J.I. (1995). Histopathology of gastroduodenal inflammation: the impact of Helicobacter pylori. *Histopathology*, Vol.26, No.1, (January 1995), pp.1-15, ISSN 0309-0167

Yanagihara K., Tsumuraya M. (1992). Transforming growth factor beta-1 induces apoptotic cell death in cultured human gastric carcinoma cells. *Cancer Res*, Vol.52, No.14, (July 1992), pp.4042-4045, ISSN 0008-5472

Zhang Ch., Yamada N., Wu Y-L., et al. (2005a). Helicobacter pylori infection, glandular atrophy and intestinal metaplasia in superficial gastritis, gastric erosion, erosive gastritis, gastric ulcer and early gastric cancer. *World J Gastroneterol*, Vol.11, No.6, (February 2005), pp. 791-796, ISSN 1007-9327

Zhang Ch., Yamada N., Wu Y-L., et al. (2005b). Comparison of Helicobacter pylori infection and gastric mucosal histological features of gastric ulcer patients with chronic gastritis patients. *World J Gastroneterol*, Vol.11, No.7, (February 2005), pp. 976-981, ISSN 1007-9327

Zverkov I.V., Isakov V.A., Aruin L.I. (1996). Helicobacter pylori, endocrine cells of the gastric mucosa, and their function in duodenal ulcer. *Arkh Patol*, Vol.58, No.1, (January-February 1996), pp.33-37, ISSN 0004-1955

6

The Role of Morphometry in Diagnostic of Chronic Gastritis

Tomasz Markiewicz[1,2], Wojciech Kozlowski[1] and Cezary Jochymski[1]
[1]Military Institute of Medicine / Pathology Department,
[2]Warsaw University of Technology,
Poland

1. Introduction

Chronic gastritis is one of the most frequent gastric diseases. The morphometry in diagnostic of chronic gastritis can as appear to be a potentially significant tool. The evaluation of the histoarchitectural structure of the gastric mucosa and quantification of the various neuroendocrine cells develop the new objective methods to describe changes caused by chronic gastritis. The development of specimen digitalization and computer image processing systems offer possibilities of automatization of this process on every high level.
Based on the endoscopic evaluation and mucosa biopsy analysis, variable numbers and various subtypes of the neuroendocrine (NE) cells have been described in association with different types of chronic gastritis. The neuroendocrine cell population, such as enterochromaffin-like cells (ECL), G cells, and D cells may occur as hyperplastic lesions, hypergastrinemia, hyperplasia, dysplasia, possibly type-1 gastric tumour or proliferation as an indirect effect of modern drugs, suppressing acid secretion (the post-pharmacotherapeutic hypo- or achlorhydric status). The wide range of methods used for evaluation of NE cells density in the histological slides from counting the number of cells per one microscopic field to shape diversity of gastric glands are frequently discussed in the literature. However, there is still a lack of acknowledged evidence on the participation of NE cells in stomach inflammation pathology and the relation between NE cells density and type of chronic gastritis require further investigation. The morphometry analysis of the mucosa specimen supported by the computerized automatic evaluation can be frequently taken into account in order to reflect the mechanism of stomach inflammation. In that analysis, other factors such as presence of Helicobacter pylori, sex and anatomical region of biopsy should be included and discussed.
In this chapter we focused on the following topics:

- Investigation of the role of different types of NE cells in chronic gastritis.
- Methodology of the evaluation of NE cells population in mucosa histological slides - different approaches and measures.
- Statistical investigation of the observed variations in the NE cells population with respect to diagnosis (type of chronic gastritis), anatomical region, Helicobacter pylori, sex, hyperplasia and other factors.
- Selected aspects of the computerization of automatic quantitative evaluation and space distribution of the NE cells, evaluation of the shape of mucosa glands and

morphometry analysis, for digital images of the selected field of view and virtual slides of the whole mucosa specimen.

2. General morphometric feature of chronic gastritis

The diagnosis of chronic gastritis is a complex problem which includes the evaluation of different clinical and histological features. This problem drew attention of many researchers, however, the consensus has not been reached. Following numerous classification systems, since the 90's of XX century the Sydney System has been used. In 1994 it was updated and added certain modifications to improve the criteria of atrophy evaluation. The commonly used criteria, presented in the chapter "Chronic gastritis" with the quality evaluation of the specimens does not give specific results in many diagnostic cases. In the light of the recent researches, the diagnostic system will be developed and improved in near future by the morphometric quantitative evaluation of different aspects of the observed changes.

Evaluation of neuroendocrine cells, which was introduced into diagnostic, provides new objective methods to extend the analysis of chronic gastritis. The first works are dated back to the 70's of XX century and focused mainly on the detection of neuroendocrine cells also in gastric mucosa. The gastric neuroendocrine cells represent the diffuse neuroendocrine cells system (DeLellis et al., 1984; Falkmer & Wilander, 1995; Lloyd, 1999; Osamura, 2002). This system contains also the APUD cells (Amine Precursors Uptake and Decarboxylation cells), first described and classified by Pearse (Pearse, 1969, 1974; DeLellis et al., 1984). All these cells originate from the stem cells of alimentary duct (Fenoglio-Preiser, 1999; Furth, 2002). Currently, according to Pears and Takor-Takor concept (Pearse & Takor-Takor, 1979) about 40 different types of the neuroendocrine cells can be distinguished.

The neuroendocrine cells of the gastric mucosa are normally located in the epithelium layer of the mucosal glands in prepyloric and oxyntic parts of stomach, sometimes in the stem part and never in the superficial epithelium of the glands of foveolar layer of gastric musoca (Dayal, 1992; Kozlowski et al., 1995; Nichols et al., 1974; Ohning et al., 1998; Portela-Gomes & Grimelius, 1986). The most numerous cells are ECL (entorechromaffin-like) cells, G (gastrinin) cells, D (somatostatin) cells and ECn (Enterochromaffin) cells. The ECL, G and D are more than 75 percent of neuroendocrine cells of gastric mucosa in oxyntic and pyloric parts (D'Adda et al., 1989; Dayal, 1992; Falkmer & Wilander, 1995; Fenoglio-Preiser , 1999). The ECL cells (this name was introduced by Hakanson et al. in 1967) are distributed in the deep 2/3 layers of gland epithelium in oxyntic and the fundus of the stomach (Bordi, 2000; Dayal, 1992; Falkmer & Wilander, 1995; Ohning et al., 1998; Solcia, 1988). They represent 30-44% of all neuroendocrine cells in these locations. Considering practical aspects, immunohistochemical methods are more valuable in detecting these cells by e.g. chromogranin-A reaction (Date et al., 2000; Dayal, 1992; Falkmer & Wilander, 1995; Whitehead, 1995). The G cells are localized only in the gland epithelium in pyloric part of gastric mucosa, mainly in the 1/3 middle region (Kozlowski et al., 1995). These cells give positive reaction not only with gastric stains, but also in chromogranin-A stain (Kinoshita et al., 1998). The D cells can be detected by anti-somatostatin reaction and ECn cells in anti-serotonin stain. The depicted monoclonal antibodies are the most specific and useful for the quantitative evaluation of several neuroendocrine cells for pathological evaluation of gastritis.

2.1 Morphometry of neuroendocrine cells

The relationship between hypergastrinemia and Helicobacter pylori colonization proved in the 90's initiated a renaissance of gastric mucosa neuroendocrine cells examinations. Initially there were examinations of mutual relations between G and D cells, later other gastric mucosa endocrine cell types were taken into the consideration. Up to now there is lack of acknowledged evidence on the participation of cells of this type in the stomach inflammation pathology. The dependence of the density of the neuroendocrine cells such as D, EC or ECL on the type of stomach disease was confirmed in previous publications (Bordi et al., 2000; Falkmer & Wilander, 1995; Kozlowski et al., 1995, 2001, 2003a, 2003b). An interesting recently published study (Peterson et al., 2009) presents the comparison between G-cells morphometry performed in three different manners: G-cell counting and presented as a ratio between its number and 1000 epithelial cells; image analysis gives the results as a ratio between the brown stained area to the total cytokeratin positive area and point counting in the superimposed grid. As far as now, there are significant differences in the used methods of morphometry. As far as these methods are concerned, we focused on the manners based on the cell recognition. They can be distinguished from other approaches either with or without consideration of the histoarchitectural structure.

2.1.1 Quantification the neuroendocrine cells in field of view

The most basic approach of the neuroendocrine cell quantification is count cells in the field of view without taking into account the observed histoarchitectural structure. As described in the study by Green et al., 1989, the neuroendocrine cells are counted in a few fields of view, with 200x magnification and results can be recalculate as the mean of cell quantity per one field. Generally, this method requires only the recognition of immunoreactivity of each cell in the field of view and counting them.

First, it should be noted that different distributions of the neuroendocrine cells in the area of the mucosa cross-section are observed. In the corpus of the stomach, the neuroendocrine cells are observed in the about 2/3 width of epithelium cross-section. Their distribution is approximately regular as it is presented in the Fig. 1.

The opposite cases are observed in the antrum where there is a high concentration of the neuroendocrine cells in the basis of foveolar region of the mucosa in cross-section (Fig. 2).

Accuracy of this approach is strongly influenced by the fact that the absolute number of the immunoreactivity cells in the field of view relates to the specimen orientation, thickness or size. As it can be seen, this quantification approach required selection of the field of view located exactly in the region with the presence of neuroendocrine cells. In the opinion of the authors, the calculation of the ratio between immunopositive and immunonegative cells in the gastric mucosa only in the region with presence of the neuroendocrine cells should be appropriate but more difficult to perform as it requires the specification of this area. A subjective opinion on location of neuroendocrine area border will have significant influence on the results.

2.1.2 Quantification the neuroendocrine cells in histoarchitectural structures.

The more complex approach, comparing to the one described above, is calculation of the number of cells per mm2 of the area of the mucosa glandular epithelium or per one gland (Aruin et al., 1984; Tzaneva & Julianov, 1999; Azzoni et al., 1996). The last proposition is particularly interesting, yet its implementation requires recognition of separate glands in the microscopic image. The benefit is additional possibilities of measuring the mucosa gland dimensionality.

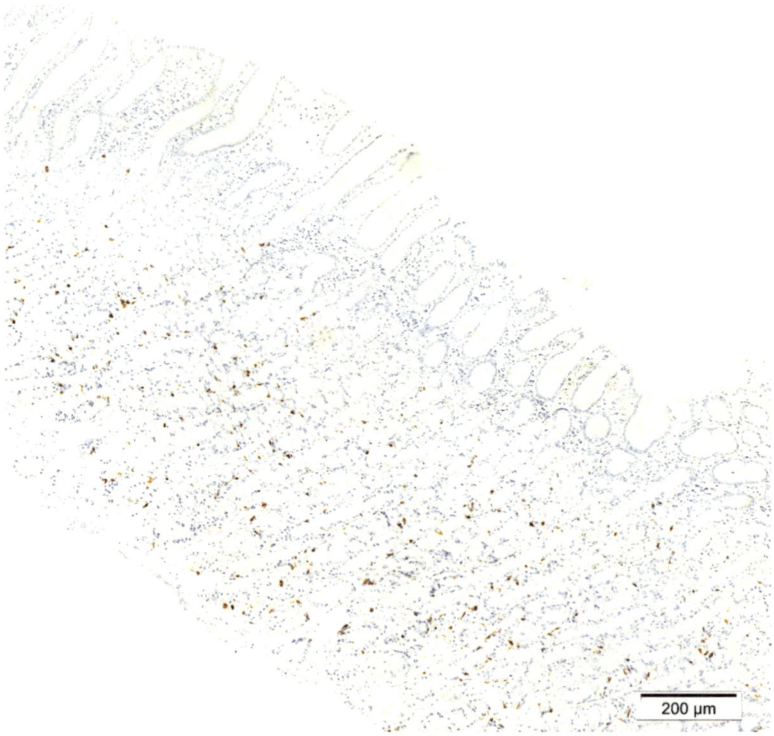

Fig. 1. The distribution of the neuroendocrine cells in the corpus mucosa (chromogranin-A, virtual slide).

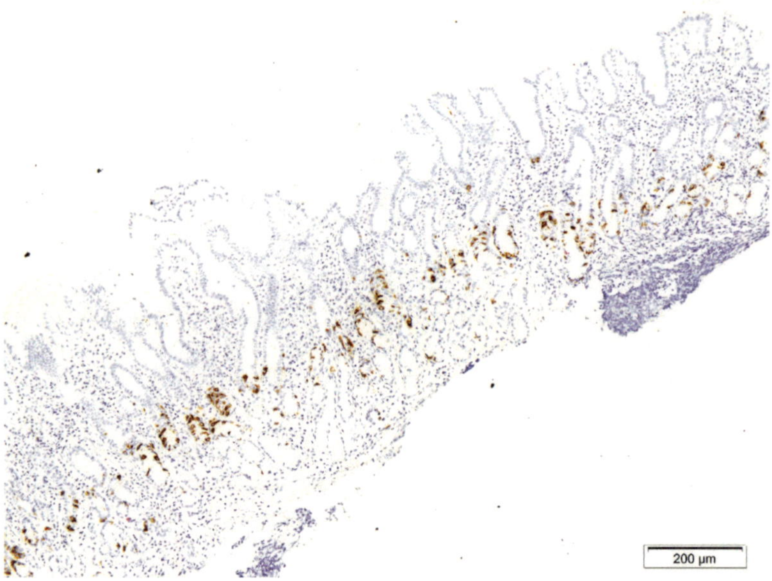

Fig. 2. The example the neuroendocrine cell localization in the antrum (chromogranin A, virtual slide)

It should be noted, that the obtained long cross-section shapes of the glands are very rare. The type of the specimen excludes efficient control over the section and as a result, the obtained shapes of gland sections located from epithelium to mucosa are rather round than ellipsoidal, as it is presented in Fig. 3.

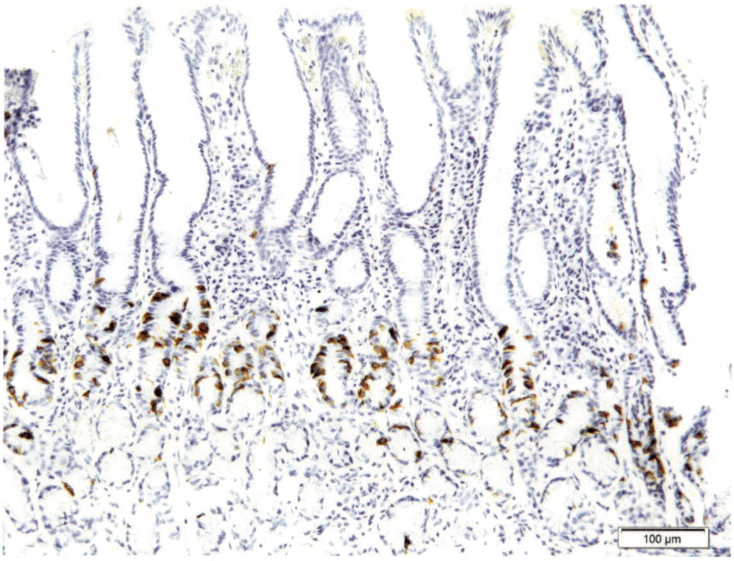

Fig. 3. Explanation of different shapes of glands (chromogranin-A, virtual slide).

Efficient evaluation of the number of neuroendocrine cells in the glands can be performed only by counting these cells in the sections of the glands. To support this evaluation, the shape of gland cross-sections should be taken into account.

This approach is connected with several problems that should be taken into account in the counting process. The first problem is to qualify particular glands for evaluation according to their cross-section. It is evident, that in the microscopic specimen some glands are cut not centrally by their lumen, but closely or exactly by their wall. In that glands the lumens are reduced to the narrow line area or only cell cluster is observed. These cases render difficult the recognition of the separate glands.

The second problem is the qualification of the glands to counting set according to its space location. This problem is illustrated in Fig 4.

Gland no. 1 is located half outside and half inside neuroendocrine region (black line outline) and its cross-section fully covers the width of this region. Gland no. 2 is fully included in the neuroendocrine area while gland no. 3 has only a small part located in this region and does not represent the full width of the measured region. For efficient counting the neuroendocrine cells in the separate glands, only glands no. 1 and 2 should be included.

The calculation of the neuroendocrine cell density based on this approach can be implemented by calculating the number of neuroendocrine cells per recognized gland, qualified for evaluation, with description of gland shape. In practice, the semi-quantitative method can be used - the glands can be divided into four groups depending on their cross-section shape: round, short ellipse, long ellipse and open. The criteria, presented in the studies (Kozlowski et al., 2009; Markiewicz et al., 2009a), are:

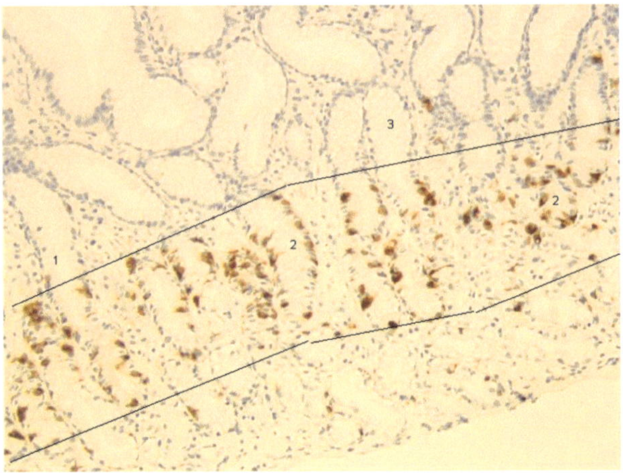

Fig. 4. Different level of inclusion of the glands in the neuroendocrine area.

- round shape – proportion between major and minor axis lengths is close to 1 (e.g. less than 1.2),
- short ellipse - proportion between major and minor axis lengths is less than 2,
- long ellipse - proportion between major and minor axis lengths is higher than 2,
- open – the gland cross-section shape is open.

The final step of the quantitative evaluation is a calculation of the number of neuroendocrine cells, detected in maximum 5 glands of any shapes described below. The recognition of the gland structures in the images gives possibility to count the ratio between numbers of neuroendocrine cells and all the cells of the mucosa glandular epithelium. Also, various geometrical features of the gland shape can be measured in these approaches.

2.2 Diagnostic influence of neuroendocrine cell morphometry

The connection between neuroendocrine cells and inflammatory disorder of the stomach is the subject of many researches. One of the observed relations deals with G cells hyperplasia in the hypochlorhydria or achlorhydria. The role of the gastrin as a regulator of the proliferation of G, ELC and D cells and their evaluation also required the morphometry of neuroendocrine cells (Calatayud et al., 2010). In another study, high correlation between age, H. pylori colonisation and atrophy of the corpus and G-cell density (Petersson et al., 2009) was reported. The degree of chronic inflammation and percentage of the G-cell was also statistically correlated. The endocrine cell hyperplasia can be developed as a consequence of functional changes and is the most prominent of autoimmune chronic gastritis. In antrum the endocrine hyperplasia is easily detected in H&E stain, but in oxyntic mucosa the immunohistochemical stains give better visualization and quantification of the changes in ECL cell population. The most detailed criteria for diagnosis and classification of gastric ECL proliferation was proposed by Solcia et al., 1995. The details are presented in table 1.

Also the changes in the number of D and G cells in atrophic gastritis were observed and several studies presented the therapy promoting the secretion of gastric acid and gastric pepsin and regulating the neuroendocrine mechanism in rats (Zhu et al., 2008; Wang et al., 2009; Czaja et al., 2008; Todorovic et al., 2008). However, as it was reported (Czaja et al., 2008), changes of serum gastrin concentration in gastric antrum in children with chronic gastritis are not statistically significantly connected with D and G cell densities.

Diagnosis	Criteria regarding increased endocrine cells	Common disorder
Simple/diffuse hyperplasia	>2x standard deviation (age/gender matched)	ZES, primary gastrin cell hyperplasia
Linear hyperplasia	Linear groups of five or more inside the glandular BM	ZES, pernicious anemia
Micronodular hyperplasia	Clusters of five or more cells within epithelium measuring <150 microns in diameter	Autoimmune atrophic gastritis
Adenomatoid hyperplasia	Aggregates of five or more micronodulares in lamina propria	Autoimmune atrophic gastritis, MEN-ZES
Dysplasias		Autoimmune atrophic gastritis, MEN-ZES
Enlarged micronodules	>150 microns	
Adenomatous micronodules	Collection(s) of at least five closely adherent micronodules, intervening BM only	
Fused micronodules	Adenomatous nicronodules with no intervening BM	
Microinfiltrative lesions	Infiltration of the lamina propria	
Carcinoids		Autoimmune atrophic gastritis, MEN-ZES
Intramucosal	Expansile/infiltrative nodules > 0.5 mm	
Invasive	Any size tumor within submucosa	

BM, Basement membrane; ZET, Zollinger-Ellison syndrome; MEN-ZET, multiple endocrine neoplasia-Zollinger-Ellison syndrome.

Table 1. Classification of ECL-cell proliferations (originally from Solcia et al., 1995).

Based on our clinical material, the authors of this chapter study the correlation between two types of chronic gastritis (superficial and deep) and neuroendocrine cells such as Chromogranin A positive cells, D cells and EC cells, identified by immunohistochemical stains. The sex and antrum/oxyntic parts are taken into account in the quantitative analysis.

3. Study of the neuroendocrine cell in chronic gastritis

3.1 Material and methods

The three types of primary antibodies has been applied:

- Monoclonal Mouse Anti-Human Chromogranin A, clone DAK-A3, code M 0869 DAKO

- Monoclonal Mouse Anti-Serotonin, clone 5HT-H209, code M 0758 DAKO
- Rabbit Polyclonal Anti-Human Somatostatin, code A0566 DAKO

Density of the following types of the cells has been further evaluated:

- Neuroendocrine cells (Chromogranin A positive cells)
- EC cells (Serotonin positive cells)
- D cells (Somatostatin positive cells)

Patients from the Military Hospital in Warsaw in Poland suffering for stomach diseases from the 1999 to 2010 were selected.

The slides used in further quantitative analysis should fulfil the following histological criteria: proper sections (automatic fixed paraffin sections, slide thickness from 3 to 5 micrometers), the right technical quality of tissue samples and the correct histo- and immunohistochemical staining, lack of any mechanical injury or any artefact (fragmentation, hemorrhages).

The morphometric evaluation of the specimens with the counting of the cell density in the field of view was performed using the acquired images of 400x magnification, at resolution of 768x576 pixels. Images were taken using Olympus BX50 microscope with the Olympus Camedia C-3030 camera and used for computer analysis. In semi-quantitative part of the studies, human experts count the number of neuroendocrine cells per one gland in five selected fields of view in each specimen.

3.2 Computerized image analysis

In the last few years many computer programs for automation of quantitative analysis of microscopic specimen, based on the image processing, have been developed (Bartels et al., 1996; Lezoray et al., 2000; Markiewicz et al., 2006, 2009b, 2010). In chronic gastritis the main task of computer automatization is the quantitative evaluation (recognition and counting) of the neuroendocrine cells. In last few years we proposed various approaches and programs used in the different types of the tissues and markers (Markiewicz et al., 2006, 2008, 2009) and our experience confirmed their accuracy. The developed programs used mainly the mathematical morphology operations, such as erosion, dilation, opening, closing or watershed method (Soille, 2003; Matlab, 2010). Counting neuroendocrine cells marked by the immunohistochemistry stains, such as chromogranin-A, serotonin, somatostatin or PCNA can be performed automatically by the program in a particular field of view. The automatization of these analyses can give an answer to the methods based on counting the cells in the field of view without taking into account any specific histological structures.

For evaluation of the density of the neuroendocrine cells the authors designed the automatic program written in Matlab language. The correct recognition of the separated nuclei and reactivity of these cells is the main task in the appropriate evaluation of the distribution density of the selected stained endocrine cells. The primary antibodies used (Chromogranin A, Serotonin and Somatostatin) stains of cytoplasmic structures. In the correct stain the nuclei are blue and only cytoplasm in the immunopositive cell is brown. The problem of recognition can be solved by the following steps: extraction of the blue nuclei of the cells and their classification into two groups - immunopositive and immunonegative cells based on the neighbouring cytoplasm. However, usually in the field of view some cells are stained fully brown. This results from the fact that cutting plane of the tissue specimen may go through any possible cutting levels of the cell. Moreover, some cells in the slide are only viewed as a part of the cytoplasm. Additionally, the nuclei are sometimes covered by the cytoplasm. According to this fact, the segmentation algorithm should posses two extraction lines: one for the cells with recognized blue nucleus and the second for recognition of the immunopositive cells without the blue nucleus.

The input image for quantitative analysis is in the form of RGB standard file. The first step is the image standardization, which means the calculation of the average RGB values of the lighter area in the field of view and linearly transformed RGB values of all pixels in the image in such a way that the lighter area will be exactly white. This step eliminates the influence of the differences in the glass transparency, lighting and other unstable values.

After standardization, the extraction of the blue nuclei as separate cells was performed. In the literature (Bartels et al., 1996; Lezoray et al., 2000; Markiewicz et al., 2006, 2008, 2009, 2010b; Kayser et al., 2006) the basic method for solving this task is the threshold operation, which is defined as follows: (Soille, 2003)

$$T_{[0,t_2]}[f(x)] = \begin{cases} 1 & \text{if} \quad 0 \le f(x) \le t_2 \\ 0 & \text{else} \end{cases} \tag{1}$$

were f(x) is the value of pixel of the image f in the x position and t_2 is the threshold value. This operation was done on the greyscale images, received by means different from the colour image, with one threshold value. Generally, this is a very difficult task because the nuclei are stained at different intensity and selecting one threshold value for this operation is problematic, and for some images even not possible.

In the papers (Markiewicz et al., 2008, 2009) the authors suggest a solution to this problem based on the threshold operation performed step by step with the increased threshold value. For the stomach specimen images we use the thresholding operation sequentially and apply an artificial neural network of Support Vector Machine (SVM) type (Vapnik, 1995; Schölkopf & Smola, 2002). The idea of this network is to create a hyperplane dividing the feature space of the input data into two separated parts with the maximum margin between them. In our case the input data are the pixels selected from the image. The input vector is composed of three colour components in RGB standard. For learning phase these data are representative for three classes: blue nuclei, brown cytoplasm and light background. Because one network recognizes only two classes, we must build three SVM networks for recognizing pixels between all pairs of classes and then use the one-against-one strategy to find the winner (Schölkopf & Smola, 2002). The learning data are manually selected from the sampled images and their quantity was 150 pixels per class. The output of the network is determined using the following formula:

$$D(\mathbf{x}) = \mathbf{w}^T \mathbf{x} + b \tag{2}$$

were w is the weight vector, **x** is the input vector and *b* is the bias. For learning process D(x) is defined as 1 for the first class and -1 for the alternative class in any pair of the classes. The learning of the network is understood as a task to find the optimal **w** and *b* values with the help of the quadratic programming with Lagrange multipliers α_k (Vapnik, 1995; Schölkopf & Smola, 2002). As a result of training we get:

$$\mathbf{w} = \sum_k \alpha_k d_k \mathbf{x}_k \tag{3}$$

and

$$b = d_k - \mathbf{w}^T \mathbf{x}_k \tag{4}$$

where d_k is 1 or -1 and α_k is the nonzero Lagrange multiplier corresponding to the k-th training data. Usually most multipliers are zero and these data points do not influence the solution.

After learning of the network the weights and bias are fixed. In the testing phase the input vectors represent the colour values of all pixels in the image. They are put to the SVM. It is evident that the output value D(**x**) will be different, depending on its relation to the respected class. For example, if the pixel is light blue, the D(**x**) signal of the SVM recognizing the nuclei will take $0<D(\mathbf{x})<1$ values. For the dark blue pixels this value will be higher than 1. Based on this relevance we use D(**x**) value as an indicator of the recognized class. In the constructed algorithm we use sequential thresholding operation starting from the minimum D(**x**) value as a threshold. Then, this threshold is increased step by step until the maximum. In any step D(**x**) for the whole image is thresholded and the separated objects, whose area are in the selected range, are added to the mask of the recognized nuclei. The result of this process will be the mask of all blue nuclei for which the area is in the preselected range. This range is selected on the basis of some knowledge and the image resolution with some margin. This process is supported by the watershed operation for the bigger cells to divide them into two cells if there is a narrow space between the two or more parts of them. This will help in the case of the overlapping nuclei of the cells.

The next step is the recognition of the immunopositive cells. This is performed with the use of the SVM and mathematical morphology operations such as closing and reconstruction. First, the brown cytoplasm is extracted by using the one-against-one strategy with three SVM networks. Next, all brown areas are closed by the structural element with the disk shape of the diameter of 7 pixels long. This operation outputs the mask of the brown cytoplasm with filled internal area of them. This filled area should be only on the internal side of the cytoplasm that is on the nuclei of the cell. If the immunopositive cell is touched with the other immunonegative cell, the second nucleus should not be selected. In practice, we can tolerance some errors in the case of overlapping.

The last process of segmentation is the extraction of still unrecognized immunopositive cells without the distinct blue nuclei. They are created from a brown mask, received in the previous step of the algorithm. Any separated brown objects that did not possess the blue nucleus and lie in the selected range of the cell area are added to the set of the immunopositive cells after a watershed operation dividing the touched items.

The final task is to count the cells according to their immunoreactivity classes. This is done in the form of simple counting of any separated objects in the masks of immunopositive and immunonegative cells, independently. Figure 5a presents a sample result of recognition in the Chromogranin stain. The immunopositive cells are marked "○", the immunonegative "+", in yellow and red colours respectively. The results for the serotonin and somatostatin stains of the same patient specimens are presented in Fig. 5b and c respectively. We evaluated more than 30 patients and the achieved accuracy was on the acceptable level. Less than 5% of the cells were unrecognized or misclassified. The developed program was written in Matlab language and tested with PC Centrino Duo 1.86 MHz, 2GB RAM. The result for one image is received in less than 1 minute. It is possible to correct the classification results of the cell manually by the intervention of a human expert.

a)

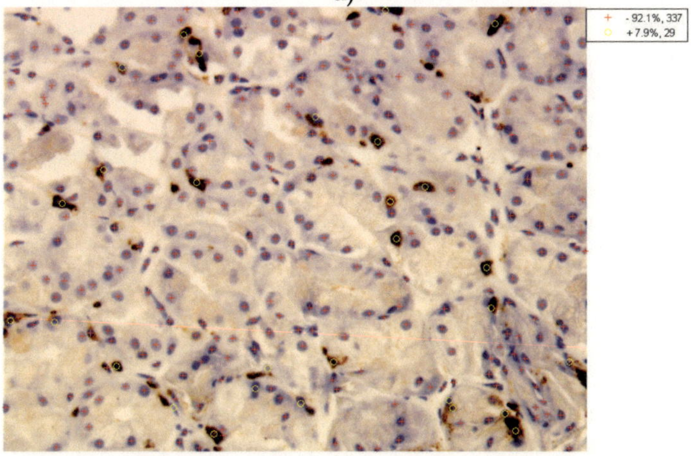

b)

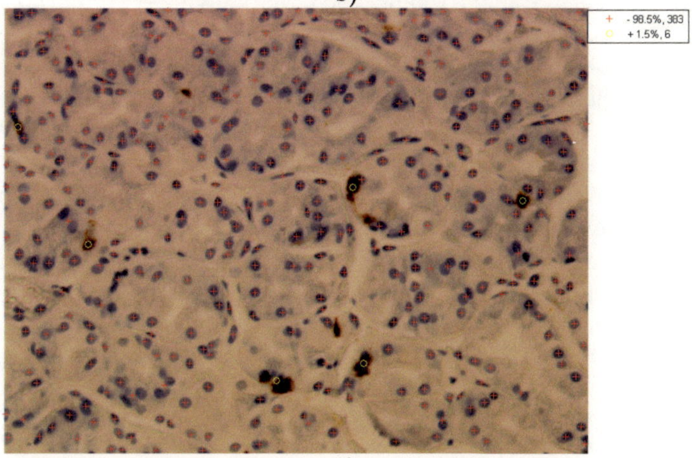

c)

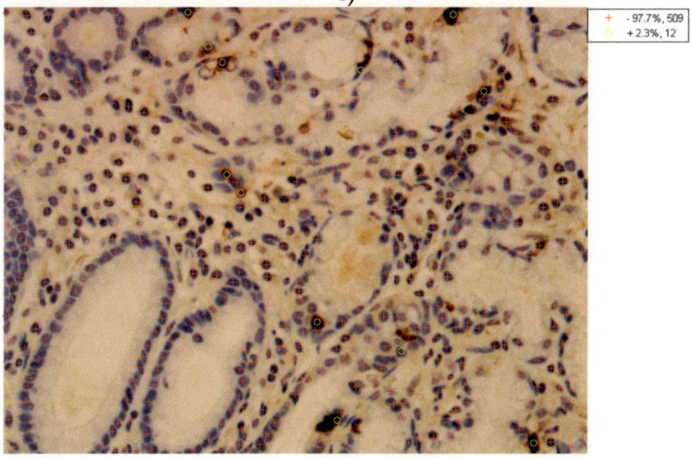

Fig. 5. The result of cell recognition in chromogranin-A (a), serotonin (b) and somatostatin (c) stains.

Calculating the number of neuroendocrine cells per one gland of the gastritis mucosa is a more complex process. The system must recognize also separate glands, measure their shape and count cells according to this histological structures. Also, based on the computerized image processing, the selected aspects of histological evaluation of the gastric mucosa can be performed. That can be gland distribution in the mucosa, proportion between gland lumen and its size. To perform the gland extraction from the image, first the cell nuclei should be recognized based on the algorithm described before. The input stage is a binary mask composed of the immunonegative and immunopositive cells. Although the contours of gland cross-section are not visible (in particular as a continuous shape), the gland face cells created the composition of the linearly bordered objects with blue stained nuclei and sometimes brown stained cytoplasm (only immunopositive cells). In comparison with other cells, the gland face cells are located more closely to each other. In practice, only gland face cells created the convex structures in the image. To reconstruct the completed gland outlining, the spaces between these cells should be filled. This task can be accomplished with the help of the Hit-or-Miss transform (HMT) with anisothropic structure element (SE) of a 35 pixels line shape (Soille, 2003; Markiewicz et al., 2009a). The based pixel of SE was a center point on the line shape, the SE foreground was formed by 3 last pixels at both ends; the rest of pixels of the line shape formed background. Because of the multipolarity and the gland contour in the image, and in the effect unconnected cell nuclei, the reconstruction process carried out by HMT should be performed in the series of SE rotation (every 5° in the scale from 0° to 175°).

Also, this operation is repeated with 23 pixels SE for obtaining the full continuous gland shape. The results of the gland face reconstruction are presented in Fig. 6. Based on the area criteria only dominant objects composed of the gland lumen and cells surrounding them should be selected as a gland cross-section planes. The recognized glands can be also categorized based on the morphometrical criteria, mainly by their major and minor axis lengths. The details of this approach were presented in the paper by Markiewicz et al., 2009a.

3.3 Results of quantitative evaluation

The evaluated specimens were taken from patients with the following diagnosis:

- chronic gastritis (CHG)
- chronic superficial gastritis (CHSG)

The specimens were divided based on oligobiopsy anatomical region – prepyloric or oxyntic part of stomach.

According to the statistical method for the ratio of immunopositive cell, the Chromogranin A, Serotonin and Somatostatin antibodies stain specimens should be evaluated. The images of them have been acquired in the manually selected regions, with the higher number of immunopositive cells in the center, mainly three per slide. As these cells are significanly more numerous in the Chromogranin A antibody stain, the regions were selected on the basis of this stain. In the Serotonin and Somatostatin stains we got images from too same regions. Based on the statistical results we found the threshold of the ratio of immunopositive cells for the selected antibody type. This threshold divided the set of patients into two groups. We evaluated the relation between this division and diagnosis (chronic gastritis and chronic superficial gastritis). Our suggestion on the dependence significance was based on the Fisher exact test (Fisher, 1922). If the returned p -value was

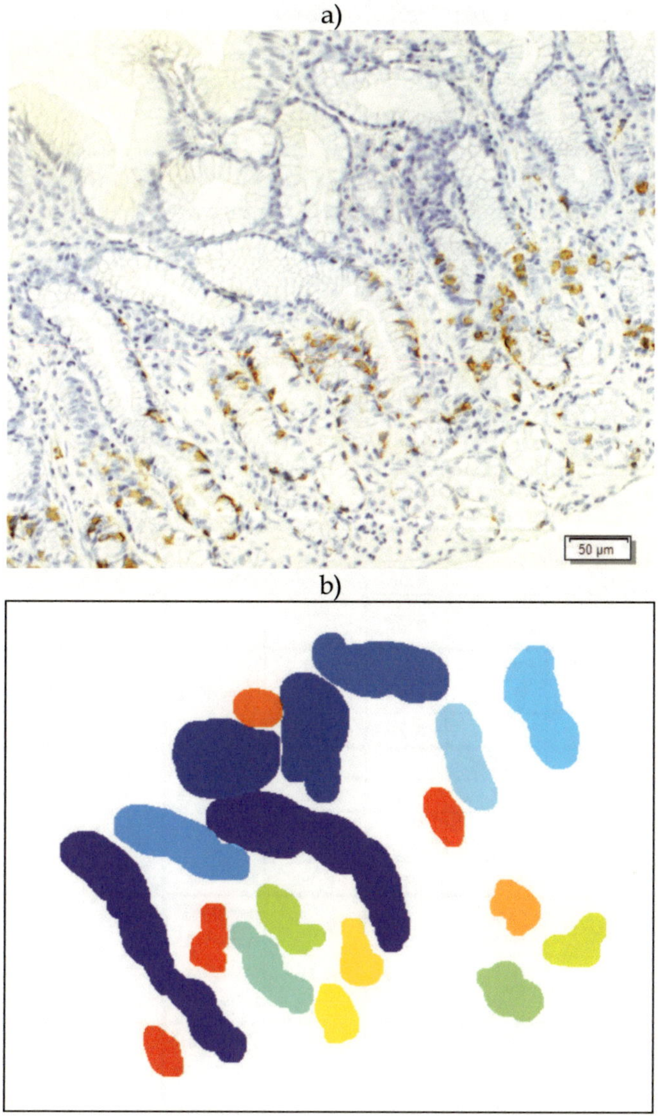

Fig. 6. The sample result of the gland cross-section plane recognition in the image.

less than 0.05, it is justified to reject the null hypothesis on lack of statistical dependence. We signed these cases as positive. The cases with p -value less than 0.07 were signed as conditionally positive with regard to restricted number of items in the data base.

To same items were evaluated with cell divided into the glands of the gastric mucosa, as was defined. The numbers of the positive cells in the recognized gland with respect to their cross-section were countered. The analysis was performed in five view fields. The returned value was calculated as the sum of the mean numbers of the positive cells in the four types of gland cross-section if they were present. Only glands with correct cutting plane were evaluated. If a field was fully packed with the cells in the gland light, this item was not useful for counting. They were divided into a set with a threshold value, similarly to the

previous manner. A difference between the number of items is the effect of the fact that some stains were too bad for automatic system but acceptable for human experts. We calculated the mean value for both examinations to illustrate scale of the difference in the cell density between types of the disease.
The results for the whole neuroendocrine cells (Chromogranin-A positive cells) are presented in table 2. The ratio of the whole neuroendocrine cells in the field of view shows that the significant dependencies with the type of disease are when:

		Ratio between NE and all cells [%]					NE cell quantity calculated in the glands			
Type of specimen	Type of disease	Threshold value and no of items		Mean of ratio	Median of ratio	Fisher test	Threshold value and no of items		Mean of cell number	Fisher test
All patients and both regions		< 5 %	>= 5 %			p=0.0965 negative	< 5.1	>=5.1		p=0.0769 negative
	CHSG	20	11	4.61	4.18		14	16	6.65	
	CHG	17	22	5.12	5.04		10	30	8.94	
Only women, both regions		< 5 %	>= 5 %			p=0.0105 positive	< 5.1	>=5.1		p=0.3175 negative
	CHSG	12	5	4.58	4.27		8	9	7.55	
	CHG	6	16	5.42	5.73		6	15	7.76	
Only men, both regions		<4.49%	>=4.49%			p=1 negative	< 6.4	>=6.4		p=0.1492 negative
	CHSG	7	6	4.65	4.18		8	5	7.35	
	CHG	10	9	4.79	3.88		6	13	10.24	
All patients, only prepy-loric		< 5 %	>= 5 %			p=0.6946 negative	< 9.6	>=9.6		p=0.4328 negative
	CHSG	6	4	5.60	4.88		6	4	10.78	
	CHG	8	10	5.26	5.0		7	11	12.29	
All patients, oxyntic		< 5.07 %	>= 5.07 %			p=0.0618 conditionally positive	< 5	>=5		p=0.0600 condi-tionally positive
	CHSG	16	5	4.14	4.18		12	8	4.58	
	CHG	10	12	5	5.15		6	16	6.19	
Only women, prepyloric		< 5 %	>= 5 %			p=0.6224 negative	< 7.8	>=7.8		p=0.3287 negative
	CHSG	3	3	5.83	5.79		3	3	8.77	
	CHG	3	6	5.03	5.00		2	7	10.68	
Only women, oxyntic		<5.07%	>=5.07%			p=0.0033 positive	< 5.1	>=5.1		p=0.2203 negative
	CHSG	10	2	3.96	3.71		7	4	4.66	
	CHG	2	10	5.71	6.02		4	8	5.57	
Only men, prepyloric		< 4%	>= 4%			p=0.5622 negative	<13.4	>=13.4		p=0.5638 negative
	CHSG	3	1	5.25	3.89		3	1	13.8	
	CHG	4	6	5.50	4.50		4	5	13.9	
Only men, oxyntic		<4.18%	>=4.18%			p=0.3698 negative	< 5	>=5		p=0.0698 condi-tionally positive
	CHSG	3	6	4.39	4.73		6	3	4.48	
	CHG	6	4	4.15	3.71		2	8	6.94	

Table 2. The dependence between the type of chronic gastritis and the neuroendocrine cells

- patient is a woman, both regions
- region is oxyntic (conditionally)
- patient is a woman and region is oxyntic

However, the results of the Fisher test synonymously indicate, that only for women and oligobiopsy from oxyntic should be considered a significant dependence. The rest of the listed cases have the positive return of the test because they included them. The evaluation of the ratio of the neuroendocrine cells in the other cases has dubious diagnostic value or does not have it.

Comparison of these results counted only in the glands epithelium of the gastric mucosa shows that there are significant differences. A conditionally positive relation was obtained in both evaluation methods only for oxyntic region and patient gender totally. By the use of this type of examination of the specimens we received additional conditionally positive dependence for male patients and mucosa oligobiopsy from oxyntic part of the stomach. A significant dependence for female patients did not reach such significance level as in the ratio method. However, some similar relations exist and this fact suggests that for the recognition of the type of gastritis diseases the ratio method is more adequate for this evaluation than the counting only in the glands epithelium of the gastric mucosa.

The next results for the EC cells (serotonin positive cells) are presented in table 3. The ratio of the EC cells in the field of view shows that the significant dependencies with the type of disease are when:

- patient is a woman, both regions
- patient is a man, both regions
- all patients and regions
- patient is a woman and region is oxyntic

However, the results of the Fisher test for all patients are not precise because there is a high inequality in the number of items in selected division. Additionally, there are significant differences in the level of the ratio between oligobiopsy region that influence the received results. Practically, only in the case of oxyntic region can we say that there are some disease dependencies, but patients must be divided in respect to their sex. For women oligobiopsy from oxyntic gastric mucosa can be considered as a significant dependence, for men it is not unequal. The results received on the set of gland shapes did not show any significant dependencies and for the recognition of the type of the disease they are not useful.

The results for the last considered type of the cells D (somatostatin positive cells) are presented in table 4. The ratio of the D cells in the field of view shows that the significant dependencies with the type of disease are when:

- patient is a woman, both regions
- all patients and regions (conditionally)
- patient is a woman and region is oxyntic

The results of the Fisher test for all patients is conditionally positive and practically only woman can speak about dependence of the ratio of the cell D with the disease. Unfortunately, in our database we have too small number of biopsies from the prepyloric for female patients (with correct somatostatin stain) to decide that this relation is for both regions. We can only think that a certain dependence is for woman patients and in the examination of the oxyntic region. We noted that for all types of staining the difference between median values for both diseases were near 100% of the level in the CHSG. This confirms well recognizable chronic gastritis and chronic superficial gastritis for this case.

		Ratio between EC and all cells [%]					EC cell quantity calculated in the glands			
Type of specimen	Type of diseases	Threshold value and no of items		Mean of ratio	Median of ratio	Fisher test	Threshold value and no of items		Mean of cell number	Fisher test
All patients and both regions		< 0.4 %	>= 0.4 %			p=0.0060 positive	< 3	>=3		p= 0.4533 negative
	CHSG	17	17	0.83	0.60		13	15	3.58	
	CHG	1	31	1.00	0.80		14	25	5.06	
Only women, both region s		< 0.4 %	>= 0.4 %			p=0.0424 positive	< 3	>=3		p= 0.3208 negative
	CHSG	10	8	0.82	0.38		8	7	3.44	
	CHG	4	16	0.8	0.70		7	13	3.89	
Only men, both regions		< 1 %	>= 1%			p=0.0325 positive	< 3	>=3		p=1 negative
	CHSG	9	4	0.86	0.70		5	8	3.76	
	CHG	5	13	1.23	1.26		7	12	3.62	
All patients, only prepyloric		< 1 %	>= 1 %			p=0.4153 negative	< 4	>=4		p= 0.6828 negative
	CHSG	5	5	1.38	1.11		5	4	5.91	
	CHG	5	12	1.29	1.37		7	10	5.03	
All patients, oxyntic		< 0.4 %	>= 0.4 %			p=0.1180 negative	< 3	>=3		p= 0.5308 negative
	CHSG	12	9	0.58	0.39		12	7	2.49	
	CHG	6	15	0.77	0.68		11	11	2.78	
Only women, prepyloric		< 1.5 %	>= 1.5 %			p=0.5805 negative	< 4	>=4		p= 0.2929 negative
	CHSG	3	3	1.52	1.31		3	2	5.69	
	CHG	6	2	1.17	1.12		2	6	5.94	
Only women, oxyntic		< 0.4 %	>= 0.4 %			p=0.0391 positive	< 3	>=3		p= 0.3811 negative
	CHSG	9	3	0.47	0.37		8	2	2.31	
	CHG	3	9	0.55	0.60		7	5	2.53	
Only men, prepyloric		< 1 %	>= 1 %			p=0.2028 negative	<3	>=3		p=1 negative
	CHSG	2	2	1.17	1.11		1	3	6.20	
	CHG	1	8	1.40	1.37		3	6	4.23	
Only men, oxyntic		< 1 %	>= 1 %			p=0.3349 negative	< 5	>=5		p=1 negative
	CHSG	7	2	0.72	0.60		4	5	2.68	
	CHG	4	5	1.05	1.11		4	6	3.07	

Table 3. The dependence between the type of chronic gastritis and the EC cells

Based on the results of morphometry of the neuroendocrine cells with recognition of the gland cross-section shape, the analysis of the correlation between the used measurements and quantity of the cells in one specific gland shape can be performed. Probably, the evaluation of the neuroendocrine cells in short ellipse-shape or long ellipse-shape glands will be representative for the whole population of the cells in a specimen. The analysis of this linear correlation gives the r coefficient equalled 0.726 and 0.809 for the short and long

		Ratio between D and all cells					D cell quantity calculated in the glands			
Type of specimen	Type of diseases	Threshold value and no of items		Mean of ratio	Median of ratio	Fisher test	Threshold value and no of items		Mean of cell nr	Fisher test
All patients and both regions		< 1.2 %	>= 1.2%			p=0.0674 conditionally positive	< 3.1	>=3.1		p= 0.0876 negative
	CHSG	18	9	1.14	0.95		21	9	3.09	
	CHG	13	19	1.51	1.33		19	21	3.50	
Only women, both regions		< 0.83%	>= 0.83%			p=0.0155 positive	< 2.1	>=2.1		p= 0.0873 negative
	CHSG	12	3	0.97	0.80		8	9	3.12	
	CHG	6	11	1.41	1.35		4	17	3.53	
Only men, both regions		< 1 %	>= 1%			p=0.7063 negative	< 3.1	>=3.1		p= 0.0751 negative
	CHSG	5	7	1.37	1.21		10	3	3.04	
	CHG	5	10	1.63	1.20		8	11	3.47	
All patients, only prepyloric		< 1 %	>= 1 %			p=0.4153 negative	< 3.1	>=3.1		p= 0.0410 positive
	CHSG	5	5	1.38	1.11		4	6	3.92	
	CHG	5	12	1.29	1.37		1	17	4.80	
All patients, oxyntic		< 0.92 %	>= 0.92 %			p=0.2049 negative	< 2.1	>=2.1		p= 0.5335 negative
	CHSG	12	7	0.96	0.80		10	10	2.67	
	CHG	8	12	1.16	1.00		8	14	2.44	
Only women, prepyloric		< 2.1 %	>= 2.1 %			p=0.1738 negative	< 4.4	>=4.4		p= 0.6084 negative
	CHSG	5	0	1.63	1.96		2	4	3.77	
	CHG	2	3	2.17	2.36		5	4	4.15	
Only women, oxyntic		< 0.83 %	>= 0.83 %			p=0.0427 positive	< 2.1	>=2.1		p= 0.4136 negative
	CHSG	8	2	0.62	0.55		6	5	2.76	
	CHG	4	8	1.09	1.12		4	8	2.37	
Only men, prepyloric		< 1.68 %	>= 1.68 %			p=0.5012 negative	<3.1	>=3.1		p= 0.0769 negative
	CHSG	2	1	1.47	1.52		2	2	4.15	
	CHG	2	5	2.03	1.83		0	9	4.53	
Only men, oxyntic		< 1 %	>= 1 %			p= 1 negative	< 3	>=3		p=1 negative
	CHSG	4	5	1.33	1.12		4	5	2.55	
	CHG	4	4	1.27	1.00		5	5	2.51	

Table 4. The dependence between the type of chronic gastritis and the D cells

ellipse-shapes respectively. Statistically, both correlations are significant (p-value less than 0.05) with R^2 equals 0.73 and 0.81 and F-statistic equals 73 and 110. The graphical illustrations of this correlations are presented in Fig. 7a and b.

The presented results suggest that it is possible to perform an appropriate evaluation of the neuroendoctine cell quantity in the gastric mucosa taking into account only one type of the gland cross-section shape. The most representative aspect for this evaluation is a long ellipse shape of the glands.

a)

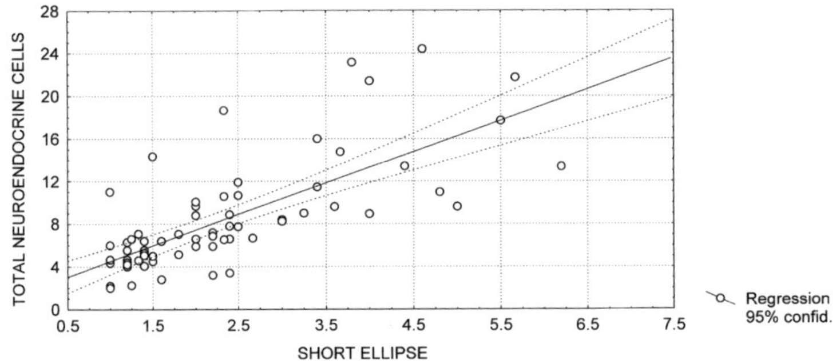

b)

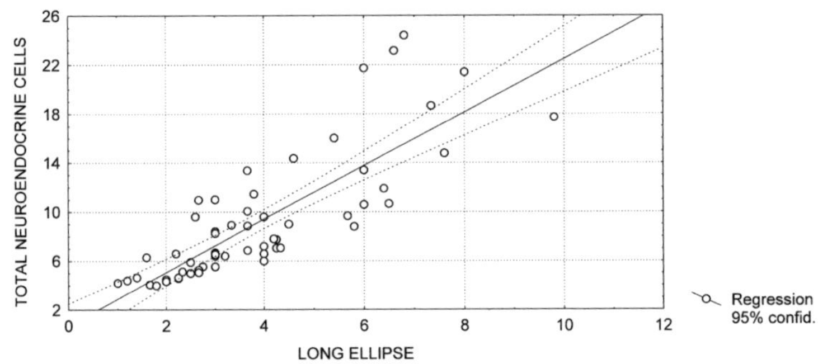

Fig. 7. Correlations between number of the neuroendocrine cells in the a) short ellipse-shape glands, or b) long ellipse-shape glands and the total number of cells in the specimen.

4. Conclusion

The presented results deal with statistical results of the density of the neuroendocrine cells in the gastric chronic diseases. The two used methods reflect some significant dependencies and possibilities of using them in the medical diagnosis. They confirm the dependence of the density of the neuroendocrine cells such as D, EC or ECL on the type of gastric disease, referred to in the previous researches. We received significant differences in the results of the used counting methods in dependence on sex of patient and oligobiopsy region. As far as recognition of type of chronic gastric diseases is concerned, we found the most significant dependence in the total neuroendocrine cells in female patients and oligobiopsy from the oxyntic part of the stomach. The Fisher test value for this case was $p=0.0033$ in the counting of all the cells in the field of view. For the EC and D cells this value was $p= 0.0391$ and $p=0.0427$ respectively. The other positive dependence received for the other groups of patients were negative or if there were positive, the evaluated group included women patients with oxyntic oligobiopsy specimens. We think that the positive test values in these

cases (indicating possible recognition of disease type) were caused only by the cases of women oxyntic specimens. This fact confirmed the negative recognition results received for the other types of specimens included in this evaluated group.
For the semi-quantitative method, based on the cell counting only in glandular epithelium of the stomach, the received results confirmed the significant dependence between number of the positive cells and type of gastritis only for D cells in the women oxyntic specimens. Additionally, very interesting results were obtained as regards counting all neuroendocrine cells in men oxyntic specimens. Contrary to the statistical counting, in this method we received conditionally positive test value $p=0.0698$. This dependence should be verified on the high number of patients.
The presented algorithm for computerized image analysis combines the mathematical morphology operations with artificial neural network of SVM type for evaluation of the ratio of the positive cells in the field of view. It can be helpful for researches in checking the endocrine cells in gastric disease and can be easily adapted to the other cytoplasm immunohistoreactivity stains. In difference to the other approaches, it imitates the human view strategy in recognition of the separated nuclei of the cells. The received accuracy is on good level and fully repeatable. In the case where we cannot use this method, the other solution is the use of semi-quantitative method with counting made manually by human experts. However, this evaluation is restricted to only few cases with a less precise method than the automatic one.
In the literature other approaches to counting neuroendocrine cell, based on grid graph, can be found (Ozkan et al., 2007). In such methods a randomly oriented parallel line-and-dot graph (grid) is superimposed on the analyzed image. The positive cells (marks in nuclear or cytoplasm staining) and negative cells coinciding with the dots on the grid are counted. This approach is oriented more on the statistics rather than on real cell recognition and in our opinion includes higher risk of counting error than full cell recognition process.
The most significant dependence between the ratio of the positive cells and type of the gastritis was in the total neuroendocrine cells in female patients and oligobiopsy from the oxyntic part of the stomach. Similar relations were found in the EC and D types of the cells. In the other type of specimens significant relations, useful for disease types recognition, were not confirmed. In the semi-quantitative evaluation performed by the human expert the diseases recognizable in female patients and oligobiopsy from the oxyntic part of the stomach were confirmed only in D cell counting. The ratio method is more effective for the recognition of the type of the disease than semi-quantitative evaluation.

5. References

Aruin L.G., Vinogradov V.A., Zverkov J.V. et al. (1984). The endocrine stomach cells containing endocrine gastrin and somatostatin in patients with duodenal ulcer. *Arkhiv Patologii*, Vol.XLVI, No.6, (1984), pp.15-20, ISSN 0004-1955

Azzoni C., Doglioni C., Viale G. et al. (1996). Involvement of BCL-2 Oncoprotein in the Development of Enterochromaffin-like Cell Gastric Carcinoids. *Am J Surg Pathol*, Vol.20, No.4,(April 1996), pp.433-441, ISSN 0147-5185

Bartels P.H., Thompson D., Montironi R. et al. (1996). Automated reasoning system in histopathologic diagnosis and prognosis of prostate cancer and its precursors. *Eur Urol*, Vol.30, No.2, (1996), pp.222-233, ISSN 0302-2838

Bordi C., D'Adda T., Azzoni C., Ferraro G. (2000). Classification of gastric endocrine cells at light and electron microscopical levels. *Microsc Res Tech*, Vol.48, No.5, (March 2000), pp. 258–271, ISSN 1097-0029

Calatayud S., Alvarez A., Victor V.M. (2010). Gastrin: An Acid-Releasing, Proliferative and Immunomodulatory Peptide? *Mini-Reviews in Medicinal Chemistry*, Vol.10, No.1, (January 2010), pp.8-19, ISSN 1389-5575

Czaja M., Szarszewski A., Kaminska B. et al. (2008). Serum gastrin concentration and changes in G and D cell densities in gastric antrum in children with chronic gastritis. *Int J Clin Pract*, Vol.62, No.7, (July 2008), pp.1044–1049, ISSN 1742-1241

D'Adda T., Bertele A., Pilato F.P., Bordi C. (1989). Quantitative electron microscopy of endocrine cells in oxyntic mucosa of normal human stomach. *Cell Tissue Res*, Vol.255, No.1, (January 1989), pp.41-48, ISSN 0302-766X

Date Y., Kojima M., Hosoda H., et al. (2000). Ghrelin, a novel growth hormone-releasing acylated peptide, is synthesized in a distinct endocrine cell type in the gastrointestinal tracts of rats and humans. *Endocrinology*, Vol.141, No.11, (November 2000), pp.4255-61, ISSN 0013-7227

Dayal Y. (1992). Hyperplastic proliferations of the ECL cells. *Yale J Biol Med*, Vol.65, No.6, (Nov-Dec 1992), pp.805-825, ISSN 0044-0086

DeLellis R.A., Tischler A.S., Wolfe H.J. (1984). Multidirectional differentiation in neuroendocrine neoplasms. *J Histochem Cytochem*, Vol.32, No.8, (August 1984), pp. 899, ISSN 0022-1554

Falkmer S., Wilander E. (1995). The endocrine cell population, In: *Gastrointestinal and oesophageal pathology (2nd ed)*, Whitehead R. (Ed.) , pp.63-71, Churchill Livingstone, ISBN 9780443047640, New York

Fenoglio-Preiser C. H. (Ed.). (1999). *Gastrointestinal Pathology: An Atlas and Text*, Lippincott-Raven, ISBN 9780397516407, Philadelphia

Fisher R.A. (1922). On the interpretation of $\chi 2$ from contingency tables, and the calculation of P. *Journal of the Royal Statistical Society*, Vol.85, No.1, (1922), pp.87-94, ISSN (current) 0964-1998

Furth E.E. (2002). Gastrointestinal tract, In: *Endocrine Pathology*, LiVolsi V.A., Asa S.L (Ed.), Churchil and Livingstone, ISBN 0443065950, Philadelphia

Green D.M., Bishop A.E., Rindi G. et al. (1989). Enterochromaffin-like cell populations in human fundic mucosa: quantitative studies of their variations with age, sex, and plasma gastrin levels. *J Pathol*, Vol.157, No.3, (March 1989), pp.235-241, ISSN 1096-9896

Hakanson R., Lilja B., Owman C. (1967). Properties of a new system of amine-storing cells in the gastric mucosa of the rat. *Eur J Pharmacol* , Vol.1, (1967), pp.188-199, ISSN 0014-2999

Kayser G., Radziszowski D., Bzdyl P. et al. (2006). Theory and implementation of an electronic, automated measurement system for images obtained from immunohistochemically stained slides. *Anal Quant Cytol Histol*, Vol.28, No.1, (February 2006), pp.27-38, ISSN 0884-6812

Kinoshita Y., Nakata H., Kishi K., et al. (1998). Comparison of the Signal Transduction Pathways Activated by Gastrin in Enterochromaffin-like and Parietal Cells. *Gastroenterology*, Vol.115, No.1, (July 1998), pp.93-100, ISSN 0016-5085

Kozlowski W., Kulig A., Czkwianianc E. et al. (1995). Morphological and immunohistochemical examinations of the dynamic changes of gastric mucosa associated with the treatment of Helicobacter pylori infection in children. *An Ac. Med Bial*,Vol.40, No.3, (1995), pp. 678-684, ISSN 1427-941X

Kozlowski W., Dabek A., Trawinski J. et al. (2001). Immunohistochemical studies of G and D cells in the mucosa of prepyloric part of the stomach in various types of inflammation. *Virchows Arch*, Vol.439, No.3, (September 2001), pp.42-43, ISSN 0945-6317

Kozlowski W., Jochymski C., Klupinska G. et al. (2003a). Chromogranin-A-plus and D cells in superficial and deep gastric mucosa inflammation. *Virchows Arch*, Vol.443, No.3, (September 2003), pp.404, ISSN 0945-6317

Kozlowski W., Jochymski C., Klupinska G. et al. (2003b). Investigation of glandular epithelium cells proliferative activity in chronic superficial and deep inflammations of gastric mucosa. *Virchows Arch*, Vol.443, No.3, (September 2003), pp.403, ISSN 0945-6317

Kozlowski W., Jochymski C., Markiewicz T. (2009). Quantitative investigation of the neuroendocrine cells in superficial and deep gastric mucosa inflammation, (22nd European Congress of Pathology, Florence). *Virchow's Archives*, Vol.455, Sup.1, (August 2009), pp.387, ISSN 0945-6317

Lezoray O., Elmoataz A., Cardot H. et al. (2000). Segmentation of color images from serous cytology for automated cell classification. *Anal Quant Cytol Histol*, Vol.22, No.4, (August 2000), pp.311-322, ISSN 0884-6812

Lloyd R.V. (1989). The Neuroendocrine and Paracrine System, In: *Diagnostic Surgical Pathology (3rd ed)*, Sternberg S.S. et al. (Ed.), pp. 435–438 Lippincott Williams and Wilkins, ISBN 978-0397587926, Philadelphia

Markiewicz T., Jochymski C., Koktysz R. et al. (2008). Automatic cell recognition in immunohistochemical Gastritis stains using sequential thresholding and SVM network. *5 International conference of biomedical imaging: From nano to macro*, pp. 971-974,ISBN 978-1-4244-2002-5,Paris, May 14-17 2008

Markiewicz T., Osowski S., Patera J. et al. (2006). Image processing for accurate recognition and counting of cells of the histological slides. *Anal Quant Cytol Histol*, Vol.28, No.5, (October 2006), pp.281-292, ISSN 0884-6812

Markiewicz T., Jochymski C., Slodkowska J. et al. (2009a). Automated recognition and counting of the immunoreactive neuroendocrine cells in chronic gastritis (the preliminary study). *Folia histochemica et cytobiologica*, Vol.47, No.4, (April 2010), pp.685-690, ISSN 0239-8508

Markiewicz T., Wisniewski P., Osowski S. et al. (2009b). Comparative analysis of the methods for accurate recognition of cells in the nuclei staining of the Ki-67 in neuroblastoma and ER/PR status staining in breast cancer. *Anal Quant Cytol Histol*, Vol.31, No.1, (February 2009), pp.49-62, ISSN 0884-6812

Markiewicz T., Grala B., Kozlowski W. et al. (2010). Computer system for cell counting in selected brain tumors at Ki-67 immunohistochemical staining., *Anal Quant Cytol Histol*, Vol.32, No.6, (December 2010), pp.323-332, ISSN 0884-6812

MATLAB. (2010). Matlab Image Processing Toolbox, user's guide. MathWorks, Nattick

Nichols D.B., Cheng H., Leblond C.P. (1974). Variability of the shape and argentaffinity of the granules in the enteroendocrine cells of the mouse duodenum. *J Histochem Cytochem*, Vol. 22, No.10, (October 1974), pp.929-44, ISSN 0022-1554

Ohning G.V., Song M., Wong H.C., et al. (1998). Immunolocalization of gastrin-dependent histidine decarboxylase activity in rat gastric mucosa during feeding. *Am J Physiol GI*, Vol.275, No.4, (October 1998), pp. G660-667, ISSN 0193-1857

Osamura R.Y. (2002). Dispersed Neuroendocrine Cells and Their Tumors, In: *Endocrine Pathology*, LiVolsi V.A., Asa S.L (Ed.), Churchil and Livingstone, ISBN 0443065950, Philadelphia

Ozcan A., Karslioglu Y., Kurt B., et al. (2007). Quantitative evaluation of immunohistochemical staining in gastrointestinal stromal tumors. *Anal Quant Cytol Histol*, Vol.29, No.3, (June 2007), pp.159-165, ISSN 0884-6812

Pearse A.G.E. (1969). The cytochemistry and ultrastructure of polypeptide hormone-producing cells of the APUD series, and the embryonic, physiologic and pathologic implications of the concept. *J Histochem Cytochem*, Vol.17, No.5, (May 1969), pp.303-13, ISSN 0022-1554

Pearse A.G.E. (1974). The APUD cell concept and its implications in pathology. *Pathol Annu* Vol.9, (1974); pp.27-41, ISSN 0079-0184

Pearse A.G.E., Takor-Takor T. (1979). Embryology of the diffuse neuroendocrine system and its relationship to the common peptides. *Fed Proc* , Vol.38, No.9, (August 1979); pp.2288-2294, ISSN 0014-9446

Petersson F., Borch K., Rehfeld J.F. et al. (2009). A Morphometric Study of Antral G-Cell Density in a Sample of Adult General Population: Comparison of Three Different Methods and Correlation with Patient Demography, Helicobacter pylori Infection, Histomorphology and Circulating Gastrin Levels. *Int J Clin Exp Patho*l, Vol.2, No.3, (2009), pp.239-248, ISSN 1936-2625

Portela-Gomes G.M., Grimelius L. (1986). Identification and characterisation of enterochromaffin cells with different staining techniques. *Acta Histochem*, Vol.79, (1986), pp.161-174, ISSN 0065-1281

Schölkopf B., Smola A. (2002). *Learning with Kernels*, MIT Press, ISBN 0-262-19475-9,Cambridge

Soille P. (2003). *Morphological image analysis, principles and application*, Springer, ISBN, Berlin.

Solcia E., Bordi C., Creutzfeldt W. et al. (1988). Histopathological classification of nonantral gastric endocrine growths in man. *Digestion*, Vol.41, No.4, (1988), pp.185-200, ISSN 0012-2823

Solcia E, Fiocca R, Villani L., et al. (1995). Hyperplastic, dysplastic, and neoplastic enterochromaffin-like-cell proliferations of the gastric mucosa: Classification and histogenesis. *Am J Surg Pathol*, Vol.19, Suppl.1, (1995), pp.S1-7, ISSN 0147-5185

Todorovic V., Koko V., Budec M. et al. (2008). G cells and gastrin in chronic alcohol-treated rats. *Alcohol*, Vol.42, No.1, (February 2008), pp.37-45, ISSN 0741-8329

Tzaneva M., Julianov A. (1999). Chromogranin A-, somatostatin- and serotonin-containing endocrine cells in the corporal gastric mucosa of patients with Helicobacter pylori associated gastritis. *Endocr Regul*, Vol.33, No.2, (1999), pp.79-82, ISSN 1210-0668

Vapnik V. (1998). *Statistical Learning Theory*, John Wiley & Sons, ISBN 0471030031, New York

Wang L.J., Zhou Q.Y., Chen Y. et al. (2009). Muscovite reverses gastric gland atrophy and intestinal metaplasia by promoting cell proliferation in rats with atrophic gastritis. *Digestion*, Vol.79, No.2, (April 2009), pp.79-91, ISSN 0012-2823

Whitehead R. (Ed.) (1995). *Gastrointestinal and oesophageal pathology*, Longman Group Ltd., ISBN 9780443047640, New York

Zhu F.S., Si J.M., Wang L.J., Wang D.F., Chen P. (2008). Effect of mica monomer powder on chief and parietal cells as well as G and D cells in gastric mucosa of chronic atrophic gastritis in rats. *Chin J Integr Med*, Vol.14, No.2, (June 2008), pp.111-116, ISSN 1993-0402

7

Molecular Pathology of Gastritis

Alejandro H. Corvalán, Gonzalo Carrasco and Wilda Olivares
Pontificia Universidad Catolica de Chile, Santiago, Chile

1. Introduction

Gastritis is an inflammation of the mucosa of the stomach, and has many etiologies. Gastritis can be classified as being acute or chronic. For the purpose of this chapter, we will focus only on chronic gastritis due to its relevance to gastric cancer. Among the causes of chronic gastritis are chronic bile reflux, stress, certain autoimmune disorders and bacterial infection, primarily *Helicobacter pylori.* Since 1870, both human and veterinary pathologists have described the presence of tiny curved bacteria within gastric mucosa, but the organisms were dismissed as irrelevant contaminants (1, 2). In 1947, when gastroscopy was first being used, Rudolf Schindler deemed gastritis as "one of the most debated diseases of the human body" and predicted that its significance would be discussed "for some time to come" (3). Schindler himself claimed that the "bacteriological etiology of chronic gastritis has not been convincingly proved in a single case" (3). In 1984, Warren and Marshall proposed that chronic "idiopathic" gastritis had a bacterial cause (i.e., *H. pylori*) (4). Their hypothesis was met with great skepticism. However, within a few years, the association between *H. pylori* gastritis, peptic ulcer, and gastric cancer came to be acknowledged and ultimately accepted (4). Subsequently, accurate morphological data were gathered by pathologic examination of autopsy material (5) and, later, of endoscopic biopsy specimens. As a result, distinct types and patterns of gastritis were recognized, which led to the conception, presentation, dismissal, and replacement of many different classification systems.

2. Histological classification and grading of gastritis

For the purpose of this chapter we decided to divided chronic gastritis in into two main categories, namely non-atrophic and atrophic gastritis (6). The main purpose of this classification is to individualize high-risk gastritis subgroup that subsequently might develop to gastric cancer. In the gastric mucosa, atrophy is defined as the loss of appropriate glands. Atrophic gastritis, resulting mainly from long-standing *H. pylori* infection, and is a major risk factor for the onset of gastric cancer. The extent and site of the atrophic changes significantly correlate with cancer risk (6, 7). Two main types of atrophic gastritis can be recognized, one characterized by the loss of glands, accompanied by fibrosis or fibromuscular proliferation in the lamina propria, and the other characterized by the replacement of the normal mucosa into an intestinal type of mucosa (i.e. intestinal metaplasia) (8). The first can be assessed with the new Operative Link for Gastritis Assessment (OLGA) staging system for atrophy risk assessment (9) which ranks the risk of gastric cancer according to the extension and severity of gastric atrophy (Fig. 1 and Table 1).

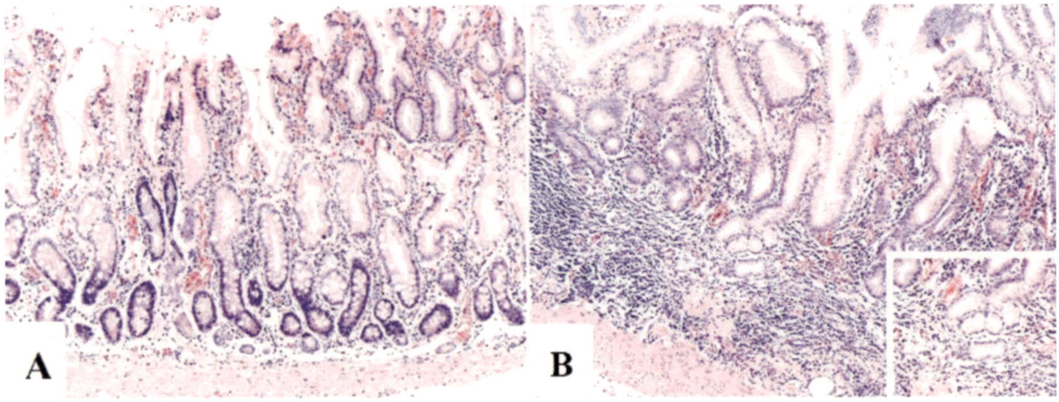

Fig. 1. Atrophy is the loss of appropriate glands. (A; H&E 10x) Antral gastric mucosa with accentuated atrophy because replacement by extensive intestinal metaplasia. (B; H&E 10x; square 20x) Fundic-corporal gastric mucosa with extensive loss of gastric glands, partially replaced by pseudo-pyloric metaplasia.

Atrophy Score		Corpus			
		No Atrophy (score 0)	Mild Atrophy (score 1)	Moderate Atrophy (score 2)	Severe Atrophy (score 3)
Antrum	No Atrophy (score 0) (including *incisura angularis*)	STAGE 0	STAGE I	STAGE II	STAGE II
Antrum	Mild Atrophy (score 1) (including *incisura angularis*)	STAGE I	STAGE I	STAGE II	STAGE III
Antrum	Moderate Atrophy (score 2) (including *incisura angularis*)	STAGE II	STAGE II	STAGE III	STAGE IV
Antrum	Severe Atrophy (score 3) (including *incisura angularis*)	STAGE III	STAGE III	STAGE IV	STAGE IV

No atrophy (0%) = score 0; mild atrophy (1–30%) = score 1 ; moderate atrophy (31–60%) = score 2; severe atrophy (>60%) = score 3. These scores (0–3) are used in the OLGA staging assessment in each compartment. Taken from Rugge et al., Dig Liver Dis 2011;43:S373-84 with permission of Elsevier.

Table 1. The OLGA staging frame. Atrophy is scored as the percentage of atrophic glands and scored on a four-tiered scale.

Cross-sectional and long-term follow-up trials conducted in various epidemiologic settings have consistently associated OLGA stages III and IV with a higher risk of gastric cancer vs. low-risk OLGA stages [ie, stages 0, I, and II]) (6). The latter can be assessed based on whether the metaplastic epithelium phenotype resembles large bowel epithelia (colonic-type intestinal metaplasia) or the small intestinal mucosa (6, 10, 11). This classification was made by determining the histochemical phenotype of intestinal metaplasia (IM) using high-iron diamine stain. Cross-sectional descriptive studies and follow-up trials have consistently supported a strong association between OLGA stages and IM histochemical phenotypes, where IM of small intestinal type (type I) significantly prevailed in low-risk atrophic stages and high-risk OLGA stages were associated with IM of types II and III (6). Accordingly, epidemiological studies have shown that degree of severity for non-metaplastic atrophy influences the prevalence of IM and that the severity of IM influences the prevalence of dysplasia (12). These results support the concept that IM and dysplasia are linked in a sequential cause-effect relationship and confirm a proposed model for the pathogenesis of gastric cancer (11). However, risk assessment for gastric cancer development has not been well defined for other premalignant conditions (13).

3. Genetics bases of gastritis

The seminal proposal of a genetic model for tumorigenesis by Fearon & Vogelstein (14) and, more recently, the categorization of different cancers types into six physiological groups proposed by Hanahan & Weinberg (15) provide a theoretical framework for understanding the genetic and epigenetic bases of gastritis as well as premalignant conditions of gastric cancer. Thus, gastritis, and gastric cancer premalignant conditions should be understood as a disturbance in the balance between tumor suppressor genes and oncogenes. p53 gene (16) and the c-erbB2 oncogene (17, 18) were the first tumor suppressor gene and oncogene to be identified in gastric cancer, respectively. From these reports, a growing number of genes have been identified (19). However, different studies have shown that mutation and/or deletion is an infrequent mechanism of inactivating well stablished tumor suppressor genes such as E-cadherin (20, 21). Similarly, loss of heterozygosity (LOH) and microsatellite instability (MSI) have been frequently found in gastric cancer (19, 22, 23). However, mutations of the DNA mismatch repair genes, hMSH2 and hMLH1, responsible for LOH and MSI, are not frequently encountered (19, 24). Taken together, these observations suggest that genetic alterations do not completely explain the accumulation of genetic damage observed in gastric cancer and premalignant conditions. In this scenario, the recent inactivation of tumor suppressor genes by a novel epigenetic mechanisms, DNA methylation, has been proposed as an alternative mechanism to mutation and/or deletions (25). The best-documented inactivation by DNA methylation in gastric cancer is the silencing of DNA mismatch repair genes hMSH2 and hMLH1 (26). This inactivation is responsible for the development of the majority of MSI-related gastric cancers. As such, this inactivation leads to subsequent mutations in simple repetitive sequences within genes that are critical to the neoplastic process (23).

4. Epigenetic bases of gastritis

Epigenetic processes control the packaging and function of the human genome and contribute to normal development and disease (27). Epigenetic mechanisms such as DNA methylation, histone modifications and microRNAs (28) virtually affects all of the pathways in the cellular network, such as DNA repair, cell cycle, and apoptosis (25). DNA methylation, a process in which cytosines acquire a methyl group in 5' position only if they are followed by a guanine (CpG site) (28) is an early event in carcinogenesis (29-31). In addition, DNA metylation has been recently considered as an excellent candidate to explain how certain environmental factors may increase the risk of cancer (32). Accordingly, an emerging catalog of specific tumor suppressor genes inactivated by DNA methylation in gastrointestinal tumors has been established (33-36). Most of these studies has been performed by Methylation Specific - Polymerase Chain Reaction (MS-PCR), the most popular assay for DNA methylation (37). In MSP sodium bisulphite is used to convert cytosine residues to uracil residues in single-stranded DNA under conditions whereby 5-methylcytosine remains non-reactive. The converted DNA is amplified with specific primers and since all the cytosine residues remaining in the sequence represent previously methylated cytosines, MSP approach allows to detect DNA isolated from fewer than 100 cells (38, 39).

5. DNA methylation and gastritis

There are limited reports on DNA methylation analysis in gastritis and premalignant lesions of gastric cancer. Kang et al (40) tested five genes (p16, hMLH1, DAP-kinase, THBS1, and TIMP-3) in a series of 64 carcinomas and 179 premalignant conditions (69 chronic gastritis, 49 IM and 61 gastric adenomas) to identify two different classes of methylation patterns, preferential methylation of THBS-1 and TIMP-3 in chronic gastritis and IM and preferential methylation of hMLH1 and p16 in intestinal metaplasia, displasia and gastric cancer. These findings suggest that DNA methylation occur early in multistep gastric carcinogenesis and specific patterns of DNA methylation on specific genes ocurr along these steps (40). A subsequent study identified specific patterns of DNA methylation associated with aging after testing 11 genes in 268 premalignant gastritis (41). DNA methylation was found in increasingly frequency as a function of aging in five genes (DAP-kinase, E-cadherin, p14, THBS1 and TIMP-3), whereas the other genes (COX-2, GSTP1, MGMT, hMLH1, p16, and RASSF1A) were rarely methylated (41). Since E-cadherin was methylated at high frequency, a further study demonstrated, for the first time, that DNA methylation of promoter region of E-cadherin was associated with *H. pylori* infection. This association was independent of the age and or type of gastritis (42). Similarly, Maekita et al (43) analyzed the effect of *H. pylori* infection on DNA methylation of several genes (HAND1, HRASLS, LOX, p16, P41ARC and THBD) by quantitative methods in *H. pylori* negative and positive healthy donors and gastric cancer patients. Among healthy donors, methylation levels were up to 300-fold higher in *H. pylori* positives than in *H. pylori* negatives (43). However, among gastric cancer patients, methylation levels were only up 30-fold higher, suggesting that *H. pylori* infection induces DNA methylation of several genes beyond E-cadherin (43). Chan et al (32) evaluate the effect or eradication of *H.pylori* on DNA methylation in gastric mucosa. Before and after the treatment DNA methylation of E-cadherin was detected in 46% and 17% of 41 patients, respectively (Fig. 2). Histological evaluation after the treatment, showed chronic inactive gastritis in most of the cases. A similar results was communicated by Leung et al (44), although they evaluated tissues from the antrum and corpus of *H. pylori*-infected subjects at baseline and after one year of successful *H. pylori* eradication. These authors identified a significant reduction in the methylation density of the promoter region and exon 1 of the E-cadherin gene by bisulfite DNA sequencing. Taken together, these results demonstrated that eradication of *H. pylori* infection reverses E-cadherin promoter hypermethylation and suggest an environmental effect on DNA methylation (32).

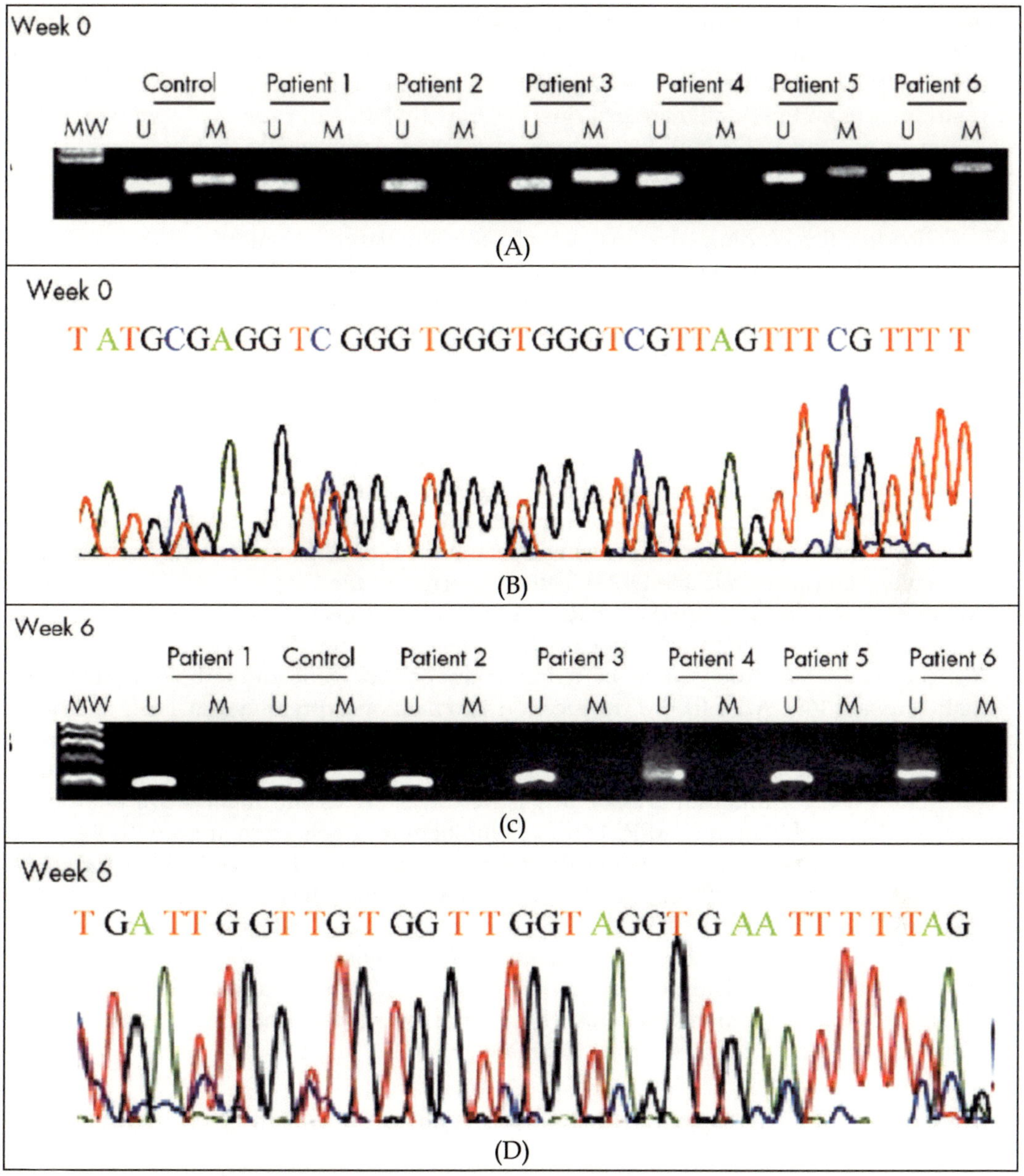

Fig. 2. CpG island methylation pattern at the E-cadherin gene in gastric mucosa from patients with dyspepsia. (A) Before eradication of *H. pylori* (week 0), methylation was present in patients 3, 5 and 6. (B) The methylated product was confirmed by sequencing using the same methylated primer. (C) After eradication of *H. pylori* (week 6), methylation was not present in any patient. (D) The methylated product was again confirmed by sequencing using the same methylated primer. No methylated cytosine was seen. MW: molecular weight marker, U: unmethylated band, M: methylated band, red color: unmethylated cytosines converted to thymidine, blue color: methylated cytosines. Taken from Chan et al., Gut 2006;55: 463-8 with permission from BMJ Publishing Group Ltd.

Recently, our group identified promotor DNA methylation of a novel gene, Reprimo (RPRM), not only in gastric mucosa but also in the plasma of gastric cancer patients (36). This methylated circulating cell-free DNA offers the opportunity for non-invasive detection of gastric cancer and premalignant gastritis. DNA methylation of promoter region of RPRM was initially identified by high-throughput microarray experiments that analyzed global changes in gene expression in pancreatic cancer cell lines treated with the demethylating agent 5-aza-2-deoxycitidine. Among 11 re-expressed genes, RPRM was highly re-expressed (45). Following this finding, the analysis of the methylation status of RPRM in clinical samples of pancreatic cancer identified a high frequency of DNA methylation of the promoter of RPRM (45). Subsequent research focused on different types of tumors (breast, esophagus, lymphoma, etc.) including gastric carcinoma (46). However, our study, not only looked into the methylation of RPRM in tumor tissues, but also in non-invasive plasma samples from the same patients (36). Interestingly, methylate circulating cell-free DNA of RPRM was found in over 90% in plasma from gastric cancer patients but less than 10% among asymptomatic controls (36). Thus, our results were the first to indicate that methylation of promoter region of RPRM might act as a potential biomarker for early detection of gastric cancer. RPRM is a downstream mediator of p53-induced G2 cell cycle arrest (47). When adenovirus expressing recombinant RPRM cDNA was infected into human colorectal cancer cell line DLD1, cell cycle arrest at the G2 phase was observed (47). However, it has been suggested that RPRM-induced cell cycle arrest is mediated by an indirect inhibition of Cdc2-CyclinB1 complex translocation to the nucleus (47). Recently, RPRM has also been proposed to be a tumor suppressor gene through in vitro colony formation assays (48). After RPRM transfection into the non-expressing renal cell carcinoma cell line SKRC39 there was a signicantly reduced number of G418 resistant colonies compared to the cell lines transfected with an empty vector control. However, it is unknown whether RPRM is a tumor suppressor in gastric cancer. A recent quantitative analysis of promoter DNA methylation of RPRM from Colombian residents from areas with high and low incidence of gastric cancer demonstrated an association with virulence factors cagA (including segments of the 30 end, encoding EPIYA polymorphisms) and vacA s1 and m1 regions of *H. pylori* strains (Fig. 3). This data suggest that cagA and vacA virulence determinants are significantly associated with DNA methylation of a specific gene, RPRM in high-risk gastritis (49). Thus, the posibility to detect DNA methylation of RPRM as a cell-free DNA in plasma in combination with *H.pylori* strains might opening the oportunity for a non-invasive detection of high-risk premalignant gastritis.

6. Integration of histological and DNA methylation features of gastritis

Although histological assessment of gastritis to search for premalignant conditions for the development of gastric cancer has been proposed (6) and epigenetic markers based on DNA methylation are associated with this progression (50), no integrative approach has been explore up to date for this two disparate fields. Recently, we have integrated histological together with *in-situ* molecular features to demonstrate that overexpression of p73 was probably the most important marker to identified high-risk premalignant gastritis (51). In that work, we analyse matched tumor/non-tumor adjacent mucosa of 91 early gastric cancer and 148 chronic gastritis cases for histological features by the Sydney and OLGA systems along with eight tissue markers to identified that overexpression of p73, severe atrophy, and OLGA stage IV were the most relevant features to identified high-risk gastritis (Fig. 4).

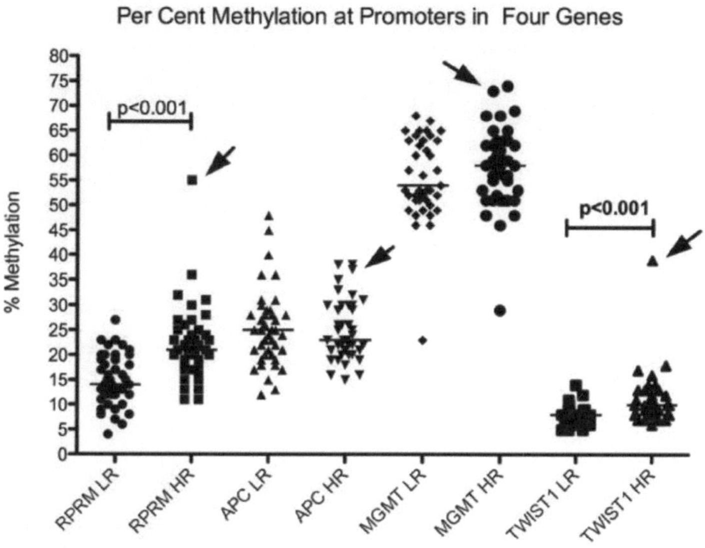

(A)

Table 3. Multivariate linear regression analysis

	Gene							
	RPRM (n = 84)		*APC* (n = 84)		*MGMT* (n = 80)		*TWIST1* (n = 82)	
Variables	Coefficient (SE)	*p*-value	Coefficient (SE)	*p*-value	Coefficient (SE)	*p*-value	Coefficient (SE)	*p*-value
Area								
Low risk for gastric cancer	0		0		0		0	
High risk for gastric cancer	6.4 (1.4)	<0.001	1.0 (1.5)	0.511	−1.5 (1.8)	0.383	3.1 (0.9)	0.001
Diagnosis								
Normal/NAG	0		0		0		0	
MAG	1.1 (2.0)	0.583	−0.6 (2.1)	0.766	1.3 (2.5)	0.594	−0.4 (1.4)	0.746
IM/DYS	0.2 (1.7)	0.926	−1.4 (1.7)	0.431	3.3 (2.1)	0.124	0.4 (1.1)	0.718
H. pylori genotypes								
Uninfected	0		0		0		0	
Other genotypes	5.6 (2.6)	0.040	−9.3 (2.9)	0.002	5.3 (3.1)	0.104	0.6 (1.7)	0.746
cagA positive, *vacA s1m1*[1]	8.3 (2.4)	0.001	−9.9 (2.6)	<0.001	11.2 (2.9)	<0.001	1.8 (1.6)	0.244
Age in years	−0.1 (0.1)	0.271	0.1 (0.1)	0.403	−0.1 (0.1)	0.598	−0.1 (0.1)	0.462
Adjusted R^2	0.3356		0.1267		0.2216		0.1281	

[1]This category includes a subject with a strain of *H. pylori* that was *cagA* positive and *vacA s1* but which repeatedly failed PCR for *vacA m*.
Abbreviations: SE: standard error; NAG: nonatrophic gastritis; MAG: multifocal atrophic gastritis; IM: intestinal metaplasia.

(B)

Fig. 3. Association between the percentage of methylation of RPRM in residents areas with low and high incidence of gastric cancer, and virulence factors CagA, VacA s1 and m1 regions of *H. pylori*. (A) Scatter plots indicate the percent methylation of each gene analysed, measured from DNA from residents of low-risk (LR) and high-risk (HR) areas. Arrows indicate the points representing the outlier subject, whose gastric histology showed widespread intestinal metaplasia and focal areas of indefinite dysplasia. (B) Multivariate regression models incorporated effects of geographic area, diagnosis, age and genotypes of the infecting *H. pylori* strain (classified as uninfected, cagA positive, vacAs1m1 and all other genotypes). Taken from Schneider et al., Int J Cancer 2010; 127: 2588-7 with permision from Wiley.

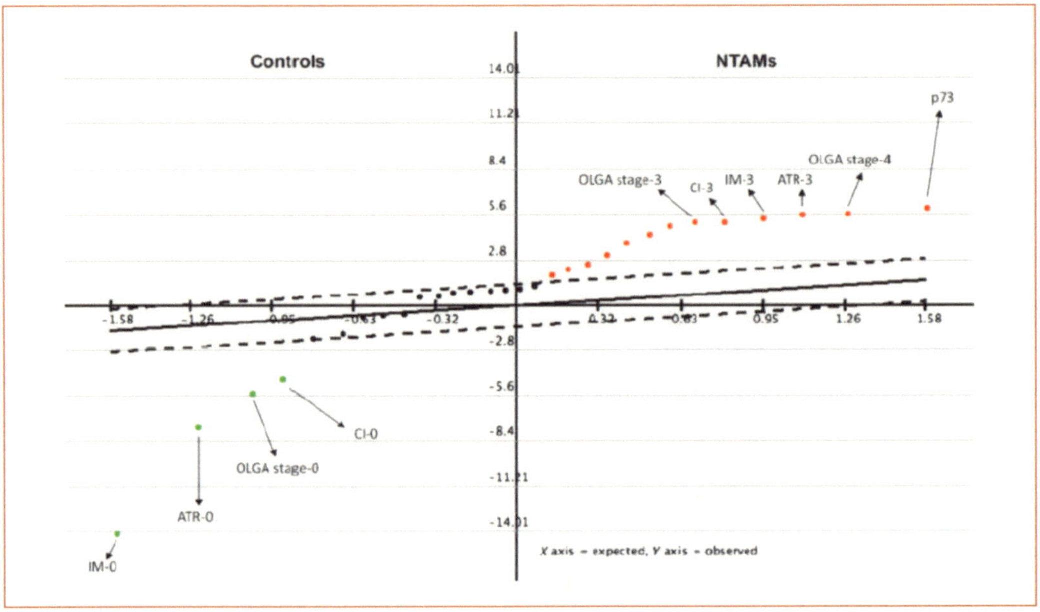

Fig. 4. Serial Analysis for Microarray from Non-tumor adjacent mucosa (NTAM) and and chronic gastritis controls. NTAM group is significantly characterized by the overexpression of p73, OLGA stages III to IV, and severe atrophy (ATR-3), intestinal metaplasia (IM-3), and chronic inflammation (CI-3) according to the Sydney System. Control group cases were significantly characterized by lack of intestinal metaplasia (IM-0), atrophy (ATR-0), and chronic inflammation (CI-0). False discovery rate = 0. Taken from Carrasco et al., 2010 Clin.Cancer Res 16:3253-9.

Interestingly, further work have shown that p73 overexpression might be associated with hypo- or demethylation of the promoter region of p73 (52). Taken together these findings suggest that DNA methylation might play a role in gastritis and premalignant condition in both ways, inactivating or activating tumor-related genes by hypermethylation or demethylation of promoter region of specific genes, respectively.

7. Conclusions

In conclusion, specific histological features with increasing risk to progress to gastric cancer can be assessed by OLGA system. Specific DNA methylation changes might play a major role in premalignant gastritis and might be associated with *H. pylori* infection. These changes are accumulative from bening to fully malignant conditions. Induced DNA methylation in specific genes by *H.pylori* might be reversible and might be associated with virulence of *H.pylori* strains. These DNA methylated genes might be detected in plasma (i.e. RPRM) as a circulating cell-free DNA. Integrative analysis of histological features of premalignant conditions with overexpression of specific genes such as p73 by demethylation might be important to identified the best biomarkers for high-risk premalignant gastritis for the development of gastric cancer.

8. Aknowledgements

We thank Natalia Saez for premium editing and proofreading of the manuscript.

9. Grant support

Grants-in-Aid for Fondo Nacional de Ciencia y Tecnologia (FONDECYT) #1111014 and Fondo de Fomento al Desarrollo Científico y Tecnológico (FONDEF) #D09i1137 to A.H. Corvalan from the Government of Chile.

10. References

[1] Figura N, Oderda G. Reflections on the first description of the presence of Helicobacter species in the stomach of mammals. Helicobacter. 1996;1:4-5.
[2] Kidd M, Modlin IM. A century of *Helicobacter pylori*: paradigms lost-paradigms regained. Digestion. 1998;59:1-15.
[3] Schindler R. Gastritis. London: William Heinmann (Medical Books); 1947.
[4] Marshall BJ, Warren JR. Unidentified curved bacilli in the stomach of patients with gastritis and peptic ulceration. Lancet. 1984;1:1311-5.
[5] Faber K. Gastritis and Its Consequences. London: Oxford University Press; 1935.
[6] Rugge M, Fassan M, Pizzi M, Pennelli G, Nitti D, Farinati F. Operative Link for Gastritis Assessment gastritis staging incorporates intestinal metaplasia subtyping. Hum Pathol. 2011.
[7] Dixon MF, Genta RM, Yardley JH, Correa P. Classification and grading of gastritis. The updated Sydney System. International Workshop on the Histopathology of Gastritis, Houston 1994. Am J Surg Pathol. 1996;20:1161-81.
[8] Rugge M, Correa P, Dixon MF, Fiocca R, Hattori T, Lechago J, et al. Gastric mucosal atrophy: interobserver consistency using new criteria for classification and grading. Aliment Pharmacol Ther. 2002;16:1249-59.
[9] Rugge M, Meggio A, Pennelli G, Piscioli F, Giacomelli L, De Pretis G, et al. Gastritis staging in clinical practice: the OLGA staging system. Gut. 2007;56:631-6.
[10] Niwa T, Tsukamoto T, Toyoda T, Mori A, Tanaka H, Maekita T, et al. Inflammatory processes triggered by *Helicobacter pylori* infection cause aberrant DNA methylation in gastric epithelial cells. Cancer Res. 2010;70:1430-40.
[11] Correa P. A human model of gastric carcinogenesis. Cancer Res. 1988;48:3554-60.
[12] Correa P, Haenszel W, Cuello C, Zavala D, Fontham E, Zarama G, et al. Gastric precancerous process in a high risk population: cross-sectional studies. Cancer Res. 1990;50:4731-6.
[13] Stemmermann GN. Intestinal metaplasia of the stomach. A status report. Cancer. 1994;74:556-64.
[14] Fearon ER, Vogelstein B. A genetic model for colorectal tumorigenesis. Cell. 1990;61:759-67.
[15] Hanahan D, Weinberg RA. Hallmarks of cancer: the next generation. Cell. 2011;144:646-74.
[16] Kim JH, Takahashi T, Chiba I, Park JG, Birrer MJ, Roh JK, et al. Occurrence of p53 gene abnormalities in gastric carcinoma tumors and cell lines. J Natl Cancer Inst. 1991;83:938-43.

[17] Falck VG, Gullick WJ. c-erbB-2 oncogene product staining in gastric adenocarcinoma. An immunohistochemical study. J Pathol. 1989;159:107-11.
[18] Yonemura Y, Ninomiya I, Yamaguchi A, Fushida S, Kimura H, Ohoyama S, et al. Evaluation of immunoreactivity for erbB-2 protein as a marker of poor short term prognosis in gastric cancer. Cancer Res. 1991;51:1034-8.
[19] Carneiro F, Oliveira C, Leite M, Seruca R. Molecular targets and biological modifiers in gastric cancer. Semin Diagn Pathol. 2008;25:274-87.
[20] Becker KF, Atkinson MJ, Reich U, Becker I, Nekarda H, Siewert JR, et al. E-cadherin gene mutations provide clues to diffuse type gastric carcinomas. Cancer Res. 1994;54:3845-52.
[21] Ascano JJ, Frierson H, Jr., Moskaluk CA, Harper JC, Roviello F, Jackson CE, et al. Inactivation of the E-cadherin gene in sporadic diffuse-type gastric cancer. Mod Pathol. 2001;14:942-9.
[22] Semba S, Yokozaki H, Yasui W, Tahara E. Frequent microsatellite instability and loss of heterozygosity in the region including BRCA1 (17q21) in young patients with gastric cancer. Int J Oncol. 1998;12:1245-51.
[23] Tamura G. Alterations of tumor suppressor and tumor-related genes in the development and progression of gastric cancer. World J Gastroenterol. 2006;12:192-8.
[24] Jankowski JA, Odze RD. Biomarkers in gastroenterology: between hope and hype comes histopathology. Am J Gastroenterol. 2009;104:1093-6.
[25] Esteller M, Herman JG. Cancer as an epigenetic disease: DNA methylation and chromatin alterations in human tumours. J Pathol. 2002;196:1-7.
[26] Fleisher AS, Esteller M, Wang S, Tamura G, Suzuki H, Yin J, et al. Hypermethylation of the hMLH1 gene promoter in human gastric cancers with microsatellite instability. Cancer Res. 1999;59:1090-5.
[27] Callinan PA, Feinberg AP. The emerging science of epigenomics. Hum Mol Genet. 2006;15 Spec No 1:R95-101.
[28] Corvalán AH, Maturana MJ. Recent Patents of DNA Methylation Biomarkers in Gastrointestinal Oncology. Recent Pat DNA Gene Seq. 2010;4:202-9.
[29] Herman JG, Baylin SB. Gene silencing in cancer in association with promoter hypermethylation. N Engl J Med. 2003;349:2042-54.
[30] Jones PA, Baylin SB. The fundamental role of epigenetic events in cancer. Nat Rev Genet. 2002;3:415-28.
[31] Kopelovich L, Crowell JA, Fay JR. The epigenome as a target for cancer chemoprevention. J Natl Cancer Inst. 2003;95:1747-57.
[32] Chan AO, Peng JZ, Lam SK, Lai KC, Yuen MF, Cheung HK, et al. Eradication of *Helicobacter pylori* infection reverses E-cadherin promoter hypermethylation. Gut. 2006; 55:463-8.
[33] Wu DL, Sui FY, Jiang XM, Jiang XH. Methylation in esophageal carcinogenesis. World J Gastroenterol. 2006;12:6933-40.
[34] Hamilton JP, Sato F, Jin Z, Greenwald BD, Ito T, Mori Y, et al. Reprimo methylation is a potential biomarker of Barrett's-Associated esophageal neoplastic progression. Clin Cancer Res. 2006;12:6637-42.
[35] Bernal C, Vargas M, Ossandón FJ, Santibáñez E, Urrutia J, Luengo V, et al. DNA methylation profile in diffuse type gastric cancer: evidence for hypermethylation of

the BRCA1 promoter region in early-onset gastric carcinogenesis. Biological research. 2008;41:303-15.
[36] Bernal C, Aguayo FR, Villarroel C, Vargas M, Diaz I, Ossandón FJ, et al. Reprimo as a potential biomarker for early detection in gastric cancer. Clin Cancer Res. 2008;14:6264-9.
[37] Fraga MF, Esteller M. DNA methylation: a profile of methods and applications. Biotechniques. 2002;33:632, 4, 6-49.
[38] Clark SJ, Harrison J, Paul CL, Frommer M. High sensitivity mapping of methylated cytosines. Nucleic Acids Res. 1994;22:2990-7.
[39] Herman JG, Graff JR, Myohanen S, Nelkin BD, Baylin SB. Methylation-specific PCR: a novel PCR assay for methylation status of CpG islands. Proc Natl Acad Sci U S A. 1996;93:9821-6.
[40] Kang GH, Shim YH, Jung HY, Kim WH, Ro JY, Rhyu MG. CpG island methylation in premalignant stages of gastric carcinoma. Cancer Res. 2001;61:2847-51.
[41] Kang GH, Lee HJ, Hwang KS, Lee S, Kim JH, Kim JS. Aberrant CpG island hypermethylation of chronic gastritis, in relation to aging, gender, intestinal metaplasia, and chronic inflammation. Am J Pathol. 2003;163:1551-6.
[42] Chan AO, Lam SK, Wong BC, Wong WM, Yuen MF, Yeung YH, et al. Promoter methylation of E-cadherin gene in gastric mucosa associated with *Helicobacter pylori* infection and in gastric cancer. Gut. 2003;52:502-6.
[43] Maekita T, Nakazawa K, Mihara M, Nakajima T, Yanaoka K, Iguchi M, et al. High levels of aberrant DNA methylation in *Helicobacter pylori*-infected gastric mucosae and its possible association with gastric cancer risk. Clin Cancer Res. 2006; 12:989-95.
[44] Leung WK, Man EP, Yu J, Go MY, To KF, Yamaoka Y, et al. Effects of *Helicobacter pylori* eradication on methylation status of E-cadherin gene in noncancerous stomach. Clin Cancer Res. 2006;12:3216-21.
[45] Sato N, Fukushima N, Maitra A, Matsubayashi H, Yeo CJ, Cameron JL, et al. Discovery of novel targets for aberrant methylation in pancreatic carcinoma using high-throughput microarrays. Cancer Res. 2003;63:3735-42.
[46] Takahashi T, Suzuki M, Shigematsu H, Shivapurkar N, Echebiri C, Nomura M, et al. Aberrant methylation of Reprimo in human malignancies. Int J Cancer. 2005;115:503-10.
[47] Ohki R, Nemoto J, Murasawa H, Oda E, Inazawa J, Tanaka N, et al. Reprimo, a new candidate mediator of the p53-mediated cell cycle arrest at the G2 phase. J Biol Chem. 2000;275:22627-30.
[48] Morris MR, Ricketts C, Gentle D, Abdulrahman M, Clarke N, Brown M, et al. Identification of candidate tumour suppressor genes frequently methylated in renal cell carcinoma. Oncogene. 2010;29:2104-17.
[49] Schneider BG, Peng DF, Camargo MC, Piazuelo MB, Sicinschi LA, Mera R, et al. Promoter DNA hypermethylation in gastric biopsies from subjects at high and low risk for gastric cancer. Int J Cancer. 2010;127:2588-97.
[50] Nakajima T, Yamashita S, Maekita T, Niwa T, Nakazawa K, Ushijima T. The presence of a methylation fingerprint of *Helicobacter pylori* infection in human gastric mucosae. Int J Cancer. 2009;124:905-10.

[51] Carrasco G, Diaz J, Valbuena JR, Ibánez P, Rodriguez P, Araya G, et al. Overexpression of p73 as a tissue marker for high-risk gastritis. Clin Cancer Res. 2010;16:3253-9.

[52] Corvalán AH, Villarroel C, Ibanez P, Carrasco G, Rodriguez C, Rodriguez P, et al. Demethylation of promoter region of p73 gene as a mechanism of overexpression of p73 protein in gastric carcinoma: Analysis by demethylation, microdissection of gastric epithelial cells and tissue microarray. AACR Meeting 2008; A4461.

Role of Natural Antioxidants in Gastritis

Mohamed M. Elseweidy
Faculty of pharmacy-zagazig university-Zagazig, Egypt

1. Introduction

Gastritis represents an inflammation of the stomach lining in response to injury. It is either acute or chronic, and has many underlying causes which can be diagnosed and classified histologically where endoscopic appearances such as redness are often misleading. Gastritis is seldom if ever symptomatic, but usually have important clinical sequelae, principally duodenal and gastric ulceration, gastric adenocarcinoma and primary gastric lymphoma (El-Zimaity, 2007; Thirumurthi & Lanza 2010). The three most important causes of gastritis are categorized as Helicobacter pylori infection, prolonged use of aspirin, non-steroidal anti inflammatory drugs (NSAIDs) and autoimmunity (Dohil & Hassall, 2011).

1.1 Acute gastritis

Acute gastritis, is usually a diffuse and intense mucosal alteration, mostly is characterized by a sudden onset of symptoms and rapid resolution after the underlying aetiological mechanisms or agents (either chemical or physical) have been corrected. The patients can present with an acute gastroenteritis-like illness, or other symptoms which may be overshadowed by their general physical condition. Broadly speaking, acute gastritis arises when there is an acute imbalance between mucosal injury and repair mechanisms (Fig. 1) and can be organized in three groups based on the aetiologies: (i) infectious gastritis (ii) secondary to caustic injury; and (iii) ulcero-haemorrhagic (Srivastava & Lauwers, 2007).

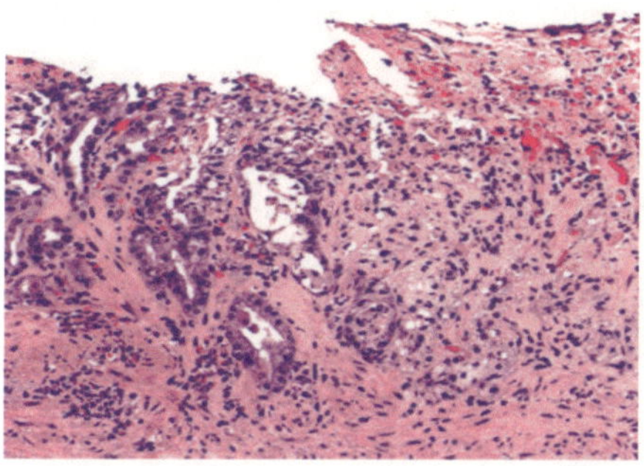

Fig. 1. Acute gastritis. Erosion and complete effacement of the epithelium is observed. The residual glands, on the left, display regenerative changes with basophilic epithelium.

No correlation may be exist between microscopic inflammation (histologic gastritis) and the presence of gastric symptoms (eg, abdominal pain, nausea, vomiting). In fact, most patients with histologic evidence of acute gastritis (inflammation) are asymptomatic. The diagnosis is usually obtained during endoscopy performed for other reasons. Acute gastritis may present with an array of symptoms, the most common being nondescript epigastric discomfort. Other symptoms include nausea, vomiting, loss of appetite, belching, and bloating. Fever, chills may be present. The diagnosis of acute gastritis may be clarified from the patient's history and can be confirmed histologically by biopsy specimens taken at endoscopy. Epidemiologic studies reflect the widespread incidence of gastritis (Ford et al., 2010).

1.1.1 Pathophysiology

Acute gastritis has a number of causes, including certain drugs; alcohol; bile; ischemia; bacterial, viral, and fungal infections; acute stress (shock); radiation; allergy, food poisoning; and direct trauma. The common mechanism of injury is an imbalance between the aggressive and the defensive factors that maintain the integrity of the gastric mucosal lining (mucosa) (Kasper et al., 2006).

Acute erosive gastritis can result from the exposure to a variety of agents or factors, referred to as reactive gastritis. These agents/factors include nonsteroidal anti-inflammatory medications (NSAIDs), alcohol, cocaine, stress, radiation, bile reflux, and ischemia. The gastric mucosa exhibits hemorrhages, erosions, and ulcers. NSAIDs, such as aspirin, ibuprofen, and naproxen, are the most common agents associated with acute erosive gastritis, mostly attributed to therapeutic. Major injury is attributed to reduced prostaglandin synthesis. Prostaglandins are chemicals responsible for maintaining mechanisms that result in the protection of the mucosa from the injurious effects of the gastric acid.

Bacterial infection is another cause of acute gastritis. The corkscrew-shaped bacterium called H. pylori is the most common cause of gastritis. Complications result from a chronic infection rather than from an acute infection. The prevalence of H. pylori in otherwise healthy individuals varies depending on age, socioeconomic class, country of origin where the infection is usually acquired in childhood. In the Western world, the number of people infected with H pylori increases with age. Evidence of H. pylori infection can be found in 20% of individuals younger than 40 years and in 50% of individuals older than 60 years. Transmission is likely from person to person through the oral-fecal route or through the ingestion of contaminated water or food. This is why the prevalence is higher in lower socioeconomic classes and in developing countries. H pylori is associated with 60% of gastric ulcers and 80% of duodenalulcers (Andersen, 2007).

H. pylori gastritis typically starts as an acute gastritis in the antrum, causing intense inflammation, and over time, it may extend to involve the entire gastric mucosa resulting in chronic gastritis. The acute gastritis encountered with H. pylori is usually asymptomatic. The bacterium imbeds itself in the mucous layer, a protective layer that coats the gastric mucosa. It protects itself from the acidity of the stomach through the production of large amounts of urease, an enzyme that catalyzes the breakdown of urea to the alkaline ammonia and carbon dioxide. The alkaline ammonia neutralizes the gastric acid in the immediate vicinity of the bacterium conferring protection. H. pylori also has flagella that enable it to move and help it to penetrate the mucous layer so that it comes into contact with gastric epithelial cells. It also has several adhesions that help it to adhere to these cells. It produces inflammation by activating a number of toxins and enzymes that activate IL-8, which eventually attracts polymorphs and monocytes that cause acute gastritis (Fig. 2) (Das & Paul, 2007).

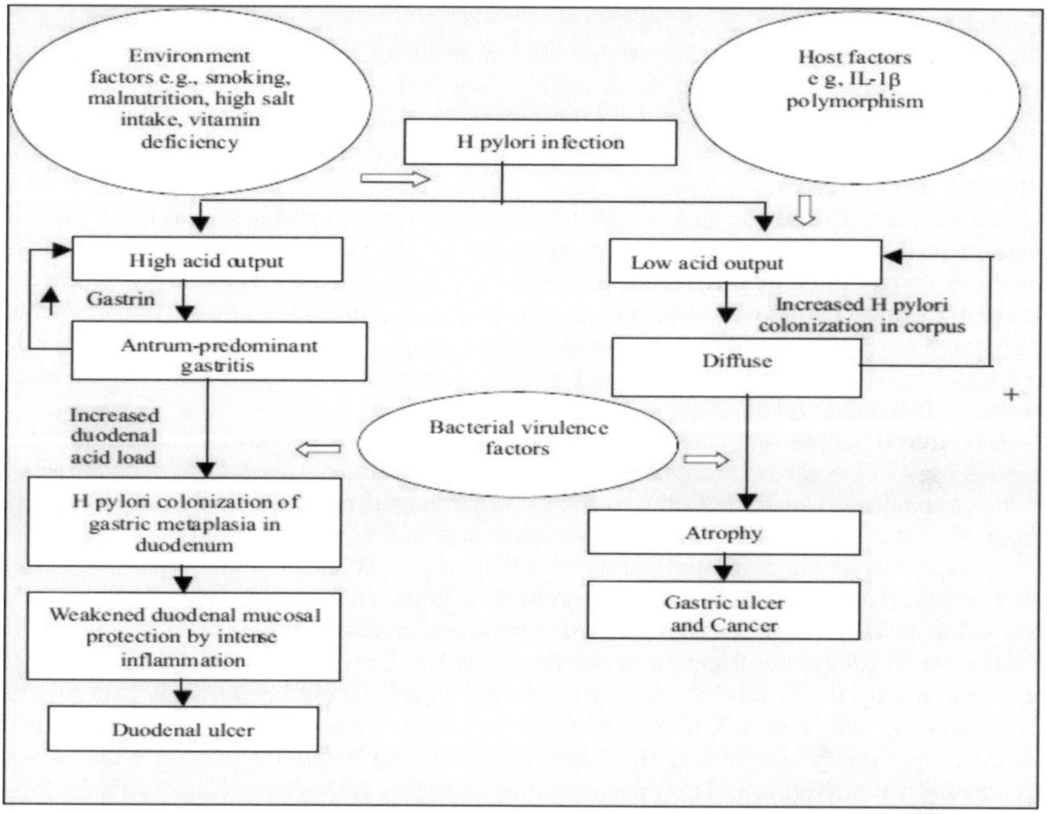

Fig. 2. Proposed interaction between host, environment and H. pylori infection in the development of gastric and doudenal ulcers.

Antigen-presenting cells activate lymphocytes and other mononuclear cells that lead to chronic superficial gastritis. The infection is established within a few weeks after the primary exposure to H. pylori. The intense inflammation can result in the loss of gastric glands responsible for the production of acid and mostly referred to as atrophic gastritis consequently production of gastric acid drops. The virulence genotype of the microbe is an important determinant for the severity of the gastritis of intestinal metaplasia transformation of gastric epithelium which can lead to gastric cancer (Soltermann et al., 2007).

Reactive gastropathy is the second most common diagnosis made on gastric biopsy specimens after H. pylori gastritis. It is now considered to represent a nonspecific response to a variety of other gastric irritants (Owen, 2003).

Tuberculosis is a rare cause of gastritis and generally associated with generally associated pulmonary or disseminated disease (Marshall, 1993) where secondary syphilis of the stomach is a rare cause of gastritis (Chen et al., 2006).

Phlegmonous gastritis is an uncommon form of gastritis (rare) caused by numerous bacterial agents, including streptococci, staphylococci, Proteus species, Clostridium species, and Escherichia coli. Phlegmonous gastritis usually occurs in individuals who are debilitated. It is associated with a recent large intake of alcohol, a concomitant upper respiratory tract infection, and AIDS. Phlegmonous means a diffuse spreading inflammation of or within connective tissue. In the stomach, it implies infection of the deeper layers of the stomach (submucosa and muscularis).

Viral infections can cause gastritis either localized or diffuse and cytomegalovirus (CMV) is a common viral cause. It is usually encountered in individuals who are immunocompromised, including those with cancer, immunosuppression, transplants, AIDS with a localized or diffuse involvement to the gastric tissuesand AIDS (Bonnet et al., 2001; Sepulveda & Patil, 2008).

Fungal infections that cause gastritis include Candida albicans and histoplasmosis. Gastric phycomycosis is another rare lethal fungal infection. The common predisposing factor is immunosuppression. C albicans rarely involves the gastric mucosa and when isolated in the stomach, the most common locations tend to be within a gastric ulcer or an erosion bed and it is generally of little consequence. Disseminated histoplasmosis can involve the stomach. The usual presenting clinical feature is bleeding from gastric ulcers or erosions on giant gastric folds (Lauwers et al., 2010).

Parasitic infections are rare causes of gastritis. Anisakidosis is caused by a nematode that embeds itself in the gastric mucosa along the greater curvature. Anisakidosis is acquired by eating contaminated sushi and other types of contaminated raw fish. It often causes severe abdominal pain that subsides within a few days and this nematode infection is associated with gastric fold swelling, erosions, and ulcers (Kim et al., 2003).

Ulcero-hemorrhagic gastritis is most commonly seen in patients who are critically ill and it is believed to be secondary to ischemia related to hypotension and shock or to the release of vaso constrictive substances but the etiology is often unknown. The gastric mucosa reveals multiple petechiae, mostly in the fundus and body, or exhibits a diffusely hemorrhagic pattern. The gross pathology may resemble that of NSAID- or other ingestion-induced gastritis except that the location of injury is different. This form of gastritis can be life-threatening if the patient experiences hemorrhaging and may even require emergency gastrectomy (Chamberlain, 1993).

Microscopic evidence of acute gastritis can be seen in patients with Crohn disease, though clinical manifestations are rare (occurring in only about 2-7% of patients with Crohn disease). Focally enhancing gastritis is now recognized as a condition seen in both Crohn disease and ulcerative colitis (Xin & Greenson, 2004).

Eosinophilic gastritis is often seen in conjunction with eosinophilic gastroenteritis but can be associated with various disorders, including food allergies (eg, cow milk, soy protein), collagen vascular diseases, parasitic infections, gastric cancer, lymphoma, Crohn disease, vasculitis, drug allergies, and H. pylori infections. An eosinophilic infiltrate is seen involving the gastric wall or epithelium (Rothenberg, 2004).

1.2 Chronic gastritis

Chronic gastritis is caused mainly by Helicobacter pylori infection, and nonatrophic gastritis progresses to atrophic gastritis for a long period. It is characterized by the presence of chronic inflammatory infiltrate in the gastric mucosa (Fig. 4). H. pylori-atrophic gastritis is strongly associated with gastric cancers, and its diagnosis is very important. It is diagnosed histologically according to the Updated Sydney System, which is now widely used in the world (Satoh et al., 2008). Chronic gastritis can be classified on the base of the underlying etiologic agent (eg, Helicobacter pylori, bile reflux, nonsteroidal anti-inflammatory drugs

[NSAIDs], autoimmunity, allergic response) and the histopathologic pattern, which may suggest the etiologic agent and clinical course (eg, H pylori -associated multifocal atrophic gastritis). Other classifications are based on the endoscopic appearance of the gastric mucosa (eg, varioliform gastritis) (Rugge & Genta, 2005).

1.2.1 Pathophysiology

The pathophysiology of chronic gastritis complicating a systemic disease, such as hepatic cirrhosis, uremia, or another infection is described in the relevant disease (Boulton et al., 2011). The pathogenesis of the most common forms of gastritis is described as follows.

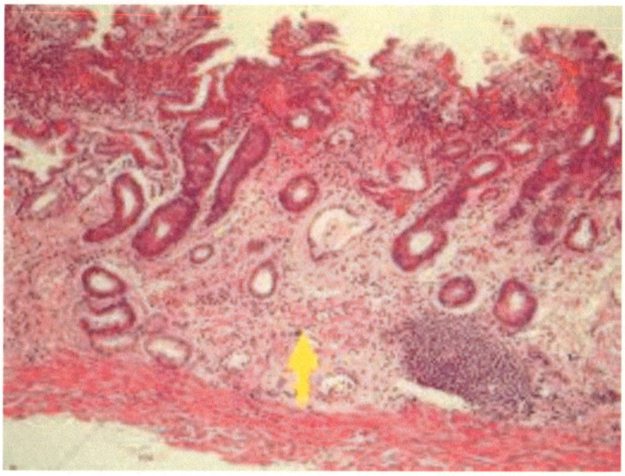

Fig. 3. Chronic gatritis showing inflammation of mucosa linning

The host response to H. pylori and bacterial products is composed of T- and B-cell lymphocytes, denoting chronic gastritis, followed by infiltration of the lamina propria and gastric epithelium by polymorphonuclear leukocytes that eventually phagocytize the bacteria. The presence of polymorphonuclear leukocytes in the gastric mucosa is diagnostic of active gastritis. The interaction of H pylori with the surface mucosa results in the release of proinflammatory cytokine interleukin (IL)-8, which leads to recruitment of polymorphonuclear cells and may begin the entire inflammatory process. Gastric epithelial cells express class II molecules, which may increase the inflammatory response by presenting H pylori antigens, leading to further cytokine release and more inflammation. High levels of cytokines, particularly tumor necrosis factor-a (TNF-α) and multiple interleukins (eg, IL-6, IL-8, IL-10), are detected in the gastric mucosa of patients with H. pylori gastritis (Zalewska-Ziob et al., 2009).

In subsequent or joining such inflammation pattern is an increase in oxidative damage due to high level of ROS and increased apoptosis level in human gastric mucosa (obst et al., 2000; cover et al., 2003). Infection also leads to the expression of inducible nitric oxide synthase (iNOS) in host macrophage and polymorphnuclear leukocytes (Tari et al., 2003). NO produced by these cells infiltrating the gastric mucosa may damage DNA. Interaction between NO and superoxide anion can form peroxinitrite, potent nitrating agent leading to apoptosis in a variety of cell types (yue et al., 2001).

Prostaglandins especially PGE2 in the stomach play an important role in the maintenance of gastric mucosal integrity via several mechanism including regulation of gastric mucosal blood flow, kinetic of epithelial cells, synthesis of mucous, inhibition of gastric acid secretion and referring to its protective potential to gastric mucosa (Takeeda et al., 2004).

Patients having Hpylori infection demonstrate significant gastremia which is mostly attributed to intragastric increase of H pylori inducing corpus atrophy and G cells damage in the antrum part. It may be also depends on alkalinization in G cells environment caused by H pylori urease (walsh et al., 1976; shacter et al., 2002).

Serum pepsinogens (1&11) are higher also and specifically in patient category having IgM positive as compared to others (IgM-ve). This may be attributed to a polypeptides secreted by HP during earlier infection which stimulates chief cells directly and promote pepsinogen synthesis (Takeeda et al., 2004; kist, 1991; Elseweidy et al., 2010 a;b).

This led certain study (Kekki et al., 1991) to consider serum pepsinogen level-as a non endoscopic blood test in the diagnosis of atrophic gastritis, HP eradication and, a screening tool for high risk subjects having atrophic gastritis rather than a test for cancer itself.

Generally known Hp infection is associated with special local and systemic immune response. Early after 18 days of infection IgM response is detectable while IgG, IgA response occurs later after 60 days of infection at which time IgG titers decline. IgG, IgA serology is widely used as an accurate test for the diagnosis of Hp infection but those 2 immunoglobulins remains detectable after eradication of HP and d'not demonstrate the infection status (acute, chronic or previously treated infection). Therefore the use of IgM test would allow for direct screening of the sample and serve as a diagnostic tool for establishing active or recent infection (Alem et al., 2002, Elseweidy et al 2010).

Accordingly many authors concluded that diagnosis of atrophic gastritis using test panel of seum gastrin 17, pepsinogen 1, HP antibodies were in good agreement with endoscopic and biopsy findings, considering such panel a non endoscopic diagnostic and screening tool (vaananen et al., 2003).

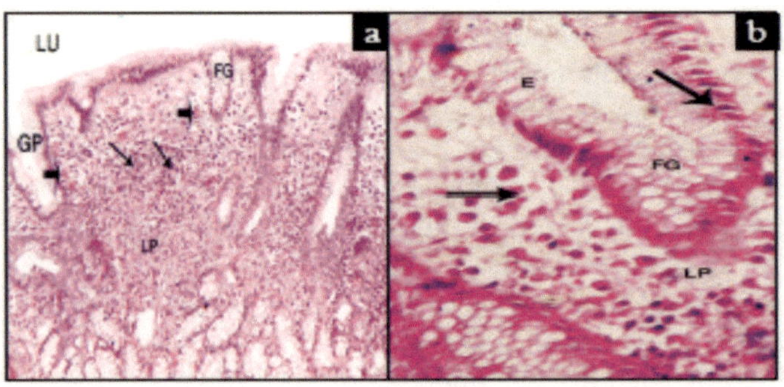

Fig. 4. Histological section of human fundic gland of patient suffering from gastritis with anti H. pylori IgM positive group showing (a) x100 irregular short fundic gland (FG), wide gastric pit (GP), multiple inflammatory cells (arrows) and blood vessels (double arrows) filling lamina propria (LP), (b) x400 showing irregular simple columnar epithelium (E), small pyknotic nuclei (arrows) of cells lyning fundic gland (FG) and multiple inflammatory cells (double arrows) filling lamina propria (LP) (Elseweidy et al., 2010 a).

2. Natural products used in treating gastritis

Phenolic compounds, which include tannins and flavonoids, are apparently related to the interesting anti-inflammatory, woundhealing, antioxidant and antiulcerogenic properties to several medicinal plants (Moleiro et al., 2009).

Tannins are potent scavengers of peroxyl radicals and can also interact with mucus proteins, improving their cytoprotective effect by forming a protein lining over the gastrointestinal mucosa (Okuda, 2005; Moleiro et al., 2009).

Fresh fruit and vegetables have been reported to exert multiple biological effects on the mucosa of the gastrointestinal tract due to their antioxidant contents (La Vecchia & Tavani, 1998). In particular, a diet rich in vegetable is associated with a lower incidence of gastric tumours (Roukos et al., 2003).

Apart from their action as radical scavengers, phenolic compounds also have several indirect effects; they can inhibit lipoxygenase (Laughton et al., 1991), reduce platelet aggregation (Ferro-Luzzi & Ghiselli, 1993) and reduce the bioavailability of food carcinogens (Stavric, 1994). Certain flavonoids or compounds with flavonoid-like properties have antiulcer activity and can prevent gastric mucosal lining lesions brought about by a number of ulcerogens (Alarcon de la Lastra et al., 2002).

Certain polyphenolics can exert a preventive action on gastric injury in rats. Research topics her have focussed on the antiulcer activity of polyphenol from grape seed (Saito et al., 1998), cacao liquor (Osakabe et al., 1998), curcuminoids and Black seed oil (Elseweidy et al., 2008) or from Opuntia ficus indica (Galati et al., 2003). This activity was mainly explained by the strong antioxidant power and/or by some other factors, such as strong protein-binding capacity (Saito et al., 1998), modulation of leukocyte function (Osakabe et al., 1998), mucus production and restoration (Galati et al., 2003). It is believed that the antioxidant activity of polyphenols is an important factor to combat the potential of free radicals.

2.1 Morinda citrifolia aqueous fruit extract

Morinda citrifolia L. (Rubiaceae), commonly known worldwide as "Noni" or so called in Thai as "Yor" is regularly consumed as food, additionally as medicinal plants used in primary health care. The decoction or infusion of roasted mature unripe fruits is recommended to relieve the symptoms of nausea and vomiting, if it is not too severe. According to the claimed efficacies in Thai traditional textbooks, the fruit is also used for treatment of various gastrointestinal disorders as a carminative, appetite stimulant, and reliever of gum diseases, heartburn or stomachache. Nevertheless, experimental studies demonstrated the preventive activity of an ethyl acetate extract of the fruit against acute gastric lesions induced by ethanol, aspirin and pyloric ligation; and acute duodenal ulcer induced by cysteamine in rats (Muralidharan & Srikanth, 2009). This extract was claimed to exhibit potent antioxidant properties and the active components are thought to be non-polar lignans (Kamiya et al., 2004). Previous studies of the effect of an aqueous fruit extract on gastrointestinal motility reported controversial results with increase (Chuthaputti et al., 1996) and delay (Pu et al., 2004) gastric emptying action.

It has been claimed also that aqueous extract have anti-inflammatory (McKoy et al., 2002) and antioxidative activities (Ikeda et al., 2009) in several in vitro test systems. Among a number of major components identified in the aqueous fruit juice, scopoletin, a coumarin derivative, as one of the main compounds that has known pharmacological activities especially an ability to control the serotonin level in the body (Levand and Larson, 1979),

together with anti-inflammatory (Deng et al., 2007; Moon et al., 2007) and antioxidative activities (Ikeda et al., 2009). Scopoletin is also recommended as a marker constituent for the quality control and pharmacokinetic study of Noni products (Samoylenko et al., 2006).
This aqueous fruit extract as well as its biomarker: scopoletin, may be beneficial as a potential preventive and therapeutic agent for gastro-esophageal inflammation. This is mainly through its antisecretory and prokinetic activities including its ability to enhance the mucosal defensive mechanisms. Their efficacy was compared with a standard potent antisecretory proton pump inhibitor (lansoprazole) and referring to its stronger prokinetic efficacy in accelerating gastric emptying and intestinal transit in rats. These observed beneficial effects of AFE may be accounted for by one of its major active biological components scopoletin (Mahattanadul et al., 2011).

2.2 Quercetin-3-O-β-D-glucuronopyranoside (QGC), isolated from Rumex Aquaticus herb

It is well known that flavonoids which have anti-inflammatory, antioxidant, antiallergic, hepatoprotective, antithrombotic, antiviral, and anticarcinogenic activities. As reported before the anti-inflammatory activities of flavonoids demonstrate their candidacy as therapeutic agents (Lewis, 1989). The flavonoids are typical phenolic compounds that act as potent metal chelators, antioxidants and free radical scavengers, which modulate intracellular signaling caused by upstream binding partners, such as, regulatory kinases and receptors (Williams et al., 2004a).
Such flavonoid is a natural flavone with various bioactivities and was found to be highly efficient to scavenge free radicals in cell-free systems (Rice-Evans et al., 1996), as compared to traditional antioxidants like vitamin C and E (Geetha et al., 2005). Gerritsen et al., (1995) found that flavonoids, especially an apigenin, blocked the cytokine-induced expressions of intercellular adhesion molecule-1 (ICAM-1), vascular cell adhesion molecule-1 (VCAM-1), and E-selectin on human endothelial cells.
Regarding gastric secretion, the oral administration of QGC reduced gastric content significantly, dose-dependently, and prevented the development of reflux esophagitis. These results suggest that QGC has inhibitory effects on reflux esophagitis and gastritis in rats. Furthermore, in feline esophageal epithelial cells, QGC was found to have a protective effect on ethanol induced cell damage by inhibiting ROS generation, activation downstream of ERK (Min et al., 2009), and downstream signal transduction induced by interleukin-1 beta (Lee et al., 2009a).

2.3 The aqueous decoction of mango flowers (Mangifera indica L.)

Mangifera indica L. (Anacardiaceae) is a large tree that grows in tropical and subtropical regions. The Caribbean population used aqueous decoction from M. indica flowers for the treatment of gastritis and gastric ulcer. Phytochemical research from different parts of M. indica has demonstrated the presence of phenolics, triterpenes, flavonoids, phytosterols and polyphenols (Selles et al., 2002; Singh et al., 2004).
Garrido et al., (2004) reported the antinociceptive and anti-inflammatory activities of Vimang®, an aqueous extract obtained from M. indica. They attributed these activities to their inhibitory influence on the prostaglandin synthesis through arachidonic acid metabolism additionally production of reactive oxygen species. Tordera et al., (1994) demonstrated the influence of several anti-inflammatory flavonoids present in M. indica on mast cell degranulation and arachidonic acid release in rats.

M. indica is also described as an antioxidant agent (Sanchez et al., 2003). Oxygen-derived free radicals have been postulated to play an important role in the pathogenesis of acute gastric mucosal injuries such as those induced by stress (Hariganesh & Prathiba, 2000), ethanol (Salim, 1990) and NSAIDs (Pihan et al., 1987) and scavenging of these radicals can stimulate the healing process. This was illustrated before in experimental model induced by acetic acid and attributed mainly to their high content of flavonoids (Naito et al., 1995).

2.4 Abarema cochliacarpos

Several medicinal plants including species of the Brazilian Cerrado biome as well as plants of the "Caatinga" biome contain phenolic compounds like tannins and flavonoids that have anti-inflammatory, antioxidant and antiulcerogenic properties (Almeida et al., 2005; Moleiro et al., 2009).

Catechins (flavan-3-ols) such as catechin, epicatechin, epigallocatechin, epicatechin gallate and epigallocatechin gallate, are particularly abundant in the bark of the species of Mimosaceae family (Santos et al., 2002). These compounds has anti-inflammatory and anti cholesterolemic effects additionally protective agent against cytotoxicity owing to their antioxidant properties (Williams et al., 2004b).

Araujo et al. (2008) studied plants with elevated levels of phenolic compounds within specific groups of plants for further therapeutic applications. They concluded that Caatinga medicinal plants, which are known and/or used for their wound-healing or anti-inflammatory properties, tend to have high tannin contents. Moreover, these compounds appear markedly elevated in some species, such as Abarema cochliacarpos, that are intensively used by the local communities (Monteiro et al., 2006).

Abarema cochliacarpos is a plant native to Brazil, occurring mainly in the Atlantic Forest and in the Caatinga biomes. It is a tree species of the legume family Mimosaceae (International Union for Conservation of Nature "IUCN", 2009), which is popularly known as "barbatimao". In this community, the decoction of the bark is utilized to wash external ulcers while its tincture, (bark immersed in white wine) "cachaca", or ingested form is used against inflammation and gastric ulcers, among other uses (Silva et al., 2006). Other authors also observed similar applications in different traditional communities (Agra et al., 2008).

As to pharmacologic effects, the hydroalcoholic extract from the bark of Abarema cochliacarpos showed antimicrobial activity. Both crude aqueous and methanol extracts also showed antinociceptive effects (Silva et al., 2009). Butanolic fraction of the methanolic extract was tested recently in a model of acute experimental trinitrobenzene sulfonic acid (TNBS)-induced colitis and showed anti-inflammatory effects (Silva et al., 2010a).

It has been suggested that Abarema cochliacarpos (Gomes) Barneby & Grimes extracts exerts gastroprotective effects and wound healing properties in the ethanol-induced ulcer model. The safety and efficacy in the healing of gastric ulcers is based on its ability to activate the expression of COX-2, vascular-endothelial growth factor (VEGF) and stimulate proliferative factors like HSP-70 that re-establish the gastric mucosa integrity (Silva et al., 2010b).

2.5 Apple polyphenol extracts

Eberhardt and colleagues (2000) illustrated the antiproliferative effect of apple extract in vitro using tumor cells and attributed such effect to the presence of phytochemicals (phenolic acids and flavonoids) other than ascorbic acid. Therefore, dietary antioxidants play a crucial role in the maintenance of gastric homeostasis by counteracting the potentially

mucosal damage exerted by ROS. This may explain the role of dietary antioxidants as scavenger of oxygen, nitrogen free radicals and breaking lipid peroxisdation reactions. Phenolic compounds are one of the major classes of dietary antioxidants and apple phenolic compounds represent 22 percent of such total (Le Marchand et al., 2000).
In vitro and in vivo studies demonstrated the protective effect of apple juice regarding gastric mucosa of rat. This was markedly observed in gastric injury model induced by aspirin and independently of its inhibition to gastric acid. Therefore it might be of therapeutic benefit in prophylaxis of aspirin- related gastropathy (D' argenio et al., 2008). Accordingly a diet rich in apple antioxidants might exert a beneficial effect in gastric diseases associated with generation of reactive oxygen species (Graziani et al., 2005).

2.6 Foeniculum vulgare (Fennel)

Foeniculum vulgare (FVE) is a well-known umbelliferous plant. For centuries, FVE fruits have been used as traditional herbal medicine in Europe and China. It is native to southern Europe and the Mediterranean area. The seeds of this plant have been used to regulate menstruation, alleviate the symptoms of female climacteric syndrome, and increase libido (Albert-Puleo, 1980). FVE also possesses emnenagague, galactagogue and antispasmodic properties additionally in folk remedies for treatment of dysmenorrheal, also as diuretic and wound dressing in Turkish traditional medicine (Savino et al., 2005).
It contains 1%-3% of a volatile oil, which is composed of 50%-85% of anethole and about 20% of d-fenchone (Dadalioglu & Evrendilek, 2004). Other compunds present in FVE are d-a-pinene, d-a-phellandrene, dipentene, methyl chavicol, feniculun, anisaldehyde, and anisic acid (Mimica-Dukic et al., 2003).
Previous studies proved that anethole possesses significant antioxidant, anti-inflammatory and ulcer healing activity in experimental models (Freire et al., 2005). Additionally, flavonoids, sterols, tannins and coumarins of some plants are also known to possess antiulcer activity (Khalil, 2006). Therefore, the presence of flavonoids content and other bioactive compounds in FVE may be beneficial in ulcer therapy. Its gastro protective effect has been also observed before in certain gastric mucosal lesion induced by ethanol, attributed mostly to its antioxidant activity and reduction of lipid peroxidation cascade.
Therefore it may be a new alternative for clinical management of gastric ulcer diseases and/or an antioxidant against oxidative stress (Birdane et al., 2007).

2.7 Flavonoids isolated from Piper carpunya Ruiz & Pav

The leaves of Piper carpunya Ruiz & Pav. (syn Piper lenticellosum C.D.C.) (Piperaceae), known with the popular name of "guaviduca" in Ecuador are widely used in folk medicine in tropical and subtropical countries of South America, as an anti-inflammatory, anti-ulcer, anti-diarrheal and anti-parasitical remedy as well as an ailment for skin irritations. The antiinflammatory activity has been confirmed in rat models like the carrageenan-induced paw edema and the results obtained can support its use in the traditional medicine of Ecuador (De las Heras et al., 1998). Recently, this plant has been shown to protect against gastric ulcers induced by non-steroidal anti-inflammatory drugs (NSAID) in rats (Trabadela et al., 2009).
Numerous plant remedies have shown to be active against Helicobacter pylori infection, such as the oil extract of Chamomilla recutita (Shikov et al., 2008), the ethanolic extract of Cuminum cyminum L., Propolis (Nostro et al., 2005) as well as the methanolic extract of

Alchornea triplinervia (Spreng.) Mull. Arg., which exhibited anti-secretory, anti-Helicobacter pylori and gastroprotective effects (Lima et al., 2008).
Several mechanisms of action have been proposed to illustrate its anti-inflammatory effects. This may be explained through other properties such as anti-oxidant activity, inhibition of eicosanoid generating enzymes or as modulator for proinflammatory molecules. Recent studies have also shown that some flavonoids are modulators of proinflammatory gene expression (Garcia-Lafuente et al., 2009). Gastro protective activity of flavonoids may be through reducing gastric acid secretion and inhibition of gastric H+, K+-ATPase. One example is Baccharis illinita D.C., which is also used in folk medicine, and whose anti-secretory activity is attributable to the flavonoid luteolin (Freitas et al., 2008).
Furthermore, some flavonoids have also demonstrated inhibitory effects on Helicobacter pylori growth and vacuolation. Helicobacter pylori induces gastric epithelial cell apoptosis via secreted mediators such as the VacA cytotoxin and lipopolysacccharides which damage epithelial acid-secreting parietal cells (Neu et al., 2002). Several flavonoids have inhibitory influence on the apoptotic signaling induced by Helicobacter pylori VacA toxin (Xiao et al., 2007). Antimicrobial compounds from plants may inhibit bacterial growth by different mechanisms and could therefore be useful in case of resistance state to antibiotics. In this way, Castillo-Juarez et al., (2007) found that the petroleum ether fraction from Amphipterygium adstringens (Schltdl.) Standl. had significant anti-microbial activity against Helicobacter pylori. From this fraction, the authors isolated a mixture of anacardic acids and three known triterpenes: masticadienonic acid, 3-alpha-hydroxymasticadienonic acid, 3-epi-oleanolic as well as the sterol ß-sitosterol.
Previous study suggested that the flavonoids (vitexin, isovitexin, rhamnopyranosylvitexin and isoembigenin), nervogenic acid and geranylbenzoate isolated from the ethanolic extract of Piper carpunya may contribute to the anti-myeloperoxidase activity, as well as to their anti-Helicobacter pylori effect. These flavonoids may also be responsible for the important inhibition of H+, K+-ATPase pathway, additionally the obtained phytosterols and phytol could be involved in these gastroprotective activities (Quilez et al., 2010).

2.8 Quassia amara

Quassia is a plant that grows typically in the American tropical regions (from Mexico to the Brazilian Amazona) below 500 m altitude, especially in the Caribbean side of Central America and the Pacific coast of Costa Rica and Panama. The plant prefers very humid environments, but it can be found in the dry forest next to a riverbank (López and Pérez, 2008).
Quassia amara L. is one of the most mentioned plants in ethnomedicine for the treatment of malaria, mainly in Surinam, Guyana and French Guyana, where tea cups are carved from the wood and the addition of hot water forms an infusion in them (Odonnea et al., 2007). There only exist a few studies on the gastrointestinal, digestive and secretagogue activity of Quassia amara L. extracts. The results point to an increase of bile secretion with a standardized extract, inhibition of ulcer induction with crude extracts, accompanied by a slight decrease in pH and peptic activity of gastric juice additionally an enhancement of cytoprotective factors like gastric mucus (Toma et al., 2002).
The biological activity of Quassia amara L. has been attributed mainly to its high content of quassinoids. These metabolites are oxygenated triterpenes derived from euphol and are exclusive to the Simaroubaceae family. The most important quassinoids in Quassia amara L. are quassin and neoquassin. Quassin is one of the most bitter substances known, it

represents 0.1% of the dried weight of wood and bark, and it is present in larger quantities when the plant is grown in the shade (Guo et al., 2005).
Quassia amara L. bark standardized extracts, Lipro® and Ligas®, which were standardized to its quassinoid content, showed an important anti-ulcerogenic and gastroprotective potential in acute ulcer induction models. Their effect was related to an increase in gastric barrier mucus and non protein sulfhydril groups (Garcia-Barrantes & Badilla, 2011). Gastric barrier mucus is an important factor in gastroprotection (Kaunitz, 1999). Animals treated with Ligas® showed substantial mucus production. Prostaglandins I2, E2 and F2 are some of the main stimuli for the production of gastric and duodenal mucus (Dharmani et al., 2005). The increase in mucus could be a signal of the role of prostaglandins in the anti-ulcerogenic properties of the extracts.

2.9 Gardenia jasminoides Ellis ethanol extract

Gardenia jasminoides Ellis (GJE), has been used in traditional oriental medicine for the treatment of jaundice, fever, hypertension, and ulcers of a skin (Tseng et al., 1995). It has been reported that the crude extract of GJE fruit has biological and pharmacological activities. In the phytochemical studies of GJE, genipin, chlorogenic acid, rutin, and ursolic acid were detected in GJE extracts (He et al., 2006). Genipin is an aglycone derived from an iridoid glycoside called geniposide present in fruit of GJE, and is an excellent natural cross-linker for proteins, collagen, gelatin, and chitosan cross-linking. It has been also used for pharmaceutical purposes, such as choleretic action for liver diseases control, and the relief of type 2 diabetes symptoms. Ursolic acid is a pentacyclic triterpene acid, used in cosmetics (Shishodia et al., 2003), and as inhibitor for various types of cancer cells by inhibiting the STAT3 activation pathway (Pathak et al., 2007) and human fibrosarcoma cells by reducing the expression of matrix metalloproteinase-9 by the glucocorticoid receptor.
Gastric cancer is the second commonest cause of death from malignant disease worldwide (Neugut et al., 1996). Antioxidant compounds, such as vitamin C and E, have a key role for prevention and termination of development of gastric cancer (Block, 1991). It has been recognized that chronic infections of the gastric mucosa by Helicobater pylori (H. pylori) plays a pivotal role in gastric carcinogenesis. Such infection usually causes acute and chronic inflammation cell infiltrate, leading to an increase of reactive oxygen species (ROS), which are highly reactive compounds. The latter may combine with DNA in a number of potentially genotoxic ways, subsequently accumulated in H. pylori gastritis. Therefore it may be possible to prevent carcinogenesis through reduction of ROS damage to cellular constituents, especially DNA, additionally the eradication of H. pylori can lead to a reduction in ROS activity in the gastric mucosa (Drake et al., 1998).
Lee et al., (2009b) in confirm indicated that the ethanolic extracts of GJE exerted protective activities against potential gastritic diseases like gastritis and gastric cancer. This action might be due to antioxidant activity, anti-H. pylori activity of ursolic acid and genipin that counteract free radicals exerting anti-ulcer activity.

2.10 Curcumin

Curcumin, the polyphenolic yellowish pigment of the rhizome Curcuma longa Linn, is known to possess anti-inflammatory, antioxidant, wound-healing, and antiallergic activities (Das& Das, 2002). Several investigators have also reported the antiulcerogenic activity of the ethanolic extract of the rhizome of C. longa in acute gastric mucosal lesion (Rafatullah et.,

1990), but not in chronic ulcer models. More recently, it has been considered that curcumin exerts a variety of pharmacological actions through inhibition of inducible nitric oxide synthase (iNOS) as well as its potential as radical scavenger (Elseweidy et al., 2008) Thus, the previously proposed mechanisms for antiulcerogenic effect of curcumin (Yano et al., 2000), such as inhibitory effect on gastric secretion, cytoprotection, antioxidant activity and inhibition of mast-cell degranulation, need to be evaluated again.

Curcumin, exerted its preventive effect on gastric lesion formation, although it possesses anti-inflammatory activity resulting from a blockade of all branches of the arachidonic acid pathway (Ammon et al., 1993). This effect is consistent with the findings reported by several authors that the inhibition of prostaglandins synthesis is unlikely to be the mechanism responsible for the inflammatory ulceration formation. Curcumin therefore may exert this through its antioxidant activity and its inhibition of nuclear factor kappa B activation which up-regulates many genes involved in inflammation and immunity, including its potent suppressive effect on mast-cell degranulation (Jobin et al., 1999). Although there is a potential increase of gastric acid secretion with a high dose of curcumin, gastric acid secretion has been found to play little role in the pathogenesis of this model (Ohta et al., 1999).

Apparent healing - promoting effect of curcumin was also observed in gastric ulcer model, induced by acetic acid with an enhancement of mucosal layer regeneration. This effect was not seen in a dose-related fashion, presumably through some curative mechanisms differently modified by curcumin dosage. Accordingly, it is conceivable that the effect of curcumin occurs at least partly through its inhibition of the cytokine-mediated inflammatory mechanism, suppression of iNOS activity and antioxidant activity as mentioned above. In addition, the curative properties and ulcer healing might result from the elevation of epidermal growth factor and transforming growth factor-beta-1, as shown in acceleration of cutaneous wound healing in rats, guinea pigs and mice (Sidhu et al., 1998). Another study attributed such preventive and curative effects of curcumin to an increase in the mucosal defensive mechanism through its antioxidant property, increase in mucin secretion and inhibition of NO or cytokine-mediated inflammation (Mahattanadul et al., 2006).

2.11 Artichoke leaf extract

Artichoke (Cynara Scolymus L.) is a plant that is widely grown in Mediterranean countries, including southern France and California in the United States. In general, the dried extract consisting of leaves and not flowering heads of artichoke has been eluted with water in European countries and the main components are caffeoylquinic acid derivatives (cynarin and chlorogenic acid), flavonoids (luteolin and apigenin) and bitters (cynaropicrin) (Joy & Haber, 2007). Artichoke leaf extract has been used for hepatoprotective and cholesterol reducing (Aktay et al., 2000) purposes. Based on in vitro (Perez-Garcia et al., 2000) and in vivo (Speroni et al., 2003) studies, it is believed that artichoke leaf extract is very effective as an antioxidant and its leaf extract contains cynaropicrin and chlorogenic acid as the main components. It is currently used in Germany and Switzerland as a remedy for indigestion. And its better compounds such as cynariopicrin as inflammatory agents due to its inhibitory influence on inflammatory mediators (Holtmann et al., 2003).

Previous results indicated that artichoke leaf extract is effective against acute hemorrhagic gastritis and its beneficial effect is due to that of cynaropicrin. The gastric mucus-increasing action of artichoke leaf extract may be, at least in part, related to the anti-gastritic action of the extract (Ishida et al., 2010).

2.12 Pear (Pyrus communis L.) procyanidins

Some European pear (Pyrus communis L.) cultivars have been reported to contain significant amounts of polyphenols, such as chlorogenic acid, flavan-3-ols and arbutin. procyanidins are reported to have many beneficial properties, such as potent antioxidant activity (Zhu et al., 2002), free radical scavenging activity (Arteel & Sies, 1999), antiinflammatory activity and anti-influenza viral activity (Hamauzu et al., 2005).

It has been shown that procyanidins extracted from pear (Winter Nelis) fruit had a very high mean degree of polymerization (mDP), indicating that these compounds may interact with mucosa proteins. Accordingly the mechanism of mucosa protection by pear procyanidins may be both physical and chemical. By binding strongly to the mucosa, procyanidins build a protective layer against injury, reducing leukocyte migration, and then exerting its local antioxidant protection against free radicals (Hamauzu et al., 2007).

2.13 Sesame lignan sesamol

Sesamol (3,4-methylenedioxyphenol), the lignan of sesame oil, is a potent antioxidant and anti-inflammatory agent in various oxidative systems, including endotoxin and iron intoxication (Hsu et al., 2007). Recent study has confirmed its effect in gastric haemorrhage model and mucosal ulcer induced in rats by aspirin. Sesamol her significantly reduced gastric mucosal lipid peroxidation, nitric oxide production, gastric mucosal proinflammatory cytokines (tumor necrosis factor-a and interleukin 1-ß levels), and the activity of gastric mucosal myeloperoxidase. This was attributed to an inhibition of neutrophil infiltration, subsequent gastric mucosal inflammation and oxidative stress in rats (Hsu et al., 2009a). It seems likely that sesamol protective influence on gastric mucosal injury may be at least partially through an inhibition of mucosal reactive nitrogen species and subsequent lipid peroxidation.

Inhibition of neutrophils activation and their infiltration into gastric mucosa may be sesamol's anti-inflammatory and antioxidative mechanism. Neutrophil activation and infiltration are crucial in the pathogenesis of NSAID-induced gastric inflammation and oxidative stress (Souza et al., 2008). Activating neutrophils results in the expression of proinflammatory genes and the overproduction of proinflammatory mediators, including TNF-α and IL-1ß, which initiates an inflammatory response (Jaeschke & Hasegawa, 2006). Overproduction of proinflammatory mediators can upregulate nitric oxide production leading to an increase of reactive nitrogen species, lipid peroxidation, and cell damage (Hayes and McLellan, 1999). Similar effect for Sesamol was also observed in the gastric mucosa of aspirin-treated rats preventing inturn gastric injury. This may be attributed to certain combination between sesamol and aspirin, inhibiting inturn neutrophil infiltration, mucosal inflammation and oxidative stress (Hsu et al., 2009a).

Daily consumption of sesame or sesame oil may be beneficial in protecting against gastric mucosal damage induced by long-term use of NSAID. Sesame lignan sesamol is one of the important antioxidative components in sesame in addition to some other antioxidants such as sesamin, sesamolin, and gamma-tocopheral (Tokusoglu et al., 2003). All of them could attenuate NSAID initiated gastric mucosal oxidative stress. Therefore, we suggested that daily consumption of sesame or sesame oil could protect against NSAID-induced gastric mucosal damage. However, more investigations will be needed to confirm this.

Also, pretreatment of sesame oil, significantly decreased acidified ethanol-induced mucosal ulcer formation and luminal hemorrhage. Sesame oil her reduced mucosal lipid peroxidation, as well as glutathione and nitric oxide production in experimental rats model attenuating in turn oxidative stress and gastric mucosal injury (Hsu et al., 2009b).

3. Conclusion

Gastritis represents an inflammation of the stomach lining in response to injury.It is either acute or chronic and has many underlying causes ,however the most important of them are Helicobacter pylori (HP) infection, Autoimmunity additionally prolonged uptake of certain drugs ,specifically aspirin and nonsteroidal antiinfilammatory drugs (NSAIDs).The common mechanism of an injury is an imbalance between the aggressive and defensive factors that maintain the integrity of the gastric lining (mucosa). In subsequent or joining such inflammation pattern an increase in oxidative damage due to high level of reactive oxygen species (ROS) , higher gastrin, pepsinogen, expression of inducible nitric oxide synthase (iNOS) leading to corpus atrophy and G cells damage. Interaction of NO and can form peroxynitrite, leading finally to apoptosis in a variety of cell types.

Tannins and flavonoids (phenolic compounds) are commonly found in several medicinal plants. Certain therapeutic properties mainly anti-inflammatory, wound healing, antioxidant and anti ulcerogenic are mostly attributed to these plant constituents.

Tannins are potent scavengers of per oxi radicals and can interact with mucus proteins, improving their cytoprotective effect by forming a protein lining over the gastrointestinal mucosa, additionally involved in wounds treatment. Fresh fruits and vegetables have been reported to exert multiple biological effects on the mucosa of gastrointestinal tract due to their antioxidants content. Certain flavonoids or compounds with flavonoid-like properties have antiulcer activity, prevent gastric mucosal lesions brought about by a number of ulcerogens. This had been illustrated before on polyphenol from grape seed, aqueous fruit extract of morinda citrifolia, Quarcetin, apple extract, curcumin, black seed oil, quassin, artichoke and others. It is conceivable that some of these plant constituents exerted their effects through the inhibition of cytokine-mediated inflammatory mechanism, suppression of iNOS, antioxidant activities and healing of the produced ulcer.

4. Acknowledgment

We acknowledge the work of Dr. Hebatallah H. Atteia, and Dr. Mona M. Taha for their technical help and Assistance.

5. References

Agra, M.F.; Silva, K.N.; Basilio, I.J.L.D.; Freitas, P.F.& Barbosa-Filho, J.M. (2008). Survey of medicinal plants used in the region northeast of Brazil. *Brazilian Journal of Pharmacognosy*, Vol. 18, No. 3, (2008), pp. 472–508, ISSN 0102-695X.

Alarcon de la Lastra, C.; Barranco, M.D.; Martin, M.J.; Herrerías, J& Motilva, V. (2002). Extra-virgin olive oil enriched diets reduce indomethacin-induced gastric oxidative damage in rats. *Dig Dis Sci*, Vol. 47, No. 12, (December 2002), pp. 2783–2790, ISSN 1573-2568.

Albert-Puleo M. (1980). Fennel and anise as estrogenic agents. J. Ethnopharmacol., Vol. 2, No. 4, (December 1980), pp. 337-344, ISSN 0378-8741.

Alem, M.; Alem, N.; Cohen, H.; England, T.; Hamedi, N.; Moussazadeh, M.; Roth, J.A.& Shen, G.Q. (2002). Diagnostic value of detection of IgM antibodies to Helicobacter pylori. *Exp Mol Pathol.*, Vol. 72, No. 1, (February 2002), pp. 77-83, ISSN 0531-5522.

Almeida, C.F.C.B.R.; Lima e Silva, T.C.; Amorim, E.L.C.; Maia, M.B.S.& Albuquerque, U.P. (2005). Life strategy and chemical composition as predictors of the selection of medicinal plants from the Caatinga (Northeast Brazil). *Journal of Arid Environments*, Vol. 62, No. 1, (July 2005), pp. 127–142, ISSN 1095-922X.

Ammon, H.P.T.; Safayhi, H.; Mack, T.& Sabieraj, J. (1993). Mechanism of anti-inflammatory actions of curcumin and boswellic acids. *J. Ethnopharmacol.*, Vol. 38, No. 2-3, (March 1993), pp. 113–119, ISSN 0378-8741.

Andersen, L.P. (2007). Colonization and infection by Helicobacter pylori in humans. *Helicobacter*, Vol. 12, No. 12, (November 2007), pp. 12-15, ISSN 1523-5378.

Arauᅇjo, T.A.S.; Alencar, N.L.; Amorim, E.L.C.& Albuquerque U.P. (2008). A new approach to study medicinal plants with tannins and flavonoids contents from the local knowledge. Journal of Ethnopharmacology, Vol. 120, No. 1, (August 2008), pp. 72–80, ISSN 0378-8741.

Arteel, G. E., & Sies, H. (1999). Protection against peroxynitrite by cocoa polyphenol oligomers. *FEBS Letters*, Vol. 462, No. (1-2), (November 1999), pp. 167–170, ISSN 0014-5793.

Binmoeller, K.F.& Benner, K.G. (1992). Emphysematous gastritis secondary to gastric infarction. *Am. J. Gastroenterol.*, Vol. 87, No. 4, (April 1992), pp. 526–529, ISSN 0002-9270.

Birdane, F.M.; Cemek, M.; Birdane, Y.O.; Gülçin, İ.& Büyükokuroğlu, M.E. (2007). Beneficial effects of Foeniculum vulgare on ethanol-induced acute gastric mucosal injury in rats. *World J. Gastroenterol.*, Vol. 13, No. 4, (January 2007), pp. 607-611, ISSN 1007-9327.

Block, G. (1991). Vitamin C and cancer prevention: the epidemiologic evidence. *Am. J. Clin. Nutr.*, Vol. 53, No. 1, (January 1991), pp. 270S–282S., ISSN 1938-3207.

Bonnet, F.; Neau, D.; Viallard, J.F.; Morlat, P.; Ragnaud, J.M.; Dupon, M.& et al. (2001). Clinical and laboratory findings of cytomegalovirus infection in 115 hospitalized non-immunocompromised adults. *Ann. Med. Interne.*, Vol. 152, No. 4, (June 2001), pp. 227-235, ISSN 0003-410X.

Boulton, R.; Hodgson, H.& Gupta, S. (2011). *Chronic gastritis*, Manson, ISBN 978-1-48067-068-2, Corringham road, London.

Castillo-Juarez, I.; Rivero-Cruz, F.; Celis, H.& Romero, I. (2007). Anti-Helicobacter pylori activity of anacardic acids from Amphipterygium adstringens. *Journal of Ethnopharmacology*, Vol. 114, No. 1, (July 2007), pp. 72–77, ISSN 0378-8741.

Chamberlain, C.E. (1993). Acute hemorrhagic gastritis. *Gastroenterol. Clin. North. Am.*. Vol. 22, No. 4, (December 1993), pp. 843–873, ISSN 0889-8553.

Chen, C.Y.; Chi, K.H.; George, R.W.; Cox, D.L.; Srivastava, A.; Rui Silva, M.& et al. (2006). Diagnosis of gastric syphilis by direct immunofluorescence staining and real-time PCR testing. *J. Clin. Microbiol.*, Vol. 44, No. 9 (September 2006), pp. 3452–3456, ISSN 1098-660X.

Chuthaputti, A.; Pattaloong, P.N.; Permpipat, U.& Techadamrongsin, Y. (1996). Study on antiemetic activity of Morinda citrifolia Fruits. *Thai Journal of Pharmaceutical Sciences*, Vol. 20, No. 3, (1996), pp. 195–202, ISSN 1948-2124.

Cover, T.L.; Krishna, U.S.; Israel, DA& Peek, R.M. Jr. (2003). Induction of gastric epithelial cell apoptosis by Helicobacter pylori vacuolating cytotoxin. *Cancer Res.*, Vol. 63, No. 5, (March 2003), pp. 951-957, ISSN 1538-7445.

Dadalioglu, I.& Evrendilek, G.A. (2004). Chemical compositions and antibacterial effects of essential oils of Turkish oregano (Origanum minutiflorum), bay laurel (Laurus nobilis), Spanish lavender (Lavandula stoechas L.), and fennel (Foeniculum vulgare) on common foodborne pathogens. *J. Agric. Food Chem.*, Vol. 52, No. 26, (December 2004), pp. 8255-8260, ISSN 1520-5118.

Dharmani, P.; Mishra, P.K.; Maurya, R.; Chauhan, V.S.& Palit, G. (2005). *Allophylus serratus*: A plant with potential anti-ulcerogenic activity. *Journal of Ethnopharmacol*, Vol. 99, No. 3, (July 2005), pp. 361-366, ISSN 0378-8741.

D'Argenio, G.; Mazzone, G.; Tuccillo, C.; Grandone, I.; Gravina, A.G.; Graziani, G.; Fogliano, V.& Romano, M. (2008). Apple polyphenol extracts prevent aspirin-induced damage to the rat gastric mucosa. *Br. J. Nutr.*, Vol. 100, No. 6, (December 2008), pp. 1228-1236, ISSN 1475-2662.

Das, K.C.& Das, C.K. (2002). Curcumin (diferuloylmethane), a singlet oxygen (1O2) quencher. *Biochem. Biophys. Res. Commun.*, Vol. 295, No. 1, (July 2002), pp. 62–66, ISSN 0006-291X.

Das, J.C.& Paul, N. (2007). Epidemiology and pathophysiology of Helicobacter pylori infection in children. Indian *Journal of Pediatrics*, Vol. 47, No., (March 2007), pp. 287-290, ISSN 0973-7693.

De las Heras, B.; Slowing, K.; Benedi, J.; Carretero, E.; Ortega, T.; Toledo, C.; Bermejo, P.; Iglesia, S.I.; Abad, M.J.; Gomez-Serranillos, P.; Liso, P.A.; Villar, A.& Chiriboga, X. (1998). Anti-inflammatory and antioxidant activity of plants used in traditional medicine in Ecuador. *Journal of Ethnopharmacology*, Vol. 61, No. 2, (June 1998), pp. 161–166, ISSN 0378-8741.

Deng, S.; Palu, A.K.; West, B.J.; Su, C.X.; Zhou, B.N.& Jensen, J.C. (2007). Lipoxygenase inhibitory constituents of the fruits of Noni (Morinda citrifolia) collected in Tahiti. *Journal of Natural Products*, Vol. 70, No. 5, (March 2007), pp. 859–862, ISSN 1520-6025.

Dohil, R.& Hassall, E. (2011). Gastritis, gastropathy and ulcer disease. In: *Pediatric Gastrointestinal and Liver Disease*, Kindle, pp. 277-292, ISBN 0721639240.

Drake, I.M.; Mapstone, N.P.; Schorah, C.J.; White, K.L.; Chalmers, D.M.; Dixon, M.F.& Axon, A.T. (1998). Reactive oxygen species activity and lipid peroxidation in Helicobacter pylori associated gastritis: relation to gastric mucosal ascorbic acid concentrations and effect of H. pylori eradication. *Gut*, Vol. 42, No. 6, (June 1998), pp. 768–771, ISSN 1468-3288.

Elseweidy, M.M.; Younis, N.N.; Amin, R.S.; Abdallah, F.R.; Fathy, A.M.& Yousif, Z.A. (2008). Effect of some natural products either alone or in combination on gastritis induced in experimental rats. *Dig Dis Sci.*, Vol. 53, No. 7, (March 2008), pp.1774-1784, ISSN 1573-2568.

Elseweidy, M.M.; Taha, M.M.; Younis, N.N.; Ibrahim, K.S.; Hamouda, H.A.; Eldosouky, M.A.; Soliman, H.& Ghate, S. (2010a). Pattern of gastritis as manipulated by current state of Helicobacter pylori infection. *International journal of biology and biomedical engineering,* Vol. 4, No. 1, (2010), pp. 1-9, ISSN 1998-4510.

Elseweidy. M.M.; Taha, M.M.; Younis, N.N.; Ibrahim, K.S.; Hamouda, H.A.; Eldosouky, M.A.& Soliman, H. (2010b). Gastritis induced by Helicobacter pylori infection in experimental rats. *Dig Dis Sci.*, Vol. 55, No. 10, (January 2010), pp. 2770-2777, ISSN 1573-2568.

El-Zimaity, H.M.T. (2007). Recent advances in the histopathology of gastritis. *Current Diagnostic Pathology,* Vol.13, No.4, (2007), pp. 340–348, ISSN 0968-6053.

Ferro-Luzzi, A.& Ghiselli, A. (1993). Protective aspects of the Mediterranean diet. *Adv. Exp. Med. Biol.*, Vol. 348, (1993), pp. 137–144, ISSN 0065-2598.

Ford, A.C.; Marwaha, A.; Lim, A.& Moayyedi, P. (2010). What is the prevalence of clinically significant endoscopic findings in subjects with dyspepsia? Systematic review and meta-analysis. *Clin. Gastroenterol. Hepatol.*, Vol. 8, No. 10, (October 2010), pp. 830-837, ISSN 1542-3565.

Freire, R.S.; Morais, S.M.; Catunda-Junior, F.E.& Pinheiro, D.C. (2005). Synthesis and antioxidant, anti-inflammatory and gastroprotector activities of anethole and related compounds. *Bioorg. Med. Chem.*, Vol. 13, No. 13, (July 2005), pp. 4353-4358, ISSN 0968-0896.

Freitas, C.S.; Baggio, C.H.; Finau, J.; Anginoni, M.; Pizzolatti, M.G.; Santos, A.R.& Marques, M.C. (2008). Inhibition of H+/K+ ATPase in the gastroprotective effect of Baccharis illinita DC. *Journal of Pharmacy and Pharmacology,* Vol. 60, No. 8, (August 2008), pp. 1105–1110, ISSN 2042-7158.

Galati, E. M.; Mondello, M. R.; Giuffrida, D.; Dugo, G.; Miceli, N.; Pergolizzi, S.& Taviano MF. (2003). Chemical characterization and biological effects of Sicilian Opuntia ficus indica (L.) Mill. fruit juice: antioxidant and antiulcerogenic activity. *Journal of Agricultural and Food Chemistry,* Vol. 51, No. 17, (August 2003), pp. 4903-4908, ISSN 1520-5118.

Garcia-Barrantes, P.M.& Badilla, B. (2011). Anti-ulcerogenic properties of *Quassia amara* L. (Simaroubaceae) standardized extracts in rodent models. *J Ethnopharmacol,* (Epub ahead of print), (February 2011), ISSN 0378-8741.

Garcia-Lafuente, A.; Guillamon, E.; Villares, A.; Rostagno, M.A.& Martinez J.A. (2009). Flavonoids as anti-inflammatory agents: implications in cancer and cardiovascular disease. *Inflammation Research,* Vol. 58, No. 3, (March 2009), pp. 537–552, ISSN 1420-908X.

Geetha, T.; Malhotra, V.; Chopra, K.& Kaur, I.P. (2005). Antimutagenic and antioxidant /prooxidant activity of quercetin. *Indian J Exp Biol,* Vol. 43, No. 1, (January 2005), pp. 61−67, ISSN 0019-5189.

Gerritsen M.E., Carley W.W., Ranges G.E., Shen C.P., Phan S.A., Ligon G.F., Perry C.A. (1995). Flavonoids inhibit cytokine-induced endothelial cell adhesion protein gene expression. *Am J Pathol,* Vol. 147, No. 2, (August 1995), pp. 278−292, ISSN 0887-8005.

Graziani, G.; D'Argenio, G.; Tuccillo, C.; Loguercio, C.; Ritieni, A.; Morisco, F.; Del Vecchio Blanco, C.; Fogliano, V.& Romano, M. (2005). Apple polyphenol extracts prevent damage to human gastric epithelial cells in vitro and to rat gastric mucosa *in vivo. Gut* Vol. 54, No. 2, (February 2005), pp. 193–200, ISSN1468-3288.

Guo, Z.; Vangapandu, S.; Sindelar, R.W.; Walker, L.A.& Sindelar, R.D. (2005). Biologically active quassinoids and their chemistry: potential lads for drug design. *Current Medicinal Chemistry*, Vol. 12, No. 2, (2005), pp. 173-190, ISSN 0929-8673.

Hamauzu, Y.; Forest, F.; Hiramatsu, K.& Sugimoto, M. (2007). Effect of pear (Pyrus communis L.) procyanidins on gastric lesions induced by HCl/ethanol in rats. *Food Chemistry*, Vol. 100, No. 1, (2007), pp. 255–263, ISSN 0308-8146.

Hamauzu, Y.; Yasui, H.; Inno, T.; Kume, C., & Omanyuda, M. (2005). Phenolic profile, antioxidant property, and anti-influenza viral activity of Chinese quince (Pseudocydonia sinensis Schneid.), quince (Cydonia oblonga Mill.), and apple (Malus domestica Mill.) fruits. *Journal of Agricultural and Food Chemistry*, Vol. 53, No. 4, (February 2005), pp. 928–934, ISSN 1520-5118.

Hariganesh, K.& Prathiba, J. (2000). Effect of dimethylglycine on gastric ulcers in rats. *Journal Pharmacy and Pharmacology*, Vol. 52, No. 12, (December 2000), pp. 1519–1522, ISSN 2042-7158.

Hayes, J. D., & McLellan, L. I. (1999). Glutathione and glutathione-dependent enzymes represent a co-ordinately regulated defense against oxidative stress. *Free Radical Research*, Vol. 31, No. 4, (October 1999), pp. 273–300, ISSN 1029-2470.

He, M.L.; Cheng, X.W.; Chen, J.K.& Zhou, T.S. (2006). Simultaneous determination of five major biological active ingredients in different parts of Gardenia jasminoides fruits by HPLC with diode-array detection. *Chromatographia*, Vol. 64, No. 11-12, (2006), pp. 713–717, ISSN 1612-1112.

Holtmann, G.; Adam, B.; Haag, S.; Collet, W.; Grunewald, E.& Windeck, T. (2003). Efficacy of artichoke leaf extract in the treatment of patients with functional dyspepsia: a six-week placebo-controlled, double-blind, multicentre trial. *Aliment. Pharmacol. Ther.*, Vol. 18, No. 11-12, (December 2003), pp. 1099-1105, ISSN 1365-2036.

Hsu, D. Z.; Chien, S. P.; Chen, K. T., & Liu, M. Y. (2007). The effect of sesamol on systemic oxidative stress and hepatic dysfunction in acutely iron-intoxicated mice. *Shock*, Vol. 28, No. 5, (November 2007), pp. 596–601, ISSN 1540-0514.

Hsu, D.-Z.; Chu, P.-Y.; Chandrasekaran, V.R.M.& Liu, M.-Y. (2009a). Sesame lignan sesamol protects against aspirin-induced gastric mucosal damage in rats. *Journal of functional foods*, Vol. 1, No. 4, 1 (2009) pp. 349–355, ISSN 1756-4646.

Hsu, D.Z.; Chu, P.Y.& Liu, M.Y. (2009b). Effect of sesame oil on acidified ethanol-induced gastric mucosal injury in rats. *JPEN J. Parenter Enteral Nutr.*, Vol. 33, No. 4, (February 2009), pp. 423-427, ISSN 1941-2444.

Ikeda, R.; Wada, M.; Nishigaki, T.& Nakashima, K. (2009). Quantification of coumarin derivatives in Noni (Morinda citrifolia) and their contribution of quenching effect on reactive oxygen species. *Food Chemistry*, Vol. 113, No. 4, (April 2009), pp. 1169–1172, ISSN 0308-8146.

Ishida, K.; Kojima, R.; Tsuboi, M.; Tsuda, Y.& Ito, M. (2010). Effects of Artichoke Leaf Extract on Acute Gastric Mucosal Injury in Rats. *Biol. Pharm. Bull.*, Vol. 33, No. 2, (February 2010), pp. 223-229, ISSN 1347-5215.

IUCN (2009). IUCN Red List of Threatened Species. Version 2009.1. <www.iucnredlist.org> (accessed 11.10.09).

Jaeschke, H., & Hasegawa, T. (2006). Role of neutrophils in acute inflammatory liver injury. *Liver International*, Vol. 26, No. 8, (October 2006), pp. 912–919, ISSN 1478-3231.

Jobin, C.; Bradham, C.A.; Russo, M.P.; Juma, B.; Narula, A.S.; Brenner, D.A.& Sartor, R.B. (1999). Curcumin blocks cytokine mediated NF-KB activation and proinflammatory gene expression by inhibiting inhibitory factor I-KB kinase activity. *J. Immunol.*, Vol. 163, No. 6, (Sep 1999), pp. 3474–3483, ISSN 1550-6606.

Joy, J.F.& Haber, S.L. (2007). Clinical uses of artichoke leaf extract. *Am. J. Health Syst. Pharm.*, Vol. 64, No. 18, (September 2007), pp. 1906-1909, ISSN 1079-2082.

Kasper, D.L.; Braunwald, E.; Fauci, A.& et al. (2006). Disorders of the gastrointestinal system. In: *Harrison's Principles of Internal Medicine: Companion Handbook*, McGraw-Hill, pp. 1855-1872, Retrieved from <http://books.mcgraw hill.com/medical/harrisons/index.html>.

Kaunitz, J.D. (1999). Barrier function of gastric mucus. *Keio Journal of Medicine*, Vol. 48, No. 2, (June 1999), pp. 63-68, ISSN 1880-1293.

Kekki, M.; Samloff, I.M.; Varis, K.& Ihamäki, T. (1991). Serum pepsinogen I and serum gastrin in the screening of severe atrophic corpus gastritis. *Scand J Gastroenterol*, Vol. 186, (1991),pp. 109-116 ISSN 1502-7708.

Khalil, M.L. (2006). Biological activity of bee propolis in health and disease. *Asian Pac. J. Cancer Prev.*, Vol. 7, No. 1, (January-March 2006), pp. 22-31, ISSN 1513-7368.

Kim, J.; Joo, H.S.; Kim, D.H.; Lim, H.; Kang, Y.H.& Kim, M.S. (2003).A case of gastric strongyloidiasis in a Korean patient. Korean. J. Parasitol., Vol. 41, No. 1, (March 2003), pp. 63–67, ISSN 0023-4001.

Kist M. (1991). Immunology of Helicobacter pylori in: Bj marshall , *HP in peptic ulceration and gastritis* . Blackwell.Sci.Boston 1991 :92-110, ISBN 04445-31815.

Laine, L.; Curtis, S.P.; Cryer, B.; Kaur, A.& Cannon, C.P. (2010). Risk factors for NSAID-associated upper GI clinical events in a long-term prospective study of 34 701 arthritis patients. *Aliment. Pharmacol. Ther.*, Vol. 32, No. 10, (November 2010), pp. 1240-1248, ISSN 1365-2036.

Lauwers, G.Y.; Fujita, H.; Nagata, K.& Shimizu, M. (2010). Pathology of non-Helicobacter pylori gastritis: extending the histopathologic horizons. *J. Gastroenterol.*, Vol. 45, No. 2, (December 2010), pp. 131–145, ISSN 1435-5922.

La Vecchia, C.& Tavani, A. (1998). Fruit and vegetables, and human cancer. *Eur. J. Cancer Prev.*, Vol. 7, No. 1, (February 1998), pp. 3–8, ISSN 1473-5709.

Lee, S.E.; Jang, H.S.; Song. H.J.; Hwang, W.K.; Sohn, U.D. (2009a). M1904 Downstream Signal Transduction Induced By Interleukin-1 Beta-Stimulated ROS Generation and Anti-Oxidative Effects of Quercetin-3-O-[beta]-D Glucuronopyranoside (QGC) in Feline Esophageal Epithelial Cells. *Gastroenterology*, Vol. 136, No. 5, (May), pp. A442−443, ISSN 0016-5085.

Lee, J.-H.; Lee, D.-U.& Jeong, C.-S. (2009b). Gardenia jasminoides Ellis ethanol extract and its constituents reduce the risks of gastritis and reverse gastric lesions in rats. *Food and Chemical Toxicology*, Vol. 47, No., 6 (February 2009), pp. 1127–1131, ISSN 0278-6915.

Le Marchand, L.; Murphy, S.P.; Hankin, J.H.; Wilkens LR, Kolonel LN. (2000). Intake of flavonoids and lung cancer. J. Natl. Cancer Inst., Vol. 92, No. 2, (January 2000), pp. 154–160, ISSN 0027-8874.

Levand, O.& Larson, H.O. (1979). Some chemical constituents of Morinda citrifolia. *Planta Medica*, Vol. 36, No. 2, (June 1979), pp. 186–187, ISSN 0032-0943.

Lewis D.A. (1989). Anti-inflammatory drugs from plant, marine sources. *Agents Actions*, Vol. 27, (1989), pp., Suppl 27: 3–373, 1989, ISSN 0065-4299.

Lima, Z.P.; Calvo, T.R.; Silva, E.F.; Pellizzon, C.H.; Vilegas, W.; Brito, A.R.; Bauab, T.M.& Hiruma-Lima, C.A. (2008). Brazilian medicinal plant acts on prostaglandin levels and Helicobacter pylori. *Journal of Medicinal Food,* Vol. 11, No. 4, (December 2008), pp. 701–708, ISSN 1557-7600.

López, J.A.& Pérez, J. (2008). Etnofarmacología y actividad biológica de *Quassia amara* (Simaroubaceae): estado de la cuestión. *Boletín Latinoamericano y del Caribe de Plantas Medicinales y Aromáticas,* Vol. 7, (2008), pp. 234-246, ISSN 0717-7917.

Mahattanadul, S.; Reanmongkol, W.; Yano, S.; Panichayupakaranant, P.; Phdoongsombut, N.& Tungsinmunkong, K. (2006). Preventive and curative effects of curcumin on the development of gastric inflammatory diseases in rats. *J. Nat. Med.,* Vol. 60, No. 3, (2006), pp. 191–197, ISSN 1861-0293.

Mahattanadul, S.; Ridtitid, W.; Nima, S.; Phdoongsombut, N.; Ratanasuwon, P.& Kasiwong, S. (2011). Effects of Morinda citrifolia aqueous fruit extract and its biomarker scopoletin on reflux esophagitis and gastric ulcer in rats. *Journal of Ethnopharmacology,* Vol. 134, No. 2, (December 2010), pp. 243-250, ISSN 0378-8741.

Marshall, J.B. (1993). Tuberculosis of the gastrointestinal tract and peritoneum. *Am. J. Gastroenterol.,* Vol. 88, No. 7, (July 1993), pp. 989–999, ISSN 0002-9270.

Mimica-Dukic, N.; Kujundzic, S.; Sokovic, M.& Couladis M. (2003). Essential oil composition and antifungal activity of Foeniculum vulgare Mill obtained by different distillation conditions. Phytother. Res., Vol. 17, No. 4, (April 2003), pp. 368-371, ISSN 1099-1573.

Min Y.S.; Lee S.E.; Hong S.T.; Kim H.S.; Choi B.-C.; Sim S.S.; Kyun W.W.& Sohn U.D. (2009). The Inhibitory Effect of Quercetin-3-O- β -D-Glucuronopyranoside on Gastritis and Reflux Esophagitis in Rats. Korean J Physiol Pharmacol., Vol. 13, No. 4, (August 2009), pp. 295-300, ISSN 1226-4512,

Moleiro, F.C.; Andreo, M.A.; Santos, R.C.S.; Moraes, T.M.; Rodrigues, C.M.; Carli, C.B.A.; Lopes, F.C.M.; Pellizzon, C.H.; Carlos, I.Z.; Bauabe, T.M.; Wagner Vilegas, W.& Hiruma-Lima, C.A. (2009). Mouriri elliptica: validation of gastroprotective, healing and anti-Helicobacter pylori effects. *Journal of Ethnopharmacology,* Vol. 123, No. 3, (April 2009), pp. 359–368, ISSN 0378-8741.

Monteiro, J.M.; Albuquerque, U.P.; Neto, E.M.F.L.; Araöujo, E.L.; Albuquerque, M.M.& Amorim, E.L.C. (2006). The effects of seasonal climate changes in the Caatinga on tannin levels in Myracrodruon urundeuva (Engl.) Fr. All. and Anadenanthera colubrina (Vell.) Brenan. *Brazilian Journal of Pharmacognosy,* Vol. 16, (2006), pp. 338–344, ISSN 0102-695X.

Moon, P.D.; Lee, B.H.; Jeong, H.J.; An, H.J.; Park, S.J.; Kim, H.R.; Ko, S.G.; Um, J.Y.; Hong, S.H.& Kim, H.M. (2007). Use of scopoletin to inhibit the production of inflammatory cytokines through inhibition of the IkB/NF-kB signal cascade in the human mast cell line HMC-1. *European Journal of Pharmacology,* Vol. 555, No. 2-3, (October 2006), pp. 218–225, ISSN 0014-2999.

Muralidharan, P.& Srikanth, J. (2009). Antiulcer activity of Morinda citrifolia Linn fruit extract. *Journal of Scientific Research,* Vol. 1, No. 2, (2009), pp. 345–352, ISSN 2070-0245.

Naito, Y.; Yoshikawa, T.; Matsuyama, K.; Yagi, N.; Arai, M.; Nakamura, Y.; Nishimura, S.; Yoshida, N.& Kondo M. (1995). Effects of oxygen radical scavengers on the quality of gastric ulcer healing in rats. *Journal of Clinical Gastroenterology*, Vol. 1, (1995), pp. S82–S86, ISSN 1539-2031.

Neu, B.; Randlkofer, P.; Neuhofer, M.; Voland, P.; Mayerhofer, A.; Gerhard, M.; Schepp, W.& Prinz, C. (2002). Helicobacter pylori induces apoptosis of rat gastric parietal cells. *American Journal of Physiology-Gastrointestinal and Liver Physiology*, Vol. 283, No. 2, (August 2002), pp. G309–G318, ISSN 1522-1547.

Nostro, A.; Cellini, L.; Di Bartolomeo, S.; Di Campli, E.; Grande, R.; Cannatelli, M.A.; Marzio, L.& Alonzo V. (2005). Antibacterial effect of plant extracts against Helicobacter pylori. *Phytotherapy Research*, Vol. 19, No. 3, (March 2005), pp. 198–202, ISSN 1099-1573.

Obst, B.; Wagner, S.; Sewing, K.F.& Beil, W. (2000). Helicobacter pylori causes DNA damage in gastric epithelial cells. *Carcinogenesis*, Vol. 21, No. 6, (June 2000), Vol. 21, No. 6, pp. 1111-1115, ISSN 1460-2180.

Odonnea, G.; Bourdy, G.; Beauchene, J.; Houel, E.; Stien, D.; Chevolot, L.& Deharo, E. (2007). From tonic-cups to bitter-cups: Kwasi bita beker from Suriname determination, past and present use of an ancient galenic artifact. *Journal of Ethnopharmacology*, Vol. 110, No. 2, (October 2006), pp. 318–322, ISSN 0378-8741.

Ohta, Y.; Kobayashi, T.& Ishiguro, I. (1999). Role of endogenous serotonin and histamine in the pathogenesis of gastric mucosal lesions in unanaesthetised rats with a single treatment of compound 48/80, a mast cell degranulator. *Pharmacol. Res.*, Vol. 39, No. 4, (April 1999), pp. 261–267, ISSN 1043-6618.

Okuda T. (2005). Systematics and health effects of chemically distinct tannins in medicinal plants. *Phytochemistry*, Vol. 66, No. 17, (September 2005), pp. 2012–2031, ISSN 0031-9422.

Osakabe, N.; Sanbongi, C.; Yamagishi, M.; Takizawa, T., & Osawa, T. (1998). Effects of polyphenol substances derived from Theobroma cacao on gastric mucosal lesion induced by ethanol. *Bioscience, Biotechnology and Biochemistry*, Vol. 62, No. 8, (August 1998), pp. 1535–1538, ISSN 1347-6947.

Owen, D.A. (2003). Gastritis and carditis. Mod. Pathol. Vol. 16, No. 4, (April 2003), pp. 325–341, ISSN 0893-3952.

Pathak, A.K.; Bhutani, M.; Nair, A.S.; Ahn, K.S.; Chakraborty, A.; Kadara, H.; Guha, S.; Sethi, G.& Aggarwal, B.B. (2007). Ursolic acid inhibits STAT3 activation pathway leading to suppression of proliferation and chemosensitization of human multiple myeloma cells. *Mol. Cancer Res.*, Vol. 5, No. 9, (September 2007), pp. 943–955, ISSN 1557-3125.

Perez-Garcia, F.; Adzet, T.& Canigueral, S. (2000). Activity of artichoke leaf extract on reactive oxygen species in human leukocytes. *Free Radic. Res.*, Vol. 33, No. 5, (November 20000), pp. 661-665, ISSN 1029-2470.

Pihan, G.; Regillo, C.& Szabo, S. (1987). Free radicals and lipid peroxidation in ethanol- or aspirin-induced gastric mucosal injury. *Digestion Disease Science*, Vol. 32, No. 12, (December 1987), pp. 1395–1401, ISSN 1573-2568.

Pu, H.F.; Huang, W.J.; Tseng, W.M.; Wang, S.W.; Liu, Y.W.; Doong, M.L.& Wang, P.S. (2004). Effects of juice from Morinda citrifolia (Noni) on gastric emptying in male rats. *Chinese Journal of Physiology*, Vol. 47, No. 4, (December 2004), pp. 169–174, ISSN 1469-7793.

Quilez, A.; Berenguer, B.; Gilardoni, G.; Souccar, C.; de Mendonca, S.; Oliveira, L.F.S.; Martin-Calero, M.J.& Vidari, G. (2010). Anti-secretory, anti-inflammatory and anti-Helicobacter pylori activities of several fractions isolated from Piper carpunya Ruiz & Pav. *Journal of Ethnopharmacology*, Vol. 128, No. 3, (February 2010), pp. 583–589, ISSN 0378-8741.

Rafatullah, S.; Tariq Al-Yahya, M.A.; Mossa, J.S.& Ageel, A.M. (1990). Evaluation of turmeric (Curcuma longa) for gastric and duodenal antiulcer activity in rats. *J. Ethnopharmacol.*, Vol. 29, No. 1, (April 1990), pp. 25–34, ISSN 0378-8741.

Rice-Evans, C.A.; Miller, N.J.& Paganga, G. (1996). Structure-antioxidant activity relationships of flavonoids and phenolic acids. *Free Radic Biol Med*, Vol. 20, No. 7, (1996), pp. 933–956, ISSN 0891-5849.

Rothenberg, M.E. (2004). Eosinophilic gastrointestinal disorders (EGID). *J. Allergy Clin. Immunol.*, Vol. 113, No. 1, (January 2004), pp. 11–28, ISSN 0091-6749.

Roukos, D.H.; Paraskevaidis, E.; Agnantis, N.J.; Kappas AM. (2003). Fruits and vegetables: do they protect from gastric cancer? *Gastroenterology*, Vol. 124, No. 7, (June 2003), pp. 2006–2007, ISSN 0016-5085.

Rugge, M.& Genta, R.M. (2005). Staging and grading of chronic gastritis. *Hum. Pathol.*,Vol. 36, No. 3, (March 2005), pp. 228-233, ISSN 0046-8177.

Saito, M.; Hosoyama, H.; Ariga, T.; Kataoka, S., & Yamaji, N. (1998). Antiulcer activity of grape seed extract and procyanidins. *Journal of Agricultural and Food Chemistry*, Vol. 46, No. 4, (March 1998), pp. 1460–1464, ISSN 1520-5118.

Salim A.S. (1990). Removing oxygen-derived free radicals stimulates healing of ethanol-induced erosive gastritis in the rat. *Digestion*, Vol. 47, No. 1, (1990), pp. 24–28, ISSN 0012-2823.

Samoylenko, V.; Zhao, J.; Dunbar, D.C.; Khan, I.A.; Rushing, J.W.& Muhammad, I. (2006). New constituents from Noni (Morinda citrifolia) fruit juice. *Journal of Agricultural and Food Chemistry*, Vol. 54, No. 17, (August 2006), pp. 6398–6402, ISSN 1520-5118.

Sanchez, G.M.; Rodriguez, H.M.A.; Giuliani, A.; Nunez Selles, A.J.; Rodriguez, N.P.; Leon Fernandez, O.S.& Re, L. (2003). Protective effect of *Mangifera indica* L. extract (Vimang) on the injury associated with hepatic ischaemia reperfusion. *Phytotherapy Research*, Vol. 17, No. 3, (March 2003), pp. 197–201, ISSN 1099-1573.

Santos, C.S.; Costa, W.F.; Ribeiro, J.P.; Guimarães, D.O.; Ferri, P.H.; Ferreira, H.D.; Seraphin, J.C. (2002). Tannin composition of barbatimao species. *Fitoterapia*, Vol. 73, No. 4, (July 2002), pp. 292–299, ISSN 0367-326X.

Satoh, K.; Osawa, H.; Yoshizawa, M.; Nakano, H.; Hirasawa, T.; Kihira, K.& Sugano K. (2008). Assessment of Atrophic Gastritis Using the OLGA System. *Helicobacter*, Vol. 13, No. 3, (June 2008), pp. 225–229, ISSN 1523-5378.

Savino, F.; Cresi, F.; Castagno, E.; Silvestro, L.& Oggero, R. (2005). A randomized double-blind placebo-controlled trial of a standardized extract of Matricariae recutita, Foeniculum vulgare and Melissa officinalis (ColiMil) in the treatment of breastfed colicky infants. *Phytother. Res.*, Vol. 19, No. 4, (April 2005), pp. 335-340, ISSN 1099-1573.

Selles, N.A.J.; Castro, H.T.V.; Aguero-Aguero, J.; Gonzalez, J.; Nadeo, F.; De Simone, F.& Rastelli, L. (2002). Isolation and quantitative analysis of phenolic antioxidants, free sugars, and polyols from mango (*Mangifera indica* L.) stem bark aqueous decoction used in Cuba as a nutritional supplement. *Journal of Agriculture Food and Chemistry*, Vol. 50, No. 4, (February 2002), pp. 762–766, ISSN 1520-5118.

Sepulveda, A.R.& Patil, M. (2008). Practical approach to the pathologic diagnosis of gastritis. *Arch. Pathol. Lab. Med.*, Vol 132, No. 10, (October 2008), pp. 1586-1593, ISSN 0003-9985.

Shacter, E.& Weitzman, S.A. (2002). Chronic inflammation and cancer. *Oncology (Williston Park)*, Vol. 16, No. 2, (February 2002), pp. 217-226, 229; discussion 230-232, ISSN 0354-7310.

Shishodia, S.; Majumdar, S.; Banerjee, S.& Aggarwal, B.B. (2003). Ursolic acid inhibits nuclear factor-kappaB activation induced by carcinogenic agents through suppression of IkappaBalpha kinase and p65 phosphorylation: correlation with down-regulation of cyclooxygenase 2, matrix metalloproteinase 9, and cyclin D1. *Cancer Res.*, Vol. 63, No. 15, (August 2003), pp. 4375–4383, ISSN 1538-7445.

Sidhu, G.S.; Singh, A.K.; Thaloor, D.; Banaudha, K.K.; Patnaik, G.K.; Srimal, R.C.& Maheshwari, R.K. (1998). Enhancement of wound healing by curcumin in animals. *Wound Repair Regen.*, Vol. 6, No. 2, (March-april 1998), pp. 167–177, ISSN 1524-475X.

Silva, M.S.; Antoniolli, A.R.; Batista, J.S.& Mota, C.N. (2006). Plantas medicinais usadas nos distuórbios do trato gastrintestinal no povoado Colônia Treze, Lagarto, SE, Brasil. *Acta botanica brasilica,* Vol. 20, (2006), pp. 815–829, ISSN 1677-941X.

Silva, N.C.B.; Esquibel, M.A.; Alves, I.M.; Velozo, E.S.; Almeida, M.Z.; Santos, J.E.S.; Campos-Buzzi, F.; Meira, A.V.& Cechinel-Filho V. (2009). Antinociceptive effects of Abarema cochliacarpos (B.A. Gomes) Barneby & J. W. Grimes (Mimosaceae). *Brazilian Journal of Pharmacognosy*, Vol. 19, No. 1A, (February 2009), pp. 46–50, ISSN 0102-695X.

da Silva, M.S.; Sanchez-Fidalgo, S.; Elena Talero, E.; Cardeno, A.; da Silva, M.A.; Vilegas, W.; Souza Brito, A.R.M.& de La Lastra, C.A. (2010a). Anti-inflammatory intestinal activity of Abarema cochliacarpos (Gomes) Barneby & Grimes in TNBS colitis model. *Journal of Ethnopharmacology*, Vol. 128, No. 18, (January 2010), pp. 467–475, ISSN 0378-8741.

da Silva, M.S.; de Almeida, A.C.A.; de Faria, F.M.; Luiz-Ferreira, A.; da Silva, M.A.; Vilegas, W.; Pellizzon, C.H.& Souza Brito A. R. M. (2010b). Abarema cochliacarpos: Gastroprotective and ulcer-healing activities. *Journal of Ethnopharmacology*, Vol. 132, No. 1, (August 2010), pp. 134–142, ISSN 0378-8741.

Shikov, A.N.; Pozharitskaya, O.N.; Makarov, V.G.& Kvetnaya, A.S. (2008). Antibacterial activity of Chamomilla recutita oil extract against Helicobacter pylori. *Phytotherapy Research*, Vol. 22, No. 2, (February 2008), pp. 252–253, ISSN 1099-1573.

Singh, U.P.; Singh, D.P.; Singh, M.; Maurya, S.; Srivastava, J.S.; Singh, R.B.& Singh, S.P. (2004). Characterization of phenolic compounds in some Indian mango cultivars. *International Journal of Food Science and Nutrition*, Vol. 55, No. 2, (March 2004), pp. 163–169, ISSN 1465-3478.

Soltermann, A.; Koetzer, S.; Eigenmann, F.& Komminoth, P. (2007). Correlation of Helicobacter pylori virulence genotypes vacA and cagA with histological parameters of gastritis and patient's age. *Mod. Pathol.*, Vol. 20, No. 8, (August 2007), pp. 878-883, ISSN 0893-3952.

Souza, M. H.; Mota, J. M.; Oliveira, R. B., & Cunha, F. Q. (2008). Gastric damage induced by different doses of indomethacin in rats is variably affected by inhibiting iNOS or leukocyte infiltration. Inflammation Research, Vol. 57, No. 1, (January 2008), pp. 28–33, ISSN 1420-908X.

Speroni, E.; Cervellati, R.; Govoni, P.; Guizzardi, S.; Renzulli, C.& Guerra, M.C. (2003). Efficacy of different Cynara scolymus preparations on liver complaints. J. Ethnopharmacol., Vol. 86, No. 2-3 , (June 2003), pp. 203-211, ISSN 0378-8741.

Srivastava, A.& Lauwers, G.Y. (2007). Pathology of non-infective gastritis. *Histopathology* Vol.50, No.1, (2007), pp. 15–29, ISSN 1365-2559.

Staroverov, V.V.; Kisel, A.T.; Sumarokov, U.A.& Kachanova, T.N. (2001). A case of phlegmonous gastritis diagnosed by echography. *Eur. J. Ultrasound.*, Vol. 13, No. 3 , (July 2001), pp. 197–200, ISSN 0929-8266.

Takeeda, M.; hayahic, Y.; murkams, M.& Takeuchi, K. (2004). roles of endogenous prostaglandins , cycloxygenase enzyme in mucosal defense of inflamed rat stomach. *J. physiology and pharmacology*, Vol. 55, No. 1, (2004), pp. 193-205, ISSN 0867-5910.

Tari, A.; Kodama, K.; Kitadai, Y.; Ohta, M.; Sumii, K.& Kajiyama, G. (2003). Is apoptosis in antral mucosa correlated with serum nitrite concentration in Japanese Helicobacter pylori-infected patients? *J Gastroenterol Hepatol.*, Vol. 18, No. 5, (May 2003), pp.498-504, ISSN 1440-1746.

Thirumurthi, S.& Lanza, F.L. (2010). Gastritis, In: *GI/Liver Secrets Plus* ,Peter R. McNally,pp. 63-67, Mosby Elsevier, ISBN 978-0-323-06397-5, Philadelphia.

Tokusoglu, O.; Yildirim, Z., & Yemis, F. (2003). Some functional properties as gelation, water and oil absorption, emulsion capacity, and foaming stability of sesame seed (Sesamum indicum L.) spreads. *Turkish Journal of Field Crops*, Vol. 8, (2003), pp. 15–21, ISSN 1303-6173.

Toma, W.; Gracioso, J.; Pezzuto, F.D.; Hiruma-Lima, C.A.; Vilegas, W.& Monteiro, A.R. (2002). Antiulcerogenic activity of four extracts obtained from the Bark Wood of *Quassia amara* L. (Simaroubaceae). *Biological & Pharmaceutical Bulletin*, Vol. 25, No. 9, (September 2002), pp. 1151-1155, ISSN 1347-5215.

Tordera, M.; Ferrandiz, M.L.& Alcaraz, M.J. (1994). Influence of antiinflammatory flavonoids on degranulation and arachidonic acid release in rat neutrophils. *Zeitschrift fur Naturforschung [C]*, Vol. 49, No. 3-4, (March-April 1994), pp. 235–240, ISSN 0932-0784.

Trabadela, C.; Sanchez-Fidalgo, S.; Mino, P.; Berenguer, B.; Quilez, A.; de la Puerta, R.& Martin, M.J. (2009). Gastroprotective effects of Piper carpunya against diclofenac-induced gastric lesions in rats. *Pharmaceutical Biology*, Vol. 46, No. 12, (February 2009), pp. 829–837, ISSN 1744-5116.

Tseng, T.H.; Chu, C.Y.; Huang, J.M.; Shiow, S.J.& Wang, C.J. (1995). Crocetin protects against damage in rat primary hepatocytes. *Cancer Lett.*, Vo. 97, No. 1, (October 1995), pp. 61–67, ISSN 0304-3835.

Väänänen, H.; Vauhkonen, M.; Helske, T.; Kääriäinen, I.; Rasmussen, M.; Tunturi-Hihnala, H.; Koskenpato, J.; Sotka, M.; Turunen, M.; Sandström, R.; Ristikankare, M.; Jussila, A.& Sipponen, P. (2003). Non-endoscopic diagnosis of atrophic gastritis with a blood test. Correlation between gastric histology and serum levels of gastrin-17 and pepsinogen I: a multicentre study. *Eur J Gastroenterol Hepatol.*, Vol. 15, No. 8, (August 2003),pp. 885-891, ISSN1440-1746.

Walsh, J.H.; Isenberg, J.I.; Ansfield, J.& Maxwell, V. (1976). Clearance and acid-stimulating action of human big and little gastrins in duodenal ulcer subjects. *J Clin Invest.*, Vol. 57, No. 5, (May 1976), pp. 1125-1131, ISSN 0021-9738.

Weck, M.N.; Gao, L.& Brenner, H. (2009). Helicobacter pylori infection and chronic atrophic gastritis: associations according to severity of disease. *Epidemiology*, Vol. 20, No. 4, (July 2009), pp. 569-574, ISSN 1531-5487 .

Williams, R.J.; Spencer, J.P.& Rice-Evans, C. (2004a). Flavonoids: antioxidants or signalling molecules? *Free Radic Biol Med*, Vol. 36, No. 7, (April 2004), pp. 838–849, ISSN 0891-5849.

Williams, R.J.; Spencer, J.P.E.& Rice-Evans Catherine (2004b). Serial review: flavonoids and isoflavones (Phytoestrogens): absorption, metabolism, and bioactivity. flavonoids: antioxidants or signalling molecules? *Free Radical Biology & Medicine*, Vol. 36, No. 11, (August 2004), pp. 838–849, ISSN 0891-5849.

Xiao, Z.P.; Shi, D.H.; Li, H.Q.; Zhang, L.N.; Xu, C.& Zhu, H.L. (2007). Polyphenols based on isoflavones as inhibitors of Helicobacter pylori urease. *Bioorganic & Medicinal Chemistry*, Vol. 15, No. 11, (June 2007), pp. 3703–3710, ISSN 0968-0896.

Xin, W.& Greenson, J.K. (2004). The clinical significance of focally enhanced gastritis. *Am. J. Surg. Pathol.*, Vol. 28, No 10., (October 2004), pp. 1347–1351, ISSN 1532-0979.

Yano, S.; Terai, M.; Shimizu, K.L.; Futagami, Y.; Horie, S.; Tsuchiya, S.; Ikegami, F.; Sekine, T.; Takamoto, K.; Saito, K.; Ueno, K.& Watanabe, K. (2000). Antiallergic activity of Curcuma longa (II) features of inhibitory actions on histamine release from mast cells. *Nat. Med.*, Vol. 54, No. 6, (2000), pp. 325–329, ISSN1861-0293.

Yue, G.; Lai, P.S.; Yin, K.; Sun, F.F.; Nagele, R.G.; Liu, X.; Linask, K.K.; Wang, C.; Lin K.T.& Wong, P.Y. (2001). Colon epithelial cell death in 2,4,6-trinitrobenzenesulfonic acid-induced colitis is associated with increased inducible nitric-oxide synthase expression and peroxynitrite production. *J Pharmacol Exp Ther.*, Vol. 297, No. 3, (June 2001), pp. 915-925, ISSN 1521-0103.

Zalewska-Ziob, M.; Adamek, B.; Strzelczyk, J.K.; Gawron, K.; Jarzab, B.; Gubala, E.; Kula, D.; Krakowczyk, Ł.; Sieroń, A.& Wiczkowski, A. (2009). TNF-alpha expression in gastric mucosa of individuals infected with different virulent Helicobacter pylori strains. *Med. Sci. Monit.*, Vol. 15, No. 6, (June 2009), pp. BR166-171, ISSN 1643-3750.

9

New Approaches in Gastritis Treatment

Guillermo Marcial, Cecilia Rodríguez,
Marta Medici and Graciela Font de Valdez
Centro de Referencia para Lactobacilos (CERELA-CONICET)
Argentina

1. Introduction

Gastritis is an inflammation of the stomach lining, which is fairly common and could have different causes. Many kind of agents may lead the stomach into an inflamed statement; in first place, it could be due to *non-steroidal anti-inflammatory drugs* (NSAID) such as aspirin, ibuprofen, naproxen, etc. (Fig. 1), which are used in different treatments to calm down some specific illness, e.g. rheumatoid arthritis; in second place, inflamation could be due to abrasive compounds (alcohol, acids and others) or unbalanced diets where the stomach is damaged by its own gastric acid; in third place, long-term physical and/or mental stress that result in the production of excessive amounts of stomach acid; in last place, the infection caused by a well-known microorganism, *Helicobacter (H) pylori*. When stomach inflammation is not treated, mainly in the latter case, the illness could end in a gastric ulcer or in the worst case, in gastric cancer.

The signs and symptoms of gastritis depend on how long the problem has existed. If it occurs suddenly is called *acute gastritis*. In acute phase, superficial inflammation of the stomach causes the classic nausea and pain or discomfort in the upper abdomen. If it develops gradually is called *chronic gastritis*, and the symptoms might vary from those of acute, with a dull pain in the upper abdomen and a feeling of fullness and loss of appetite after a few bites of food. However, in some cases, people with chronic gastritis could not feel any of these symptoms. Another type is the *reactive or chemical gastritis*, which is defined as a foveolar elongation, tortuosity, and hypercellularity of the gastric surface epithelium, together with edema, vasodilatation, congestion of gastric lamina propria, and a paucity of inflammatory cells. This type of gastritis has been thought to result from duodenogastric bile reflux or the use of NSAIDs (Voutilainen et. al., 2002).

Clinicians differ on classification of the less common and specific forms of gastritis, particularly since there are so much overlap with *H. pylori* in development of chronic gastritis and its complications. Other types of gastritis that may be diagnosed include: a) *Acute stress gastritis*, the most serious form of gastritis which usually occurs in critical ill patients, such as those in intensive care, where stress erosions may develop suddenly as a result of severe trauma or stress to the stomach lining; b) *Atrophic gastritis*, resulting from chronic gastritis which is leading to atrophy, or decrease in size and wasting away of the gastric lining. Gastric atrophy is the final stage of chronic gastritis and may be a precursor of gastric cancer; c) *Superficial gastritis* is a term often used to describe the initial stages of chronic gastritis; d) *Uncommon specific forms of gastritis* include granulomatous, eosiniphilic and lymphocytic gastritis (Sipponen & Price, 2011).

A recent advance in the histopathology of gastritis is the replacement of the traditional definition of gastric atrophy, "loss of glands", with the new definition of gastric atrophy as the "loss of appropriate glands". By this definition, intestinalized glands represent atrophy when the metaplastic change involves the entire length of the original glandular unit and is considered as metaplastic atrophy. The application of the new definition has resulted in a high level of agreement among gastrointestinal pathologists trained in different cultural contexts. As there is obvious evidence that the severity and the extent of gastric atrophy relate to different risk levels of gastric cancer, an international group of gastroenterologists and pathologists, *Operative Link on Gastritis Assessment* (OLGA), has developed a system of histologically reporting gastritis by combining the semi-quantitative scoring scale of the updated Sydney system (Stolte & Meining, 2001) with the new definition of gastric atrophy. This system expresses the extent of gastric atrophy in terms of gastritis staging (Quach et. al., 2011).

Nowadays, one of the most important cases of gastritis is the infection by *H. pylori* strains. This affection was the attention focus that led to many researchers in the last years to study different branches of the infection process (Chenoll et. al.; 2011; Cui et. al., 2010; Ko et. al., 2010; Wittschier et. al., 2009; Wolle & Malfertheiner, 2007). However, equal important is the gastritis associated to the consumption of NSAIDs since these drugs are widely used to treat some pains. The chronic use of NSAIDs is a common cause of gastroduodenal erosions and peptic ulcers resulting, in many cases, in fatal haemorrhage. Aspirin, a famous NSAID, is thought to cause gastric damage by both, topical irritant effects on the gastric epithelium and systemic effects related to suppression of mucosal prostaglandin synthesis (Fig. 1). Inhibition of prostaglandin synthesis reduces mucosal defenses, including mucus and bicarbonate secretion, blood flow, epithelial cell turnover and repair, and mucosal immunocyte function. NSAIDs can also interfere with the healing of preexisting lesions and cause a fast drop in pH within the mucus cap (Shiotani et. al., 2008). In clinical practice, a prostaglandin E_1 derivative, misoprostol, and anti-acids, including proton pump inhibitors (PPIs) are routinely used for the treatment and prevention of NSAID enteropathy (Peura, 2004). The authors previously reported the usefulness of PPIs for healing the small intestinal mucosal injury in experimental animal models treated with NSAID; however, there are no clinical data on the usefulness of PPIs in such injuries. Some studies indicated the efficacy of misoprostol on NSAID-induced intestinal injuries (Kuroda et. al., 2006) whereas others reported no effectiveness (Davies et. al., 1993).

Among the most conventional drugs employed, PPIs such as omeprazole (OPZ) and its derivates are the most common although most of these drugs produce undesirable side effects and drug interactions (Pali-Schöll et. al., 2010, 2011). OPZ is available over-the-counter and in inexpensive generic formulations. It is promoted as a therapy for a range of disease states, from mild heartburn to aggressive *H. pylori* gastritis (40 mg can suppress over 80% of gastric acid secretion) being also one component of the triple-agent therapy (clarithromycin, amoxicillin, omeprazole) that is commonly used to eradicate *H. pylori* infection (Logan et. al., 1995). However, it is increasingly well-recognized that OPZ may also contribute to gastric gland toxicity, effect demonstrated by Kohler et. al. (2010) in rabbit gastric gland at physiologically relevant doses. Data suggest that thiol oxidation negatively affects intracellular proteins, which are susceptible to this chemical reaction. Authors also evinced that OPZ toxicity can be reversed with Vitamin C, thus providing an explanation for the previously observed benefits of Vitamin C co-administrated with OPZ in *H. pylori* gastritis (Kohler et. al., 2010).

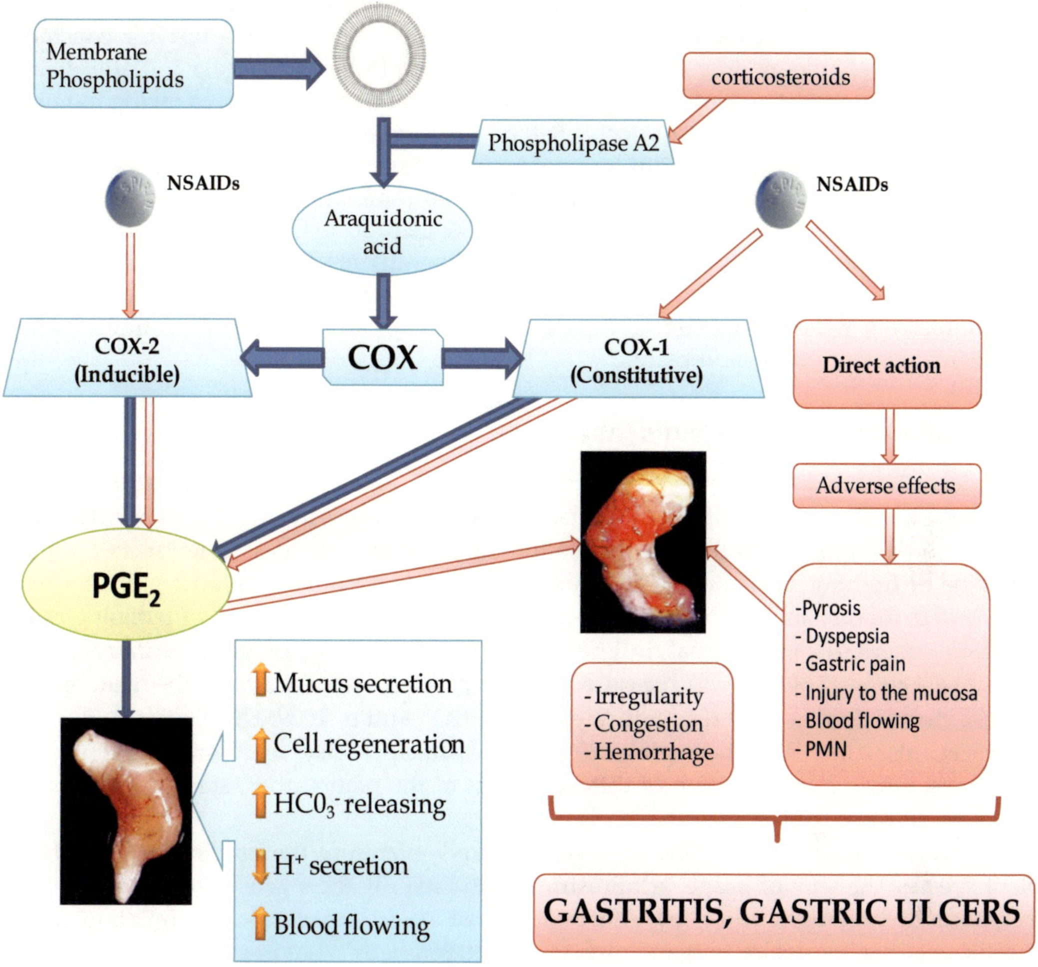

Fig. 1. Deleterious effects of NSAIDs after administration for long periods. Normal levels of PGE_2 helps gastric mucosa in keeping its normal characteristics. The intake of NSAIDs for long periods blocks the PGE_2 generating unbalance in the process and situations of cytotoxicity. These conditions lead gastric mucosa to be unhealthy and to come into gastritis process.

Anti-ulcer drugs are useful co-medications to protect the gastric mucosa from damage due to steroidal and non-steroidal drugs. This is especially relevant during long-term pain and anti-inflammatory therapies, e.g. in management of rheumatoid arthritis or inflammatory bowel disease. Inhibition or neutralization of gastric acid with so-called anti-ulcer drugs is necessary to treat gastritis and peptic ulcers, e.g. drugs such as PPIs, histamine type-2 receptor antagonist, sucralfate, or acid neutralizers like bismuth compounds (co-prescribed to protect the gastric mucosa). The therapy goal is to reach gastric pH levels above 4.5 (Julapalli & Graham, 2005) also for children (Tofil et. al., 2008) or even above 6.0 for treating bleeding

peptic ulcers (Pali-Schöll et. al., 2010). Avoidance of acid is needed to stop autodigestive processes and support mucosal healing in the extreme environment of the gastric lumen.
The success rate of conventional eradication of triple therapy is *ca.* 80% but it is constantly decreasing worldwide, mainly due to *H. pylori* antibiotic resistance (Wolle & Malfertheiner, 2007). In addition to the cost of the treatment, this kind of therapy involves taking too many drugs, which might cause side effects. Before the recognition of *H. pylori* as the main ethiological agent of chronic gastritis and peptic ulcer disease, research studies were focused on the gastroprotective, and/or anti-acid, and/or anti-inflammatory effects of traditional medicinal plants and their mode of action (Borrelli & Izzo, 2000; Castillo-Juarez et. al., 2009). Nowadays, studies of natural products in gastritis therapy have become the main research area around the world. The novel therapies include natural compounds or their derivates co-administered whith conventional drugs. These biological and natural products include beneficial microorganisms and plants.

2. Phytotherapy on gastric diseases

Plant derivates had been employed by population to prevent different kind of diseases for centuries. The knowledge of plant properties was acquired by ancient civilization that passed down from generation to generation until today and it is known as "popular medicine or traditional medicine" (Al-Qura´n, 2009). The number of plants species around the world is infinite and medicinal plants are used to treat different kind of pathologies like infection, internal and external inflammatory process, dermatological, urinary/genital, parasitosis, hemorrhoids, blood pressure, diabetic problems, etc., although the main usage is against gastrointestinal and respiratory problems (Al-Qura´n, 2009; De la Cruz et. al., 2007; Neves et. al., 2009; Rehecho et. al., 2010). The principal way of administration is like beverages, infusion or decoction of different parts of the plants (root, stem, seed, rhizome, bark, leaf, flowers, fruit or mixtures).
The surveys of popular medicine are useful to understanding the application of different plant species, the way of usage, administration and mainly their properties. In some cases, this kind of beverages could be effective against gastric mucosal inflammation (active chronic gastritis, erosive or not) and also against *H. pylori*, thus having antimicrobial activity besides anti-inflammatory effects. *Asteraceae* and *Lamiaceae* families are mainly used as gastroprotector, but at the same time they are also used against other diseases as wound healing, analgesic and anti-inflammatory. Most studies addressed the gastroprotector effect of different plants extracts in experimental models, e.g., gastritis (mucosal inflammation and mucosal infectious model), ulcers and even advanced processes like cancer model (De la Cruz et. al., 2007; Nergard et. al., 2004).
Beverages are known in different cultures as "tea". The *tea* is the extract obtained after maintaining raw plant materials in contact with hot water during certain time (the methodology could change if it is infusion or decoction, where decoction is an aggressive process of extraction). In this extract it is possible to find different compounds like polyphenols, flavonoids (glycosilated or not) and polysaccharides among others, that could interact with the mucosal barrier cells by changing the cell metabolism and modifying the cellular regulation; they could also display anti-*H. pylori* activity (Coşkun et. al., 2004; Formica & Regelson, 1995; Kahraman et. al., 2003; Lengsfeld et. al., 2004). Examples of some medicine plants against gastric disorders are presented in Table 1.

MEDICINAL PLANTS USED IN GASTRIC DISEASES AROUND THE WORLD							
Family	**Plant species**	**Common name**	**Part used**	**Mode of using**	**Traditional uses**	**Country/ region**	**References**
Acanthaceae	*Dicliptera peruviana* (Lam.) Juss.	Chuncho-chuncho (Q)	Leaves	Infusion	Stomachache	Perú (Canta, Lima)	De la Cruz et. al., 2007
Asteraceae	*Ageratum conyzoides* L.	-	Leaves	Infusion/ Decoction	Purgative, gastric ulcers, wound healing	West Africa, Asia and South America	Shirwaikar et. al., 2003
	Carlina acaulis L.	Caroelina (I)	Roots	Decoction	Stomachache	Italy (Valvestino)	Vitalini et. al., 2009
	Tagetes elliptica Smith	Chinche (S)	Leaves	Decoction	Stomachache, intestinal pain, digestive	Perú (Canta, Lima)	De la Cruz et. al., 2007
	Tagetes filifolia Lag.	Anis Serrano (S)	Aerial parts	Decoction	Stomachache, intestinal pain	Perú (Ancash)	Hammond et. al., 1998
	Vernonia kotschyana Sch.	-	Roots	Decoction, cold macerate	Gastrointestinal disorders, gastritis and gastroduodenal ulcers	Mali	Nergard et. al., 2004
Brassicaceae	*Brassica carinata* A. Braun.	Koza (ET)	Leaves	-	Gastritis	Ethiopia (Sheko)	Giday et. al., 2010
	Brassica nigra (L.) W.D.J.Koch	-	Seeds	-	Stomachache	Ethiopia (Sheko)	Giday et. al., 2010
Celastraceae	*Maytenus ilicifolia* Mart.	Espinheira santa (P)	Leaves	Infusion	Contraceptive, abortifacient, emenagogue, stomach disorders	Argentina, Brazil, Paraguay	Hatsuko Baggio et. al., 2007
Compositae	*Achillea tomentosa* L.	Mifoil (E)	Aerial parts	Infusion	Stomachache	Jordan (Showbak)	Al-Qura'n et. al., 2009
	Croton cajucara Benth	Sacaca (P)	Leaves barks	Infusion	Antiulcerogenic, gastrointestinal disorders	Brazil	Hiruma-Lima et. .al., 2000
Euphorbiaceae	*Jatropha isabelli* Muell.	Yagua rova (G)	Rhi-zome	Infusion/ Decoction	Gastroprotective	Paraguay, Argentina	Pertino et. al., 2007
Geraniaceae	*Geranium molle* L.	Erva de S. Roberto, Bico de pinga amor (P)	Aerial parts, roots	-	Stomach acidity and stomachache, cancer treatment, uterus inflammation	Portugal (Trás-os-Montes)	Neves et. al., 2009
	Pelargonium sidoides DC	Umckaloabo (A)	Roots	-	Antimicrobial effects	Southern Africa	Wittschier et. al., 2007
	Pelargonium roseum (Andrews)	Geranio (S)	Leaves	Infusion/ decoction	Digestive, carminative, gastritis,	Perú (Nor-Yauyos)	Elmann et. al. 2010; Rehecho et. al., 2010

MEDICINAL PLANTS USED IN GASTRIC DISEASES AROUND THE WORLD							
Family	**Plant species**	**Common name**	**Part used**	**Mode of using**	**Traditional uses**	**Country/ region**	**References**
	W.T.Aiton				amigdalitis, hemorrhagias of the gastro-intestinal tube, others		
Krameriaceae	*Krameria lappacea* (dombey) Burdet et B. Simpson	Ratanya or Ratiñay (Q)	Roots, stems	Decoction	Diarrhea, inflammation, treatment of stomach cancer	Perú (Ancash)	Hammond et. al., 1998; De la Cruz et. al., 2007
Lamiaceae	*Glechoma hederacea* L.	Malvela, redondinha (P)	Aerial parts	-	Cough, stomach pain, gastritis and acidity, diarrhoea, renal problems, others	Portugal (Trás-os-Montes)	Neves et. al., 2009
Lamiaceae	*Melissa officinalis* L.	Cidreira (P)	Aerial parts	-	Intestinal gases and pain, digestion and bile stimulation, stomachache and gastritis, others.	Portugal (Trás-os-Montes)	Neves et. al., 2009
	Mentha piperita L.	Hortelão, Piperita, Pimenta (P); Menta (S)	Green leaves	Infusion	Digestive and antiflatulence to relieve gastritis, dyspepsia and biliar disorders, analgesic, rheuma, others	Portugal (Trás-os-Montes); Perú (Nor-Yauyos)	Neves et. al., 2009; Rehecho et. al., 2010
	Minthostachys mollis (Kunth.) Griseb.	Muña (S)	Leaves	Infusion	Digestive, carminative, emolient ,diuretic, to treat diarrhea, gastritis and colics, others	Perú (Nor-Yauyos)	Rehecho et. al., 2010; Schmidt-Lebuhn, 2008; De la Cruz et. al., 2007
	Marrubium vulgare L.	Mala mujer (S)	Leaves, stems	Infusion	Stomachache	Perú (Canta, Lima)	De la Cruz et. al., 2007
	Ocimun suave Willd	Olomora (A)	Leaves	Oil	Gastric ulcers, anti-cathartic, fever, stomachache	Tropical Asia ; west and east Africa	Tan et. al., 2002
Fabaceae	*Glycyrrhiza glabra* L.	Liquorice (E)	Roots	Syrup	Diuretic, gastric ulcer, expectorant	Mediterranean region, Asia Minor and Middle East	Al-Qura'n et. al., 2009; Wittschier et. al., 2009
Malvaceae	*Althaea rosea* (L.) Cav.	Rose mallow (E); Alteia (P)	Aerial parts, roots	Infusion	Abdominal inflammation, cough, colitis and	Jordan (Showbak); Portugal	Al-Qura'n et. al., 2009; Neves et. al.,

MEDICINAL PLANTS USED IN GASTRIC DISEASES AROUND THE WORLD							
Family	**Plant species**	**Common name**	**Part used**	**Mode of using**	**Traditional uses**	**Country/ region**	**References**
					gastritis, pleura infection, dental growth and development, others	(Trás-os-Montes)	2009
	Abelmoschus esculentus (L.) Moench.	Okra	Fruits	Fresh fruits	Cholesterol reduction hypoglycemic, gastric irritation	Africa, Asia and America	Lengsfeld et. al., 2004
Papaveraceae	*Papaver rhoeas* L.	Poppy(E)	Leaves, stems	Decoction	Antidysenteric, antispasmodic	Jordan (Showbak)	Al-Qura'n et. al., 2009;
Piperaceae	*Peperomia galioides* HBK var *gladioides*	Congona (Q)	Aerial parts	Crushed/ Juice	Wounds healing, juice is swallowed to treat gastric ulcers	Perú (Ancash)	Hammond et al., 1998
Poaceae	*Cynodon dactylon* L.	Grama (P)	Dried roots	-	Diuretic, depurative, gastric inflammation	Portugal (Trás-os-Montes)	Neves et. al., 2009
Polygalaceae	*Polígala paniculata* Linneau	Barba-de-são-joão,vasso urinha branca or mimosa (P)	Aerial parts	-	Gastrprotector , asthma, bonchitis, stomach pain, diarrhea, anti-inflammatory, anti-spasmodic	Brazilian Atlantic coast	Rocha Lapa et. al., 2007
Punicaceae	*Punica granatum* L.	Pomegranate (E)	Fruits	Fresh fruits	Ulcer, hepatic damage, tonic fever, heart and gastric diseases, others	Europe, Indo-China, South Africa	Ajaikumar et. al., 2005
Rosaceae	*Sarcopetertum spinosum* (L.) Spach.	Thorny burnet (E)	Roots, fruits	Soaking	Renal calculi, antidiabetic, gastric diseases	Jordan (Showbak)	Al-Qura'n et. al., 2009;
Scrophulariaceae	*Calceolaria bicolor* Ruiz & Pav.	Zapatito or globo-globo (S)	Leaves, flowers	Infusion	Stomachache	Perú (Canta, Lima)	De la Cruz et. al., 2007
	Calceolaria lobata Cav.	Globo-globo (S)	Leaves, flowers	Infusion	Stomachache	Perú (Canta, Lima)	De la Cruz et. al., 2007
Solanaceae	*Hyoscyamus aureus* L.	Handbane (E)	Aerial parts	Decoction	Narcotic, hypnotic, stomachache	Jordan (Showbak)	Al-Qura'n et. al., 2009
Verbenaceae	*Lippia siodides* Cham.	-	Aerial parts	Hydro-alcoholic tincture	Wounds, mycoses, stomachache	Northeast Brazil	Barros Monteiro et. al., 2007
	Lippia integrifolia (Gris.) Hieron.	Incayuyo (S)	Aerial parts	Infusion/ Decoction	Dyspepsia, diuretic, cough treatment, indigestion, stomachache	Central and Northwest Argentina	Gorzalczany et. al., 2008

MEDICINAL PLANTS USED IN GASTRIC DISEASES AROUND THE WORLD							
Family	**Plant species**	**Common name**	**Part used**	**Mode of using**	**Traditional uses**	**Country/ region**	**References**
Vochyslaceae	*Vochysla tucanorum*	Pau-tucano or pau-doce (P)	Leaves, barks	Infusion	Stomach inflammation, asthma, pulmonary congestion	South America	Camargo Gomes et al., 2009
Zingiberaceae	*Amomum subulatum* Roxb. N. O.	Heel kalan, Bari ilaichi (I)	Fruits	Infusion	Stomacheache, digestive, anti-emetic, carminative	India	Jafri et al., 2001

Table 1. Medicinal plants used for treatment gastric disorders according to native population of different areas around the world. The names of the species are given according to the regional language: (Q) *quechua*, an indigenous language from Bolivia, Perú, north-western of Argentina and Chile; (I) Italian; (S) Spanish; (E) English; (ET) Ethiopian; (P) Portuguese; and (G) *Guaraní*, a native language from Paraguay, south-western of Brazil and north-eastern of Argentina.

2.1 Effects of phenolic compounds of medicinal plants on gastritis

Gastritis troubles led to researchers to study the gastric mucosa in different animal model (rat, mouse, pig, rabbit, among others) where mucosal damage was induced by either chemical compounds (aspirin, HCl, ethanol, acetic acid, ibuprofen and more), stress (hypothermia), pylorus ligation or by microbiological agents (*H. pylori*). These *in vivo* experimental assays are useful to resemble gastric diseases as gastritis or ulcers, and help us to understand the way of action of natural compounds or complex extract of medicinal plants. These compounds acts at different levels, e.g., immune mucosal response, H^+/K^+ pumping block, histamine release from mast cell, mucus wall structure, or prostaglandin (PG), myeloperoxidase (MPO) and nitric oxide (NO) regulation. Results obtained in the framemark of pre-clinical studies may be extrapolated to human cases (Elseweidy et. al., 2008; Hatsuko Baggio et. al., 2007; Wittschier et. al., 2007).

Flavonoids are phenolic compounds widely distributed in a wide variety of edible plants including leafy vegetables, fruits (strawbery, apple, etc.) and beverages (tea, red wine, beer, etc.). They have been reported to exert multiple biological effects, including antiviral, antithrombotic, anti-ischemic, anti-inflammatory, antihistaminic, antioxidant and free-radical scavenging abilities (Kahraman et. al., 2003). The phenolic compounds, widely distributed in plants, are the major compounds associated to human health and beneficial effects on gastritis, ulcer and cancer. The gastroprotective effect seems to be related to increase in endogenous PG, reduction in histamine secretion, scavenging oxygen-derived free radicals and even to gastric mucus stimulation (Rocha Lapa et. al., 2007; Tan et. al., 2002). The importance of such effects is to assure the gastric mucosal integrity by a dynamic balance and homeostasis between epithelial cell renewal and cellular apoptosis. In normal mammalian stomach, gastric mucosal cells have a rapid rate of turnover, being entirely replaced within 3–5 days as the result of rapid proliferation of progenitor cells at the isthmus and rapid cell death at the gastric surface (Park et. al., 2004).

However, treatment of gastric trouble with phenolic compounds is not always beneficial to gastritis condition. On one hand, the main effect is associated to anti-inflammatory response due to PG and NO inhibition; on the other hand, PG is responsible for the integrity of gastric mucosa through activation of a cascade of mechanisms that include inhibition of gastric acid secretion, stimulation of mucus-bicarbonate secretion and apoptosis, as well as modulation of the blood flow (Atay et. al., 2000) while NO is also involved in regulation of gastric motility, mucus and acid secretion (Uchida et. al., 2001).

Different medicinal plants gave good results in gastric trouble treatments, effects that were related to the anti-inflammatory and antioxidant activity of phenolic compounds. As an example, the ethanol extract of *Ageratum conyzoides* L. (Asteraceae) exhibited DPPH (2,2-diphenyl-1-picrylhydrazyl, and stable radical) scavenging activity and NO generation in a concentration dependent manner, displaying greater gastroprotector effect (at dose levels of 500 and 750 mg/kg) than conventional drugs as misoprostol and famotidine, which are used in gastritis treatment (Shirwaikar et. al., 2003). Flavonoids including quercetin (3,5,7,3′,4′-pentahydroxyflavone) and catechins (belonging to the flavan-3-ols group) were identified in *Maytenus ilicifolia* Mart. (Celastraceae) named in Brazil as "espinheira santa"; these compounds are related to antiulcerogenic activity and/or inhibition of gastric acid secretion, both *in vivo* and *in vitro* models. The effective gastric protection of *M. ilicifolia* flavonoid-rich fraction seems to be related to inhibition of gastric acid secretion (cyclooxygenase-prostaglandin system) rather than to glutathione and mucus regulation. The arabinogalactan fraction of this plant proved to be more effective than the flavonoid-rich fraction (Hatsuko Baggio et. al., 2007).

Quercetin is a common flavonoid distributed in a broad variety of vegetables, fruits and beverages as tea, red wine, beer, etc. It is known for its vasoactive properties but it also prevented gastric mucosal ulcers induced in rats by the administration of ethanol. The flavonoid prevented the increase of MPO activity (associated to this experimental model) thus protecting gastric mucosa from the deleterious effects of activated neutrophil infiltration (Kahraman et. al., 2003). Besides, its antioxidant property may reduce the lipid peroxidation and protein carbonyl compounds, increasing the superoxide dismutase activity which may play a role on gastric inflammation (Coskun et. al., 2004; Kahraman et. al., 2003, as cited in Serrano et. al., 1999). A novel natural product isolated from the *Scutellaria baicalensis* Georgi (Lamiaceae) roots (traditionally used against inflammation related diseases) is *Wogonin* (5,7-dihydroxy-8-methoxyflavone) which displayed similar effects of rebamipide (a well-known drug prescribed clinically for the treatment of gastritis and gastric ulcer) in the prevention of alcohol stomach injury (Park et. al., 2004). The target of these compounds would be the araquidonic acid metabolism including suppression of 5-*lipooxigenase* (LOX) and induction of ciclooxigenase-2 (COX-2), thus displaying strong anti-inflammatory activity on alcohol-related gastric disease (Cellotti & Laufer, 2001).

Besides phenolic compounds, terpenes from essential oil (EO) were also tested with outstanding results. Solidagenone is a labdane diterpene synthesized in rhizomes of *Solidago chilensis* Meyen (Asteraceae); it was used to treat symptomatologies related to inflammation. Solidagenone and its derivative solidagen-6β-ol on the HCl/ethanol-induced gastric lesions in mice was assessed at 100 mg/kg, being as active as lansoprazole at 20 mg/kg, but the mode of action remains to be elucidated (Schmeda-Hirschmann et. al., 2002). Oral pre-treatment of mice with EO from *Lippia sidoides* Cham. (Verbenaceae) caused inhibition of gastric lesions but did not stimulate mucus production; similar results were obtained with OPZ. Consequently, the gastroprotective mechanism induced by the *Lippia sidoides* EO would not be related with cytoprotection (Barros Monteiro et. al., 2007). The EO of *Croton sonderianus* (Muell. Arg), *Amomum sublatum* (Jafri et. al., 2001), *Nigela sativa* (El-Abhar et. al., 2002) and *Croton cajucara* (Hiruma-Lima et. al., 2000) also showed protective activities on gastric mucosa. On the other hand, Anethole, a constituent present in many essential oils and its derivatives 1-hydroxy-1-(4-methoxyphenyl)-propane and 1-hydroxy-1-(4-methoxyphenyl)-2-*m*-chlorobenzoyl-propane seemed to have gastroprotector effect against ethanol-induced gastric lesions without modifying the mucus secretion (Freire et. al., 2005).

OPZ is an effective inhibitor of leukocyte infiltration, over-expression of adhesion molecules, IL-1a, and TNF-α production. When rats received OPZ, the lipid-peroxidation (expressed in terms of malondialdehyde and NO) decreased and pepsinogen secretion is stimulated, so its therapeutic effect could be related to its antioxidant property. On the other hand, authors compare the OPZ with natural compounds as curcuminoids; curcuminoids are isolated from dried roots of turmeric (*Curcuma longa;* Zingiberaceae) and when are administered in rats with induced gastritis the serum NO level tend to decrease compared to control group (without treatment). This effect could be associated to some mechanisms: Reduction of iNOS expression or scavenging of NO molecule. The free radicals scavenging properties of curcuminoids and maintaining cellular glutathione (GSH) stores in glandular stomach are factors acting to inhibit lipid peroxidation. Although curcuminoids significantly decreased serum gastrin level, it failed to stimulate pepsinogen release from chief cells (Elseweidy et. al., 2008).

2.2 Effectiveness of plants glycoside derivate compounds on *H. pylori* infection

Phenolic compounds as flavonoids and their derivates have also antimicrobial effects as it was demonstrated in cases of H. *pylori* infection (Atherton, 2006; Wittschier et. al., 2007, as cited in Warren and Marhall, 1983). Thus, catechins the main component of green tea, may inhibit the *H. pylori* urease (Matsubara et. al., 2003) and also when it is used together with sucralfate in Mongolian gerbils (Takabayashi et. al., 2004). The *green tea* has confirmed its bactericidal and bacteriostatic effects *in vitro* assays while *in vivo* studies demonstrated that its consumption when is taken before infection prevents gastric mucosal inflammation, and when is taken after infection diminishes the magnitude of gastritis. On the other hand, Castillo-Juarez et. al., (2009) studied the anti-*H. pylori* activity of 53 plants used in Mexican traditional medicine for gastrointestinal disorders. On the whole, about 77% of the assayed plants are active, having from moderate to strong antibacterial activity against *H. pylori.* Since some of these medicinal plants are used as condiments or food ingredients (e.g., *Ocimum basiliscum, Persea americana, Lippia berlandieri, Teloxys graveolens*), it seems that a frequent consumption could have a preventive effect in controlling the *H. pylori* population on infected people.

It has been suggested that the best way to prevent *H. pylori* infections is to eliminate the pathogen from its most common habitat, the gastric mucus layer but nowadays research is focused on a new property of some natural compounds, i.e., the anti-*H. pylori* adhesion. The adhesive process of *H. pylori* is based on bacterial adhesins located on its outer cell wall, which are responsible for interaction with mucosal glycoproteins and epithelial mucins; in this way the infection is established. Certain compounds, e.g. polysaccharides, may interact with the bacterial adhesins before adhesin-mucin adhesion avoiding the infection process. Studies on the complex nature of these adhesins are reported by Evans & Evans, (2000), Kusters et. al. (2006), and Wittschier et. al. (2009).

Adhesion to epithelial cells has been recognized as an essential step of the infectious process for virtually all bacterial pathogens and therefore many efforts are aimed to develop anti-adhesion therapy. Sialyllactose (NeuAc[K2-3]Gal[L1-4]Glc), an inhibitor of the sialic acid-specifc adhesin of *H. pylori*, significantly reduced the load of the bacteria in monkeys (Burger et. al., 2000, as cited in Glaser, 1997). Accordingly, it would seem appropriate to target such therapy against *H. pylori* toward its association with the mucus before the pathogen adheres to the underlying epithelial cells and causes disease. However, the bulk production of oligosaccharides specific for the *H. pylori* lectins as anti-adhesion therapeutic agents is still a problem to be solved. As an alternative approach, dietary inhibitors might be the solution for certain infections, e.g. the inhibition of sialic acid-specific adhesion of *H. pylori* to human gastric mucus and to human erythrocytes by cranberry juice (Burger et. al., 2000). Another example is the root extracts of *Pelargonium sidoides* DC (Geraniaceae) a medicinal specie used to treat acute respiratory infections, which contains a polysaccharide fraction, EPs 7630, with anti-adhesive activity against *H. pylori* (Wittschier et. al., 2007). The roots of *Glycyrrhzia glabra* L. contain a raw polysaccharide fraction mainly composed of arabinose, galactose, glucose and glucuronic acid, which interacts with the outer-membrane surface adhesins of *H. pylori* avoiding its adhesion to mucus (Wittschier et. al., 2009). Authors consider this anti-adhesive effect an advantage to prevent re-infection by *H. pylori* after antibiotic eradication therapy.

These beneficial effects lead us to conclude that natural inhibitors of bacterial growth and inflammation may offer alternatives to antibiotic therapy for bacterial eradication and may be used as supplements to conventional eradication therapy in populations at high risk for gastric cancer (Stoicov et. al., 2009).

3. Lactic acid bacteria in gastritis

Lactic acid bacteria (LAB) are a group of *Gram*-positive, non-sporulating bacteria that include species of *Lactobacillus, Leuconostoc, Pediococcus* and *Streptococcus*. Dietary LAB refers to those species and strains that are used in food- and feed-fermentation processes. The term LAB is a group of organisms that are defined by their ability to produce a common end product, lactic acid, from the fermentation of sugar. LABs have limited biosynthetic abilities, and require pre-formed amino acids, B vitamins, purines, pyrimidines and, usually, a sugar as a carbon and energy source. LABs occupy a range of niches, including milk, plant surfaces and the oral cavity, gastrointestinal tract and vagina of vertebrates. Since ancient times, dietary LABs have been used to ferment a range of raw materials such as milk, which is used to produce cheese (species of *Lactococcus*) and yoghurts (species of *Streptococcus* and *Lactobacillus*). Consumed for centuries, LABs have a long and safe association with humans and their food (Wells & Mercenier, 2008).

Probiotic foods containing LAB have been proposed as a natural alternative to improve the general health status, preventing various gastrointestinal disorders such as gastric ulcers and inflammation related to *H. pylori* infection, gastrointestinal infections (Lebeer et. al., 2010) or antibiotic-associated diarrhea (Chen et. al., 2009; Gill & Guarner, 2004; Penner et. al., 2005) providing beneficial effects to the host by modulating immune functions, e.g. systemic cytokine production (Borchers et. al., 2009).

Different LAB species were tested in gastritis models mainly in treatment of *H. pylori* infection. Some reports suggested that certain species of exogenous lactobacilli have inhibitory effects on gastric infection (Cui et. al., 2010; Ryan et. al., 2008), e.g., *Lactobacillus (L.) reuteri* ATCC 55730 displayed ability to colonize the gastrointestinal tract and at the same time, to generate an inmune response when it was administered to human volunteers.

After administration, *L. reuteri* was detected by fluorescence in situ hybridization (FISH) in stomach and duodenum in some volunteers. According to these results it was suggested that stimulation of T-helper cells in human ileum could be a central mechanism of symbiosis for improving the health of the host gut (Valeur et. al., 2004). Similar results were obtained with a commercial product (Lacidofil®) containing *L. acidophilus* R0052 and *L. rhamnosus* R0011 (Johnson-Henry et. al., 2004). The probiotic mixture exhibits bactericidal activity in a dose-dependent manner by altering normal *H. pylori* morphology and thereby inhibiting its growth. Authors (Johnson-Henry et. al. 2004) suggested that probiotics are an attractive option for counteracting the effects caused by *H. pylori* infection for many reasons: LABs are able to resist acid and bile, to transiently remain under the harsh stomach conditions, and to competitively exclude pathogenic bacteria. *In vitro* studies showed that certain LAB strains and their cell-free cultures are able to inhibit or kill *H. pylori* (Michetti et. al., 1999; Sgouras et. al., 2005) as well as to reduce urease activity in the human gastric epithelial cells (AGS) by exclusion effect (Lin et. al., 2011). Likely, Ko et. al. (2010) evinced that *L. casei* ATCC 393-loaded chitosan microspheres inhibited *H. pylori* growth in *in vitro* assays.

B. bifidum CECT 7366 is also a promising microorganism against *H. pylori* infection. Results from *in vitro* and *in vivo* models (BALB/c mice) indicated that the strain partially relieves damage of gastric tissues caused by the pathogen and also decreases the *H. pylori* pathogenicity ratio (Chenoll et al., 2011).

The inclusion of probiotics in a conventional therapy (triple therapy: antibiotics and PPI) for *H. pylori* eradication was also evaluated (Kim et. al., 2008). *H. pylori*-infected patients were administered with yogurt (*Will* yogurt) containing *L. acidophilus* HY2177, *L. casei* HY2743, *Bifidobacterium longum* HY8001 and *Streptococcus thermophilus* B1; at the same time, they were treated according to the triple therapy. As a conclusion, the addition of yogurt did not reduce the side-effects of the therapy but increased the *H. pylori* eradication rate. Similar results had been reported using fermented milks with *L. acidophilus* and *L. casei* (M.J. Park et. al., 2001). Recently, Shirasawa et. al. (2010) evinced that the probiotic strain *B. bifidum* BF-1 is able to suppress IL-8 induction by *H. pylori* through inhibition of the genes related to the NF-κB signaling pathways. Other LAB strains were also effective against *H. pylori* in gastritis cases, e.g., *L. johnsonii* La1 displayed a pronounced anti-inflammatory effect on *H. pylori*-associated neutrophilic and lymphocytic infiltration in animal model by reducing pro-inflammatory chemokine levels in the gastric mucosa during the early stages of infection (Sgouras et. al., 2005). The markers for gastric inflammation such as prostaglandin I/II ratio (Sakamoto et. al., 2001) or ornithine decarboxylase activity (Linsalata et. al., 2004) also decreased in patients treated with probiotics, effects that persisted for several weeks after cessation of the treatment. Likely, Cui et. al. (2010) demonstrated that *L. fermenti* (CCTCC M 206110) and *L. acidophilus* LC, isolated from gastric biopsy materials of patients, could alleviate the gastric inflammation in *H. pylori*-infected BALB/c mice after oral administration. These results would indicate that specific lactobacilli strains may colonize the gastric mucosa, which may be related to their capacity to survive and develop in acidic environments (Cats et. al., 2003; Cui et. al., 2010; Gotteland & Cruchet, 2003; Mater et. al., 2005; Mozzi et. al., 2009; Valeur et. al., 2004; Wang et. al., 2004).

The effect of LAB on acute gastric lesions induced by chemical agents in experimental models was also reported. The administration of probiotic lactobacilli as *L. gasseri* OLL2716, *L. casei* GG, *L. paracasei* subsp. *paracasei* NTU 101 and *L. plantarum* NTU 102 to rats inhibits the gastric mucosa injury in HCl/ethanol-induced ulcer and pyloric ligation models (Lam et. al., 2007; Liu et. al., 2009; Uchida & Kurakazu, 2004).

Researchs on the functional properties of metabolites produced in food by LAB during fermentation such as exopolysaccharides (EPS) increased in recent years by assigning to biopolymers potential beneficial effects on human health. These effects include prebiotic effects (Dal Bello et. al., 2001; Korakli et. al., 2002; Salazar et. al., 2009), hypocholesterolemic effect (Pigeon et. al., 2002) and immunomodulatory and anti-tumor activity (Chabot et. al., 2001; Kitazawa et. al., 1998;) as well as other immune functions such as proliferation of T-lymphocytes (Forsén et. al., 1987), activation of macrophages and induction of cytokine production (Kitazawa et. al., 1991, 1996). The EPS could remain attached to the cell wall (capsular EPS) or be excreted into the environment in the form of slime or ropy EPS and its structure may vary depending, mainly, on the strain (van Hijum et. al., 2006). LABs produce two different kinds of EPS by using distinct biosynthetic pathways. The homo-polysaccharide (HoPS) are synthesized by extracellular glycansucrases and contain only one type of sugar (generally glucose) and the hetero-polysaccharide (HePS) that are assembled by cell wall-bound glycosyl-transferases from intracellular sugar nucleotide precursors, which may be constituted by 3 to 8 different monosaccharides (de Vuyst et. al., 2001). There are many EPS-producing LABs, e.g., *L. acidophilus, L. sakei, L. delb.* subsp. *bulgaricus, L. helveticus, L. paracasei, L. pentosus, L. plantarum, L., rhamnosus, L. reuteri, L. casei, Leuconostoc mesenteroides* and *Streptococcus thermophilus* although it is a strain-dependent property (Mozzi et. al., 2006; Ruas-Madiedo et. al., 2002).

It is known that the EPS of LAB have many functional properties; they have effect on the mucosal immune system, could avoid the *H. pylori* adhesion to the mucus layer, and could make the mucus layer stronger, among others. Despite these beneficial properties, there are few studies in the literature concerning the protection of gastric epithelium by EPS-producing LAB or the role they could play in the gastric injury. Ruas-Madiedo et. al. (2006) suggested that the biopolymers are involved in the mechanism of competitive exclusion of probiotics through adherence to the mucus and Nagaoka et. al. (1994) reported anti-ulcer effects of the cell wall polysaccharide of bifidobacteria, lactobacilli and streptococci strains, which were attributed to the high rhamnose content of the polymers (> 60%).

Rodríguez et al. (2009, 2010) reported the first evidences on the beneficial effects of both the EPS-producing LAB strains and the biopolymer on gastritis experimental animal models using acetyl salicylic acid (ASA) as gastritis inductor. Authors demonstrated the gastroprotector effect of fermented milk with the EPS-producing strain *S. thermophilus* CRL 1190 on superficial chronic gastritis in BALB/c mice as preventive and therapeutic treatment. Other EPS-producing strains *S. thermophilus* CRL 804 and CRL 638, and *L. casei* CRL 87 were also evaluated *in vivo* assays but with unsuccessful results. The biopolymers had different physical-chemical properties: *S. thermophilus* CRL 1190 produced a high molecular mass EPS (1500 kDa) composed of D-glucose and D-galactose; *S. thermophilus* CRL 638, a high EPS (1200 kDa) composed of D-glucose, D-galactose and N-acetilglucosamine; *S. thermophilus* CRL 804 produced a low EPS (95 kDa) composed of D-galactose and L-rhamnose, and at last, *L. casei* CRL 87 produced a low EPS (800 kDa) composed of D-glucose, D-galactose and L-rhamnose. The strains CRL 1190 and CRL 87 also produced capsular polysaccharide in addition to the slime EPS in milk and was able to form ropy milk cultures similar to CRL 638, while the strain CRL 804 was negative for both the capsular and ropy phenotypes (Mozzi et. al., 2006).

The fermented milk with *S. thermophilus* CRL 1190 (FM-1190) as well as the EPS (EPS-1190) suspended in milk (but not in water) was the only one effective in both the therapeutic and preventive treatment of chronic gastritis in animal models. Results obtained were similar to that of OPZ but with the advantage of not having side effects. The FM-1190 also activated the synthesis of mucin, which in turn led to an increase in the thickness of the mucus layer and in the amount of mucus of the body and antrum that were decreased after ASA administration. The recovery of the gastric defensive systems and the mucus-bicarbonate layer in animals fed FM-1190 favored the recovery of the damaged gastric mucosa. These evidences support previous reports obtained in rats with acute gastric damage which were fed with probiotic lactobacilli (Nam et. al., 2005; Lam et. al., 2007).

The fermented milk FM-1190 and the EPS-1190 were able to modulate the gastric inflammatory response at the immune system level (decrease in the number of cells producing pro-inflammatory cytokines, INF-γ and TNF-α, and increase in the number of cells producing regulatory cytokines, such as IL-10). These promising results, however, can not be ascribed to all EPS-producing LABs because of the complexity of the phenomenon. The fermented milk with the strain *S. thermophillus* CRL 804 which produced an EPS formed by rhamnose and galactose did not display any anti-gastritis effect in contrast to the results obtained by Nagaoka et. al. (1994) with cell wall polysaccharides containing rhamnose. In contrast to the FM-1190, the fermented milk with *S. thermophilus* CRL 638 generated a great stomach inflammation in animal model, without gastritis induction, after 7d of feeding.

Studies of scanning electronic microscopy (SEM) confirmed a greater secretion of gastric mucus after oral administration of FM-1190; they also put in evidence the presence of the strain CRL 1190 in the stomach at least 15 days after finishing the administration of the fermented milk. These confirmed previous reports concerning the ability of *S. thermophilus* strains to survive the passage through the gastrointestinal tract and to exert the beneficial effects on various gastrointestinal disorders (Brigidi et. al., 2003; Delorme, 2008; Guarner et. al., 2005; Mater et. al., 2005; Vinderola & Reinheimer, 2003). Studies performed in *in vitro* gastric system evinced a partially degradation of the EPS-1190 when subjected to this harsh conditions (Mozzi et. al., 2009). From results from *in vivo* and *in vitro* studies, it is assumed that the biopolymer may still exert its beneficial properties in the stomach even partially degraded.

Several studies reported that high molecular mass-polysaccharides of different sources (herbs, marine microalgae and fungi) have anti-ulcer, anti-inflammatory or inmuno-stimulatory effects related to anti-secretory activity of acid and pepsin, inmuno-stimulation, stimulation of gastric mucus, increase in gastric prostaglandin levels and partially suppression of TNF-α genes (Gao et. al., 2002, 2004; Yamada, 1995; Yim et. al., 2005). However, the beneficial effects can not be only attributed to the size of the polymer. The different effect obtained with the strains CRL 1190, CRL 804 and CRL 638 evinced that the phenomenon is strongly strain-dependent and complex.

Whey proteins as α-lactalbumin would also have gastroprotector effect (Matsumoto et. al., 2001; Rosaneli et. al., 2004; Ushida et. al., 2003, 2007); so, the interaction of EPS-producing LAB or the EPS with milk proteins may be a key factor in gastroprotection. Studies on the interaction between EPS and milk proteins is complex since EPS are gradually produced during fermentation, and the characteristics of the proteins such as charge and hydrophobicity may change during fermentation and consequently the interaction between them. The EPSs bind water and increase the moisture in the non-fat portion, interfere with protein-protein interactions reducing the rigidity of the protein network, and increase the viscosity of the serum phase (Hassan, 2008). Similar research was carried out by Ayala-Hernandez et. al. (2008) who studied the interaction between milk proteins and the EPS produced by *Lactococcus lactis* ssp. *cremoris* using SEM techniques. They observed that EPS

molecules clearly interact not only with caseins but also with whey proteins and play an active role in the formation of the aggregates.
Considering these statements, it is assumed that in fermented milks, e.g., FM-1190, the LAB strains and the EPS together with the milk and whey proteins perform a stable three-dimensional complex network, which is attached to the gastric mucosa preferably to the mucus layer, when it is administered to animals. Thus, the EPS could interact with the mucosal tissue exerting an inmunomodulador effect, thus avoiding inflammation and or making the mucus barrier stronger, which could also affect *H. pylori* adhesion. The mode of action of probiotic LAB strains and their EPS in gastritis has not yet been completely elucidated.

4. Conclusion

Gastritis is the most common illness associated to the stomach, and it is the beginning of different complication that led to ulcers and, in the worst case, gastric cancer. The disease is due to different causes as an imbalanced diet, intake of aggressive agents, or stress process (related to neurological condition) which is very common nowadays due to the population rhythm of life. However, the most aggressive case is due to *H. pylori* infection. Allopathic treatment of gastritis includes different conventional drugs acting as inhibitors of the proton pump and of the acid gastric production, thus helping the stomach to balance the acid condition when there is an inflammation, infection or injury. The increase in gastric pH is a necessary condition to stop autodigestive processes and support mucosal healing in the extreme environment of the gastric lumen; this effect is mainly required in the treatment of peptic ulcer. Other drugs are also used, which exert different effects on the gastric mucosa tissue to alleviate the inflamed condition, e.g., by stimulation of the mucus synthesis, inhibition of the stomach motility, or by displaying anti-*H. pylori* effects, among other properties. The disadvantages of employing these drugs for long periods, such as ranitidine, OPZ and derivates, and antibiotics in the case of *H. pylori* infection, is that many of them could have side effects.
Medicinal plants and their effect in different kind of diseases, on the basis of ancient knowledge and supported by scientific evidences, emerge as an alternative therapy to cure or prevent gastric disorders. The beneficial effects are mainly related to anti-inflammatory activity and the ability to maintain a balance in the mucus barrier and mucosal renovation. Phenolic compounds, polysaccharides and derivates in different combinations are mainly involved in gastric protection, effect associated in some cases to modulation of the immune system (cytokine regulation) and mucus stimulation.
Probiotic lactic acid bacteria and probiotic foods, which beneficial effects on the gut health are strongly supported by scientific evidences, also appear as a novel and promising bio-alternative for gastritis treatment. Recent evidences indicate that some exopolysaccharide (EPS)-producing lactic acid bacteria are able to regulate and to revert the gastritis process prompted by NSAIDs, a property that is mainly related to the EPS produced by specific strains. The biopolymers could also interact with *H. pylori* and inhibit its adhesion to mucus barrier thus avoiding the infection process. The mode of action of probiotics and their EPS, which involves modulation of the immune system, increase in gastric pH, and stimulation of mucus production, among other cascade reactions, is under study.
Considering the beneficial effects of these bio-treatments in gastritis processes, it would be advisable to include them as adjunct in conventional treatments programs to reduce the side effect derived from the intake of drugs during long periods.

5. References

Ajaikumar, K.; Asheef, M.; Babu, B. & Padikkala, J. (2005). The inhibition of gastric mucosal injury by *Punica granatum* L. (pomegranate) methanolic extract. *Journal of Ethnopharmacology*, Vol.96, No.3, (January 2005), pp. 171-176, ISSN: 0378-8741.

Al-Qura'n, S. (2009). Ethnopharmacological survey of wild medicinal plants in Showbak, Jordan. *Journal of Ethnopharmacology*, Vol.123, No.1, (May 2009), pp. 45-50, ISSN: 0378-8741.

Atay, S.; Tarnawski, A. & Dubois, A. (2000). Eicosanoids and the stomach. *Prostaglandins & Other Lipid Mediators*, Vol.61, No.3-4, (May 2000), pp. 105–124, ISSN: 1098-8823.

Atherton, J.C. (2006). The pathogenesis of *Helicobacter pylori*–induced gastro-duodenal diseases. *Annual Review of Pathology: Mechanisms of Disease*, Vol.1, (February 2006), pp. 63-96, ISSN: 1553-4006.

Ayala-Hernández, I.; Goff, H.D. & Corredig, M. (2008). Interactions between milk proteins and exopolysaccharides produce by *Lactococcus lactis* observed by scanning electron microscopy. *Journal of Dairy Science*, Vol.91, No.7, (July 2008), pp. 2583-2590, ISSN: 1525-3198.

Barros Monteiro, M.V.; Rocha de Melo Leite, A.K.; Medeiros Bertini, L.; de Morais, S.M. & Sousa Nunes-Pinheiro, D.C. (2007). Topical anti-inflammatory, gastroprotective and antioxidant effects of the essential oil of *Lippia sidoides* Cham. leaves. *Journal of Ethnopharmacology*, Vol.111, No.2, (May 2007), pp. 378-382, ISSN: 0378-8741.

Borchers, A.T.; Selmi, C.; Meyers, F.J.; Keen, C.L. & Gershwin, M.E. (2009). Probiotics and immunity. *Journal of Gastroenterology*, Vol.44, No.1, (January 2009), pp. 26-46, ISSN: 0944-1174.

Borrelli, F. & Izzo, A. (2000). The plant kingdom as a source of antiulcer remedies. *Phytotherapy Research*, Vol.14, No.8, (December 2000), pp. 581-591, ISSN: 0951-418X.

Brigidi, P.; Swennen, E.; Vitali, B.; Rossi, M. & Matteuzzi, M. (2003). PCR detection of *Bifidobacterium* strains and *Streptococcus thermophilus* in feces of human subjects after oral bacteriotherapy and yoghurt consumption. *International Journal of Food Microbiology*, Vol.81, No.3, (March 2003), pp. 203-209, ISSN: 0168-1605.

Burger, O.; Ofek, I.; Tabak, M.; Weiss, E.I; Sharon, N. & Neeman, I. (2000). A high molecular mass constituent of cranberry juice inhibits *Helicobacter pylori* adhesion to human gastric mucus. *FEMS Immunology and Medical Microbiology*, Vol.29, No.4, (December 2000), pp. 295-301, ISSN: 0928-8244.

Camargo Gomes, R.; Bonamin, F.; Darin, D.D.; Seito, L.N.; Di Stasi, L.C.; Dokkedal, A.L.; Vilegas, W.; Souza Brito, A.R. & Hiruma-Lima, C.K. (2009). Antioxidative action of methanolic extract and buthanolic fraction of *Vochysia tucanorum* Mart. in the gastroprotection. *Journal of Ethnopharmacology*, Vol.121, No.3, (January 2009), pp. 466-471, ISSN: 0378-8741.

Castillo-Juárez, I.; González, V.; Jaime-Aguilar, H.; Martínez G.; Linares, E.; Bye, R. & Romero, I. (2009). Anti-*Helicobacter pylori* activity of plants used in Mexican traditional medicine for gastrointestinal disorders. *Journal of Ethnopharmacology*, Vol.122, No.2, (March 2009), pp. 402-405, ISSN: 0378-8741.

Cats, A.; Kuipers, E.J.; Bosschaert, M.A.R.; Pot, R.G.J.; Vandenbroucke-Grauls, C.M.J.E. & Kusters, J.G. (2003). Effect of frequent consumption of a *Lactobacillus casei*-containing milk drink in *Helicobacter pylori*-colonized subjects. *Alimentary Pharmacology & Therapeutics*, Vol.17, No. 3, (February 2003), pp. 429–435, ISSN: 0953-0673.

Cellotti, F. & Laufer, S. (2001). Anti-inflammatory drugs: New multi-target compounds to face an old problem. The dual inhibition concept. *Pharmacological Research*, Vol.43, No.5, (May 2001), pp. 429–436, ISSN: 1043-6618.

Chabot, S.; Yu, H.L.; De Léséleuc, L.; Cloutier, D.; van Calsteren, M.R.; Lessard, M.; Roy, D.; Lacroix, M. & Oth, D. (2001). Exopolysaccharide from *Lactobacillus rhamnosus* RW-9595M stimulate TNF, IL-6 and IL-12 in human and mouse cultured inmunocompetent cells, and IFN-γ in mouse splenocytes. *Le Lait*, Vol.81, No.6, (November 2001), pp. 683–697, ISSN: 0023-7302.

Chen, L.L.; Wang, X.H.; Cui, Y.; Lian, G.H.; Zhang, J.; Ouyang, C.H. & Lu, F.G. (2009). Therapeutic effects of four strains of probiotics on experimental colitis in mice. *World Journal of Gastroenterology*, Vol.15, No.3, (January 2009), pp. 321-327, ISSN: 1007-9327.

Chenoll, E.; Casinos, B.; Bataller, E.; Astals, P.; Echevarría, J.; Iglesias, J.R.; Balbarie, P.; Ramón, D. & Genovés, S. (2011). Novel probiotic *Bifidobacterium bifidum* CECT 7366 strain active against the pathogenic bacterium *Helicobacter pylori. Applied & Environmental Microbiology*, Vol.77, No.4, (February 2011), pp. 1335-1343, ISSN: 0099- 2240.

Coşkun, Ö.; Kanter, M.; Armutçu, F.; Çetin, K.; Kaybolmaz, B. & Yazgan, Ö. (2004). Protective effects of quercetin, a flavonoid antioxidant, in absolute ethanol-induced acut gastric ulcer. *European Journal of General Medicine*, Vol.1, No.3, (July 2004), pp. 37-42, ISSN: 1304-3897.

Cui, Y.; Wang, C.L.; Liu, X.W.; Wang, X.H.; Chen, L.L.; Zhao, X.; Fu, N. & Lu, F.G. (2010). Two stomach-originated lactobacillus strains improve *Helicobacter pylori* infected murine gastritis. *World Journal of Gastroenterology*, Vol.16, No.4, (January 2010), pp. 445-452, ISSN: 1007-9327.

Dal Bello, F.D.; Walter, J.; Hertel, C. & Hammes, W.P. (2001). In vitro study of prebiotic properties of levan-type exopolysaccharides from lactobacilli and non-digestible carbohydrates using denaturing gradient gel electrophoresis. *Systematic & Applied Microbiology*, Vol.24, No.2, (July 2001), pp. 232–237, ISSN: 0723-2020.

Davies, G.; Wilkie, M. & Rampton, D. (1993). Effects of metronidazole and misoprostol on indomethacin-induced changes in intestinal permeability. *Digestive Diseases & Sciences*, Vol.38, No.3, (March 1993), pp. 417–425, ISSN: 0163-2116.

De la Cruz, H.; Vilcapoma, G. & Zevallos, P.A. (2007). Ethnobotanical study of medicinal plants used by the Andean people of Canta, Lima, Perú. *Journal of Ethnopharmacology*, Vol.111, No.2, (May 2007), pp. 284-294, ISSN: 0378-8741.

de Vuyst, L.; de Vin, F.; Vanigelgem, F. & Degeest, B. (2001). Recent developments in the biosynthesis and applications of heteropolysaccharides from lactic acid bacteria. *International Dairy Journal*, Vol.11, No.9, pp. 687-707, ISSN: 0958-6946.

Delorme, C. (2008). Safety assessment of dairy microorganisms: *Streptococcus thermophilus*. *International Journal of Food Microbiology*, Vol.126, No.3, (September 2008), pp. 274-277, ISSN: 0168-1605.

El-Abhar, H.S.; Abadía, D.M. & Saleh, S. (2002). Gastroprotective activity of *Nigella sativa* oil and its constituent, thymoquinone, against gastric mucosal injury induced by ischaemia/reperfusion in rats. *Journal of Ethnopharmacology*, Vol.84, No.2-3, (February 2003), pp. 251-258, ISSN: 0378-8741.

Elmann, A.; Mordechay, S.; Rindner, M. & Ravid, U. (2010). Anti-neuroinflammatory effects of geranium oil in microglial cells. *Journal of Functional Foods*, Vol.2, No.1, (January 2010), pp. 17–22, ISSN: 1756-4646.

Elseweidy, M.M.; Younis, N.N.; Amin, R.S.; Abdallah F.R.; Fathy, A.M. & Yousif, Z.A. (2008). Effect of some natural products either alone or in combination on gastritis induced in experimental rats. *Digestive Diseases and Sciences,*Vol.53, No.7, (July 2008), pp. 1774-1784, ISSN: 0163-2116.

Evans, D.J. & Evans, D.G. (2000). *Helicobacter pylori* adhesins: review and perspectives. *Helicobacter,* Vol.5, No.4, (December 2000), pp. 183–195, ISSN: 1083-4389.

Formica, J. & Regelson, W. (1995). Review of the biology of quercetin and related bioflavonoids. *Food & Chemical Toxicology,* Vol.33, No.12, (December 1995), pp. 1061-1080, ISSN: 0278-6915.

Forsén, R.; Keiska, E.; Herva, E. & Arvilommi, H. (1987). Immunobiological effects of *Streptococcus cremoris* from cultured milk "villi"; application of human lymphocyte culture techniques. *International Journal of Food Microbiology,* Vol.5, No.1, (September 1987), pp. 41-47, ISSN: 0168-1605.

Freire, R.S.; Morais, S.M.; Catunda-Junior, F.E.A. & Nunes-Pinheiro, D.C.S. (2005). Synthesis and antioxidant, anti-inflammatory and gastroprotector activities of anethole and related compounds. *Bioorganic & Medicinal Chemistry,* Vol.13, No.13, (July 2005), pp. 4353-4358, ISSN: 0968-0896.

Gao, Y.; Zhou, S.; Wen, J.; Huang, M. & Xu, A. (2002). Mechanism of the antiulcerogenic effect of *Ganoderma lucidum* polysaccharides on indomethacin-induced lesions in the rat. *Life Sciences,* Vol.72, No.6, (December 2002), pp. 731-745, ISSN: 0024-3205.

Gao, Y.; Tang, W.; Gao, H.; Chan, E.; Lan, J. & Zhou, S. (2004). *Ganoderma lucidum* polysaccharide fractions accelerate healing of acetic acid-induced ulcers in rats. *Journal of Medicinal Food,* Vol.7, No.4, (Winter 2004), pp. 417-421, ISSN: 1096-620X.

Giday, M.; Asfaw, Z. & Woldu, Z. (2010). Ethnomedicinal study of plants used by Sheko ethnic group of Ethiopia.*Journal of Ethnopharmacology,* Vol.132, No.1, (October 2010), pp. 75-85, ISSN: 0378-8741.

Gill, H.S. & Guarner, F. (2004). Probiotics and human health: a clinical perspective. *Postgraduate Medical Journal,* Vol.80, No.947, (February 2004), pp. 516–26, ISSN: 0032-5473.

Gorzalczany, S.; Sülsen, V.; Redko, F.; Vescina, C.; Muschietti, L.; Martino, V.; Acevedo, C. (2008). Choleretic and antispasmodic effects of *Lippia integrifolia* aqueous extract. *Revista Brasileira de Farmacognosia,* Vol.18, No.1, (Mach 2008), pp. 16-20, ISSN 0102-695X.

Gotteland, M. & Cruchet, S. (2003). Suppressive effect of frequent ingestion of *Lactobacillus johnsonii* La1 on *Helicobacter pylori* colonization in asymptomatic volunteers. *Journal of Antimicrobial Chemotherapy,* Vol.51, No.5, (May 2003), pp. 1317-1319, ISSN: 0305-7453.

Guarner, F.; Perdigon, G.; Corthier, G.; Salminen, S.; Koletzko, B. & Morelli, L. (2005). Should yogurt cultures be considered probiotic?. *British Journal of Nutrition,* Vol.93, No.6, (June 2005), pp. 783–786, ISSN: 0007-1145.

Hammond, G.B.; Fernández, I.D.; Villegas, L.F. & Vaisberg, A.J. (1998). A survey of traditional medicinal plants from the Callejón de Huaylas, Department of Ancash, Perú. *Journal of Ethnopharmacology,* Vol.61, No.1, (May 1998), pp. 17-30, ISSN: 0378-8741.

Hassan, A.N. (2008). ADSA Foundation Scholar Award: Possibilities and challenges of exopolysaccharide-producing lactic cultures in dairy foods. *Journal of Dairy Science,* Vol.91, No.4, (April 2008), pp. 1282-1298, ISSN: 1525-3198.

Hatsuko Baggio, C.; Freitas, C.; Martini Otofuji, G.; Cipriani, T.; de Souza, L.; Lanzi Sassaki, G.; Iacomini, M.; Andrade Marques, M. & Mesia-Vela, S. (2007). Flavonoid-rich fraction of *Maytenus ilicifolia* Mart. ex. Reiss protects the gastric mucosa of rodents through inhibition of both H+,K+-ATPase activity and formation of nitric oxide. *Journal of Ethnopharmacology*, Vol.113, No.3, (September 2007), pp. 433-440, ISSN: 0378-8741.

Hiruma-Lima, C.A.; Gracioso, J.S.; Rodríguez, J.A.; Haun, M.; Nunes, D.S. & Souza Brito, A.R.M. (2000). Gastroprotective effect of essential oil from *Croton cajucara* Benth. (Euphorbiaceae). *Journal of Ethnopharmacology*, Vol.69, No.3, (March 2000), pp. 229-234, ISSN: 0378-8741.

Jafri, M.A.; Farah, J.K. & Singh, S. (2001). Evaluation of the gastric antiulcerogenic effect of large cardamom (fruits of *Amomum subulatum* Roxb). *Journal of Ethnopharmacology*, Vol.75, No.2-3, (May 2001), pp. 89-94, ISSN: 0378-8741.

Johnson-Henry, K.C.; Mitchell, D.J.; Avitzur, Y.; Galindo-Mata, E.; Jones, N.L. & Sherman, P.M. (2004). Probiotics reduce bacterial colonization and gastric inflammation in *H. pylori*-infected mice. *Digestive Diseases & Sciences*, Vol.49, No.7-8, (August 2004), pp. 1095-1102, ISSN: 0163-2116.

Julapalli, V. & Graham, D. (2005). Appropriate use of intravenous proton pump inhibitors in the management of bleeding peptic ulcer. *Digestive Diseases & Sciences,*Vol.50, No.7, (July 2005), pp. 1185–1193, ISSN: 0163-2116.

Kahraman, A.; Erkasap, N.; Köken, T.; Serteser, M.; Aktepe, F. & Erkasap, S. (2003). The antioxidative and antihistaminic properties of quercetin in ethanol-induced gastric lesion. *Toxicology*, Vol.183, No.1-3, (February 2003), pp. 133-142, ISSN: 0300-483X.

Kim, M.N.; Kim, N.; Lee, S.H.; Park, Y.S.; Hwang, J.H.; Kim, J.W.; Jeong, S.H.; Lee, D.H.; Kim, J.S.; Jung, H.C. & Song, I.S. (June 2008). The effects of probiotics on PPI-triple therapy for *Helicobacter pylori* eradication. *Helicobacter*, Vol.13, No.4, pp. 261–268, ISSN: 1083-4389.

Kitazawa, H. Toba, T.; Itoh, T.; Kumano, N.; Adachi, S. & Yamaguchi, T. (1991). Antitumoral activity of slime-forming encapsulated *Lactococcus lactis* subsp. *cremoris* isolated from Scandinavian ropy sour milk, "viili." *Animal Science & Technology*, Vol.62, pp. 277–283, ISSN: 0377-8401.

Kitazawa, H.; Itoh, T.; Tomioka, Y.; Mizugaki, M. & Yamaguchi, T. (1996). Induction of IFN-γ and IL-1 alpha production in macrophages stimulated with phosphopolysaccharide produced by *Lactococcus lactis* ssp. *cremoris*. *International Journal of Food Microbiology*, Vol.31, No.1-3, (August 1996), pp. 99-106, ISSN: 0168-1605.

Kitazawa, H.; Harata, T.; Uemura, J.; Saito, T.; Kaneko, T. & Itoh, T. (1998). Phosphate group requirement for mitogenic activation of lymphocytes by an extracellular phosphopolysaccharide from *Lactobacillus delbrueckii* spp. *bulgaricus*. *International Journal of Food Microbiology*, Vol.40, No.3, (April 1998), pp. 169- 175, ISSN: 0168-1605.

Ko, J.A.; Lim, H.J. & Park, H.J. (2010). Effect of microencapsulated precipitants of *Lactobacillus casei* ATCC 393 on *Helicobacter pylori* eradication. *Process Biochemistry*, Vol.46, No.3, (March 2011), pp. 631-635, ISSN: 1359-5113.

Kohler, J.; Blass, A.; Liu, J.; Kaniza, T. & Soybel, D. (2010). Antioxidant pre-treatment prevents omeprazole-induced toxicity in an *in vitro* model of infectious gastritis. *Free Radical Biology & Medicine*, Vol.49, No.5, (June 2010), pp. 786-791, ISSN: 0891-5849.

Korakli, M.; Gänzle, M.G. & Vogel, R.F. (2002). Metabolism by bifidobacteria and lactic acid bacteria of polysaccharides from wheat and rye, and exopolysaccharides produced by *Lactobacillus sanfranciscensis*. *Journal of Applied Microbiology*, Vol.92, No.5, (April 2002) pp. 958–965, ISSN: 1364-5072.

Kuroda, M.; Yoshida, N.; Ichikawa, H.; Takagi, T.; Okuda, T. & Naito, Y. (2006). Lansoprazole, a proton pump inhibitor, reduces the severity of indomethacin-induced rat enteritis. *International Journal of Molecular Medicine*, Vol.17, No.1, (January 2006), pp. 89–93, ISSN: 1107-3756.

Kusters, J.G.; van Vliet, A.H.M. & Kuipers, E.J. (2006). Pathogenesis of *Helicobacter pylori* infection. *Clinical Microbiology Reviews*, Vol.19, No.3, (July 2006), pp. 449–490, ISSN: 0983-8512.

Lam, E.K.Y.; Tai, E.K.K.; Koo, M.W.L.; Wong, H.P.S.; Wu, W.K.K.; Yu, L.; So, W.H.L.; Woo, P.C.Y. & Cho, C.H. (2007). Enhancement of gastric mucosal integrity by *Lactobacillus rhamnosus* GG. *Life Sciences*, Vol.80, No.23, (May 2007), pp. 2128–2136, ISSN: 0024-3205.

Lebeer, S.; Vanderleyden, J. & De Keersmaecker, S.C.J. (2010). Host interactions of probiotic bacterial surface molecules: comparison with commensals and pathogens. *Nature Reviews Microbiology,* Vol.8, (March 2010), pp. 171-184, ISSN: 1740-1526.

Lengsfeld, C.; Titgemeyer, F.; Faller, G. & Hensel, A. (2004). Glycosylated compounds from okra inhibit adhesion of *Helicobacter pylori* to human gastric mucosa. *Journal of Agricultural & Food Chemistry*, Vol.52, No.6, (February 2004), pp. 1495-1503, ISSN: 0021-8561.

Lin, W.H.; Wu, C.R.; Fang, T.J.; Guo, J.T.; Huang, S.Y.; Lee, M.S. & Yang, H.L. (2011). Anti-*Helicobacter pylori* activity of fermented milk with lactic acid bacteria. *Journal of the Science of Food & Agriculture, Vol.-*, No.-, (March 2011), pp.-, ISSN: 0022-5142 (IN PRESS).

Linsalata, M.; Russo, F.; Berloco, P.; Caruso, M.L.; Matteo, G.D.; Cifone, M.G.; Simone, C.D.; Ierardi, E. & Di Leo, A. (2004). The influence of *Lactobacillus brevis* on ornithine decarboxylase activity and polyamine profiles in *Helicobacter pylori*-infected gastric mucosa. *Helicobacter*, Vol.9, No.2, (April 2004), pp. 165-172, ISSN: 1083-4389.

Liu, C.F.; Hu, C.L.; Chiang, S.S.; Tseng, K.C.; Yu, R.C. & Pan, T.M. (2009).Beneficial preventive effects of gastric mucosal lesion for soy-skim milk fermented by lactic acid bacteria. *Journal of Agricultural & Food Chemistry*, Vol.57, No.10, (May 2009), pp. 4433-4438, ISSN: 0021-8561.

Logan, R.; Walker, M.; Misiewicz, J.; Gummett, P.; Karim, Q. & Baron, J. (1995). Changes in the intragastric distribution of *Helicobacter pylori* during treatment with omeprazole. *Gut*, Vol.36, No.1, (April 1994), pp. 12–16, ISSN: 0017-5749.

Mater, D.D.; Bretigny, L.; Firnesse, O.; Flores, M.J.; Mogenet, A.; Bresson, J.L. & Carthier, G. (2005). *Streptococcus thermophilus* and *Lactobacillus delbrueckii* subsp. *bulgaricus* survive gastrointestinal transit of healthy volunteer consuming yogurt. *FEMS Microbiology Letters*, Vol.250, No.2, (September 2005), pp. 185–187, ISSN: 0378-1097.

Matsubara, S.; Shibata, H.; Ishikawa, F.; Yokokura, T.; Takahashi, M.; Sugimura, T. & Wakabayashi, K. (2003). Suppression of *Helicobacter pylori*-induced gastritis by green tea extract in Mongolian gerbils. *Biochemical and Biophysical Research Communications*, Vol.310, No.3, (October 2003), pp. 715–719, ISSN: 0006-291X.

Matsumoto, H.; Shimokawa, Y.; Ushida, Y.; Toida, T. & Hayasawa, H. (2001). New biological function of bovine α-lactalbumin: Protective effect against ethanol and stress-induced gastric mucosal injury in rats. *Bioscience Biotechnology & Biochemistry*, Vol. 65, No.5, (May 2001), pp. 1104-1111, ISSN: 0916-8451.

Michetti, P.; Dorta, G.; Wiesel, P.H.; Brassart, D.; Verdu, E.; Herranz, M.; Felley, C.; Porta, N.; Rouvet, M.; Blum, A.L. & Corthesy-Theulaz, I. (1999). Effect of whey-based culture supernatant of *Lactobacillus acidophilus* (*johnsonii*) La1 on *Helicobacter pylori* infection in humans. *Digestion*, Vol.60, No.3, (October 2008), pp. 203–209, ISSN: 0012-2823.

Mozzi, F.; Vaningelgem, F.; Hébert, E.M.; Van der Meulen, R.; Foulquié Moreno, M.R.; Font de Valdez, G. & De Vuyst, L. (2006). Diversity of heteropolysaccharide-producing lactic acid bacterium strains and their biopolymers. *Applied & Environmental Microbiology*, Vol.72, No.6, (June 2006), pp. 4431-4435, ISSN: 0099- 2240.

Mozzi, F.; Gerbino, E.; Font de Valdez, G. & Torino, M.I. (2009). Functionality of exopolysaccharides produced by lactic acid bacteria in an *in vitro* gastric system. *Journal of Applied Microbiology*, Vol.107, No.1, (July 2009), pp. 54-64, ISSN: 1364-5072.

Nagaoka, M.; Hashimoto, S.; Watanabe, T.; Yokokura, T. & Mori, Y. (1994). Anti-ulcer effects of lactic acid bacteria and their cell wall polysaccharides. *Biological & Pharmaceutical Bulletin*, Vol.17, No.8, (August 1994), pp. 1012-1017, ISSN: 0918-6158.

Nam, S.Y.; Kim, N.; Lee, C.S.; Choi, K.D.; Lee, H.S.; Jung, H.C. & Song, I.S. (2005). Gastric mucosal protection via enhancement of MUC5AC and MUC6 by geranylgeranylacetone. *Digestive Diseases & Sciences*, Vol.50, No.11, (November 2005), pp. 2110-2120, ISSN: 0163-2116.

Nergard, C.S.; Diallo, D.; Michaelsen, T.E.; Malterud, K.E.; Kiyohara, H.; Matsumoto, T.; Yamada, H. & Paulsen, B.S. (2004). Isolation, partial characterisation and immunomodulating activities of polysaccharides from *Vernonia kotschyana* Sch. Bip. ex Walp. *Journal of Ethnopharmacology*, Vol.91, No.1, (March 2004), pp. 141-152, ISSN: 0378-8741.

Neves, J.; Matos, C.; Moutinho, C.; Queiroz, G. & Gomes, L. (2009). Ethnopharmacological notes about ancient uses of medicinal plants in Trás-os-Montes (northern of Portugal). *Journal of Ethnopharmacology*, Vol.124, No.2, (May 2009), pp. 270-283, ISSN: 0378-8741.

Pali-Schöll, I.; Herzog, R.; Wallmann, J.; Szalai, K.; Brunner, R.; Lukschal, A.; Karagiannis, P.; Diesner, S. & Jensen-Jarolim, E. (2010). Antacids and dietary supplements with an influence on the gastric pH increase the risk for food sensitization. *Clinical &Experimental Allergy*, Vol.40, No.7, (July 2010), pp. 1091–1098, ISSN: 0954-7894.

Pali-Schöll, I. & Jensen-Jarolim, E. (2011). Anti-acid medication as a risk factor for food allergy. *Allergy*, Vol.66, No.4, (December 2011), pp. 469–477, EISSN: 1398-9995.

Park, M.J.; Kim, J.S.; Yim, J.Y.; Jung, H.C.; Song, I.S.; Yu, E.S.; Lee, J.J.; Huh, C.S. & Baek, Y.J. (2001). The suppressive effect of a fermented milk containing *Lactobacilli* on *Helicobacter pylori* in human gastric mucosa. *Korean Journal of Gastroenterology*, Vol.38, No.4, (October 2001), pp. 233-240, ISSN: 1598-9992.

Park, S.; Hahm, K.; Oh, T.; Jin, J. & Choue, R. (2004). Preventive effect of the flavonoid, wogonin, against ethanol-induced gastric mucosal damage in rats. *Digestive Diseases and Sciences*,Vol.49, No.3, (March 2004), pp. 384-394, ISSN: 0163-2116.

Penner, R.; Fedorak, R.N. & Madsen, K.L. (2005). Probiotics and nutraceuticals: non-medicinal treatments of gastrointestinal diseases. *Current Opinion in Pharmacology*, Vol.5, No.6, (December 2005), pp. 596-603, ISSN: 1471-4892.

Pertino, M.; Schmeda-Hirschmann, G.; Rodríguez, J.A. & Theoduloz, C. (2007). Gastroprotective effect and cytotoxicity of terpenes from the Paraguayan crude drug "yagua rova" (*Jatropha isabelli*). *Journal of Ethnopharmacology*, Vol.111, No.3, (May 2007), pp. 553-559, ISSN: 0378-8741.

Peura, D. (2004). Prevention of non-steroidal anti-inflammatory drug associated gastrointestinal symptoms and ulcer complications. *The American Journal of Medicine,* Vol.117, No.5, (Suppl.1), (September 2004), pp. 63–71, ISSN: 0002-9343.

Pigeon, R.M.; Cuesta, E.P. & Gilliland, S.E. (2002). Binding of free bile acids by cells of yogurt starter culture bacteria. *Journal of Dairy Science,* Vol.85, No.11, (November 2002), pp. 2705-2710, ISSN: 1525-3198.

Quach, D.; Le, H.; Nguyen, O.; Nguyen, T. & Uemura N. (2011). The severity of endoscopy gastric atrophy could help to predict Operative Link on Gastritis Assessment gastritis stage. *Journal of Gastroenterology & Hepatology,* Vol.26, No.2, (January 2011), pp. 281–285, ISSN: 0815-9319.

Rehecho, S.; Uriarte-Pueyo, I.; Calvo, J.; Vivas, L. & Calvo, M. (2010). Ethnopharmacological survey of medicinal plants in Nor-Yauyos, a part of the Landscape Reserve Nor-Yauyos-Cochas, Perú. *Journal of Ethnopharmacology,* Vol.133, No.1, (January 2011), pp. 75-85, ISSN: 0378-8741.

Rocha Lapa, F.; Freitas, C.; Hatsuko Baggio, C.; Missau, F.; Pizzolatti, M.; Santos, A. & Marques, M. (2007). Gastroprotective activity of the hydroalcoholic extract obtained from *Polygala paniculata* L. in rats. *Journal of Pharmacy & Pharmacology,* Vol.59, No.10, (October 2007), pp. 1413-1419, ISSN: 0022-3573.

Rodríguez C.; Medici, M.; Rodríguez, A.V.; Mozzi, F. & Font de Valdez, G. (2009). Prevention of chronic gastritis by fermented milks made with exopolysaccharide-producing *Streptococcus thermophilus* strains. *Journal of Dairy Science,* Vol.92, No.6, (June 2009), pp. 2423-2434, ISSN: 1525-3198.

Rodríguez, C.; Medici M.; Mozzi, F. & Font de Valdez, G. (2010). Therapeutic effect of *Streptococcus thermophilus* CRL 1190-fermented milk on chronic gastritis. *World Journal of Gastroenterology,* Vol.16, No.13, (April 2010), pp. 1622-1630, ISSN: 1007-9327.

Rosaneli, C.F.; Bighetti, A.E.; Antônio, M.A.; Carvalho, J.E. & Sgarbieri, V.C. (2004). Protective effect of bovine milk whey protein concentrate on the ulcerative lesions caused by subcutaneous administration of indomethacin. *Journal of Medicinal Food,* Vol.7, No.3, (Fall 2004), pp. 309-314, ISSN: 1096-620X.

Ruas-Madiedo, P.; Hugenholtz, J. & Zoon, P. (2002). An overview of the functionality of exopolysaccharides produced by lactic acid bacteria. *International Dairy Journal,* Vol.12, No.2-3, pp. 163-171, ISSN: 0958-6946.

Ruas-Madiedo, P.; Gueimonde, M.; Margolles, A.; de los Reyes-Gavilán, C.G. & Salminen, S. (2006). Exopolysaccharides produced by probiotic strains modify the adhesion of probiotics and enteropathogens to human intestinal mucus. *Journal of Food Protection,* Vol.69, No.8, (August 2006), pp. 2011-2015, ISSN: 0362-028X.

Ryan, K.A.; Daly, P.; Li, Y.; Hooton, C. & O'Toole, P.W. (2008). Strain specific inhibition of *Helicobacter pylori* by *Lactobacillus salivarius* and other lactobacilli. *Journal of Antimicrobial Chemotherapy,* Vol.61, No.4, (April 2008), pp. 831-834, ISSN: 0305-7453.

Sakamoto, I.; Igarashi, M.; Kimura, K.; Takagi, A.; Miwa, T. & Koga, Y. (2001). Suppressive effect of *Lactobacillus gasseri* OLL2716 (LG21) on *Helicobacter pylori* infection in humans. *Journal of Antimicrobial Chemotherapy,* Vol.47, No.5, (December 2001), pp. 709-710, ISSN: 0305-7453.

Salazar, N.; Prieto, A.; Leal, J.A.; Mayo, B.; Bada-Gancedo, J.C.; de los Reyes-Gavilán, C.G. & Ruas-Madiedo, P. (2009). Production of exopolysaccharides by *Lactobacillus* and *Bifidobacterium* strains of human origin, and metabolic activity of the producing bacteria in milk. *Journal of Dairy Science,* Vol.92, No.9, (September 2009), pp. 4158-4168, ISSN: 1525-3198.

Schmeda-Hirschmann, G.; Rodriguez, J. & Astudillo, L. (2002). Gastroprotective activity of the diterpene solidagenone and its derivatives on experimentally induced gastric lesions in mice. *Journal of Ethnopharmacology*, Vol.81, No.1, (June 2002), pp. 111-115, ISSN: 0378-8741.

Schmidt-Lebuhn, A.N. (2008). Ethnobotany, biochemistry and pharmacology of *Minthostachys* (Lamiaceae). *Journal of Ethnopharmacology*, Vol.118, No.3, (August 2008), pp. 343-353, ISSN: 0378-8741.

Sgouras, D.N.; Panayotopoulou, E.G.; Martinez-Gonzalez, B.; Petraki, K.; Michopoulos, S. & Mentis, M. (2005). *Lactobacillus johnsonii* La1 attenuates *Helicobacter pylori*-associated gastritis and reduces levels of pro-inflammatory chemokines in C57BL/6 Mice. *Clinical and Diagnostic Laboratory Immunology*, Vol.12, No.12, (December 2005), pp. 1378-1386, ISSN: 1071-412X.

Shiotani, A.; Kamada, T. & Haruma K. (2008). Low-dose aspirin induced gastrointestinal diseases: past, present, and future. *Journal of Gastroenterology*, Vol.43, No.8, (April 2008), pp. 581-588, ISSN: 0944-1174.

Shirasawa, Y.; Shibahara-Sone, H.; Iino, T. & Ishikawa, F. (2010). *Bifidobacterium bifidum* BF-1 suppresses *Helicobacter pylori*-induced genes in human epithelial cells. *Journal of Dairy Science*, Vol.93, No.10, (October 2010), pp. 4526-4534, ISSN: 1525-3198.

Shirwaikar, A.; Bhilegaonkar, P.; Malini, S. & Sharath Kuma J. (2003). The gastroprotective activity of the ethanol extract of *Ageratum conyzoides*. *Journal of Ethnopharmacology*, Vol.86, No.1, (May 2003), pp. 117-121, ISSN: 0378-8741.

Sipponen, P. & Price, A. (2011). The Sydney system for classification of gastritis: 20 years ago. *Journal of Gastroenterology & Hepatology*, Vol.26, No.l, (January 2011), pp. 31–34, ISSN: 08159319.

Stoicov, C.; Saffari, Z. & Houghton, J.M. (2009). Green tea inhibits *Helicobacter* growth *in vivo* and *in vitro*. *International Journal of Antimicrobial Agents*, Vol.33, No.5, (May 2009), pp. 473-478, ISSN: 0924-8579.

Stolte, M. & Meining A. (2001). The updated Sydney system: Classification and grading of gastritis as the basis of diagnosis and treatment. *The Canadian Journal of Gastroenterology*, Vol. 15, No. 9, (September 2001), pp. 591-598, ISSN: 08357900.

Takabayashi, F.; Harada, N.; Yamada, M.; Murohisa, B. & Oguni, I. (2004). Inhibitory effect of green tea catechins in combination with sucralfate on *Helicobacter pylori* infection in Mongolian gerbils. *Journal of Gastroenterology*, Vol.39, No.1, (January 2004), pp. 61–63, ISSN: 0944-1174.

Tan, P.; Nyasse, B.; Dimo, T. & Mezui, C. (2002). Gastric cytoprotective anti-ulcer effects of the leaf methanol extract of *Ocimum suave* (Lamiaceae) in rats. *Journal of Ethnopharmacology*, Vol.82, No.2-3, (October 2002), pp. 69-74, ISSN: 0378-8741.

Tofil, N.; Benner, K.; Fuller, M. & Winkler, M. (2008). Histamine 2 receptor antagonists vs intravenous proton pump inhibitors in a pediatric intensive care unit: a comparison of gastric pH. *Journal of Critical Care*, Vol.23, No.3, (September 2008), pp. 416–421.

Uchida, M.; Matsueda, K.; Shoda, R.; Muraoka, A. & Yamato, S. (2001). Nitric oxide donating compounds inhibit HCl-induced gastric mucosal lesions mainly via prostaglandin. *Japanese Journal of Pharmacology*, Vol.85, No.2, (February 2001), pp. 133–138, ISSN: 0021-5198.

Uchida, M. & Kurakazu, K. (2004). Yogurt containing *Lactobacillus gasseri* OLL2716 exerts gastroprotective action against acute gastric lesion and antral ulcer in rats. *Journal of Pharmacological Sciences*, Vol.96, No.1, (September 2004), pp. 84-90, ISSN: 1347-8613.

Ushida, Y.; Shimokawa, Y.; Matsumoto, H.; Toida, T. & Hayasawa, H. (2003). Effects of bovine α-lactoalbumin on gastric defense mechanisms in naive rats. *Bioscience Biotechnology & Biochemistry*, Vol.67, No.3, (March 2003), pp. 577-583, ISSN: 0916-8451.

Ushida, Y.; Shimokawa, Y.; Toida, T.; Matsui, H. & Takase, M. (2007). Bovine α-lactoalbumin stimulates mucus metabolism in gastric mucosa. *Journal of Dairy Science*, Vol.90, No.2, (February 2007), pp. 541-546, ISSN: 1525-3198.

Valeur, N.; Engel, P.; Carbajal, N.; Connolly, E. & Ladefoged, K. (2004). Colonization and immunomodulation by *Lactobacillus reuteri* ATCC 55730 in the human gastrointestinal tract. *Applied & Environmental Microbiology*, Vol.70, No.2, (February 2004), pp. 1176-1181, ISSN: 0099- 2240.

van Hijum, S.; Kralj, S.; Ozimek, L.K.; Dijkhuizen, L. & van Geel-Schutten, I.G. (2006). Structure-function relationships of glucansucrase and fructansucrase enzymes from lactic acid bacteria. *Microbiology & Molecular Biology Reviews*, Vol.70, No.1, (March 2006), pp. 157-176, ISSN: 1092-2172.

Vinderola C.G & Renheimer, J.A. (2003). Lactic acid starter and probiotic bacteria: a comparative *"in vitro"* study of probiotic characteristics and biological barrier resistance. *Food Research International*, (September 2003) Vol.36, No.9, pp. 895-904, ISSN: 0963-9969.

Vitalini, S.; Tomè, F. & Fico, G. (2009). Traditional uses of medicinal plants in Valvestino (Italy). *Journal of Ethnopharmacology*, Vol.121, No.1, (January 2009), pp. 106-116, ISSN: 0378-8741.

Voutilainen, M.; Juhola, M.; Färkkilä, M. & Sipponen, P. (2002). Foveolar hyperplasia at the gastric cardia: prevalence and associations. *Journal of Clinical Pathology*, Vol.55, No.5, (November 2001), pp. 352–354, ISSN: 0021-9746.

Wang, K.Y.; Li, S.N.; Liu, C.S.; Perng, D.S.; Su, Y.C.; Wu, D.C.; Jan, C.M.; Lai, C.H.; Wang, T.N. & Wang, W.M. (2004). Effects of ingesting *Lactobacillus*- and *Bifidobacterium*-containing yogurt in subjects with colonized *Helicobacter pylori*. *American Journal of Clinical Nutrition*, Vol.80, No.3, (September 2004), pp. 737–741, ISSN: 0002-9165.

Wells, J.M. & Mercenier, A. (2008). Mucosal delivery of therapeutic and prophylactic molecules using lactic acid bacteria. Nature Reviews Microbiology, Vol.6, (May 2008), pp. 349-362, ISSN: 1740-1526.

Wittschier, N.; Faller, G. & Hensel, A. (2007). An extract of *Pelargonium sidoides* (EPs 7630) inhibits in situ adhesion of *Helicobacter pylori* to human stomach. *Phytomedicine*, Vol. 14, No. 4, (April 2007), pp. 285-288, ISSN: 0944-7113.

Wittschier, N.; Faller, G. & Hensel, A. (2009). Aqueous extracts and polysaccharides from Liquorice roots (*Glycyrrhiza glabra* L.) inhibit adhesion of *Helicobacter pylori* to human gastric mucosa. *Journal of Ethnopharmacology*, Vol.125, No.2, (September 2009), pp. 218-223, ISSN: 0378-8741.

Wolle, K. & Malfertheiner, P. (2007). Treatment of *Helicobacter pylori*. *Best Practice & Research Clinical Gastroenterology*, Vol.21, No.2, (April 2007), pp. 315-324, ISSN: 1521-6918.

Yamada, H. (1995). Structure and pharmacological activity of pectic polysaccharides from the roots of *Bupleurum falcatum* L. *Nippon Yakurigaku Zasshi,* Vol.106, No.3, (September 1995), pp. 229-237, EISSN: 0015-5691.

Yim, J.H.; Son, E.; Pyo, S. & Lee, H.K. (2005). Novel sulfated polysaccharide derived from red-tide microalga *Gyrodinium impudicum* strain KG03 with immunostimulating activity *in vivo*. *Marine Biotechnology* (New York), Vol.7, No.4, (Julio 2005), pp. 331-338, ISSN: 1436-2228.

Part 3

Helicobacter Pylori Infection in Gastritis and Gastric Cancer

10

Gastric Cancer Risk Diagnosis and Prevention in Subjects with *Helicobacter pylori*-related Chronic Gastritis

Shotaro Enomoto, Mika Watanabe, Chizu Mukoubayashi, Hiroshi Ohata, Hirohito Magari, Izumi Inoue, Takao Maekita, Mikitaka Iguchi, Kimihiko Yanaoka, Hideyuki Tamai, Jun Kato, Masashi Oka and Masao Ichinose
Second Department of Internal Medicine, Wakayama Medical University
Japan

1. Introduction

Helicobacter pylori (HP) is recognized as a major pathogenic factor for persistent inflammation in the human stomach (Dooley et al., 1989; Marshall & Warren, 1984). In 1994, the International Agency for Research on Cancer (IARC) classified HP infection as a definite class I carcinogen (International Agency for Research on Cancer (IARC), 1994). HP triggers chronic inflammation of the infected stomach mucosa and is considered a major risk factor for gastric cancer (GC) and associated precursor lesions. Long-lasting inflammation in the stomach mucosa leads to a cascade of molecular and morphological changes, representing the gastritis-atrophy-metaplasia-dysplasia-cancer sequence (Correa, 1992). The HP infection rate is higher in Japan than in Western countries, with nearly all cases of GC occurring in subjects with underlying HP-related chronic gastritis. HP infection is widely accepted as a major risk factor for the development of GC and its precursor lesions, based on extensive evidence derived from many studies (Blaser et al., 1995; EUROGAST Study Group, 1993; Forman et al., 1991; Hirayama et al., 1999; Honda et al., 1998; Huang et al., 1998; Nomura et al., 1991; Parsonnet et al., 1991; Shimizu et al., 1999; Sipponen et al., 1992; Sugiyama et al., 1998; Talley et al., 1991; Tokieda et al., 1999; Uemura et al., 2001; Watanabe et al., 1998; Zheng et al., 2004).
However, in countries such as Japan, where the HP infection rate is high, prediction of GC risk based solely on the presence or absence of HP infection does not offer sufficient specificity. Elucidation of groups at high risk based on the natural history of GC is clearly necessary. The identification of useful markers of GC risk is thus hoped for. Evaluating HP-related chronic gastritis and determining which subjects are at high risk for developing GC is very important, and would likely increase the efficacy of GC screening by endoscopic or other examinations (Enomoto et al., 2010a; Mukoubayashi et al., 2007; Ohata et al., 2005), and strategic approaches to metachronous multiple GC after endoscopic mucosal resection (EMR) or endoscopic submucosal dissection (ESD) performed as minimally invasive treatment for early GC (Gotoda, 2007; Kakushima & Fujishiro, 2008; Nakajima et al., 2006). In addition, in terms of GC prevention, it has become clear that HP-related chronic gastritis cannot be ignored as an origin of carcinogenesis.

Here, we discuss the significance of serum pepsinogen (PG) as a marker of GC risk and GC high-risk groups based on HP-related chronic gastritis. We also discuss the prevention for individuals with HP-related chronic gastritis.

2. GC risk diagnosis based on the natural history of HP-related chronic gastritis

Novel risk markers to identify GC high-risk groups based on a detailed natural history of HP-related chronic gastritis have long been awaited. In this section, we discuss the emerging significance of serum PG as a GC risk marker for more precise identification of GC high-risk groups.

2.1 Serum PG test

HP-related chronic gastritis usually starts in the antrum and expands proximally towards the body of the stomach (Kimura, 1972; Tatsuta et al., 1973). As several studies dealing with endoscopic biopsies or chromoendoscopic testing have found that progression of chronic atrophic gastritis (CAG) increases the risk of cancer (Meister et al., 1979; Sipponen et al., 1985; Siurala et al., 1966; Tatsuta et al., 1993; Testoni et al., 1987), accurate and reliable evaluation of the extent of CAG is considered important for identifying individuals at high risk of cancer. However, accurately diagnosing the extent of CAG based on a few biopsy samples is difficult, because CAG together with intestinal metaplasia is a multifocal process. Furthermore, histological diagnosis of gastric atrophy depends on subjective judgment without a gold standard (Guarner et al., 1999; Plummer et al., 1997). A test for CAG progression that is more convenient, free of discomfort or risk, economical and based on objective parameters is needed.

PG is the inactive precursor of pepsin, a digestive enzyme specifically produced in the stomach. Immunologically, two isozymes exist (Kageyama, 2003). PGI is produced by chief cells and mucus neck cells of the gastric fundic glands. In contrast, PGII is produced not only by chief cells and mucus neck cells, but also in cardiac glands, pyloric glands, and Brunner's glands, with localization of producing cells in a wide range from the stomach to the duodenum. The majority of PG produced (about 99%) is secreted in the stomach lumen and functions as a digestive enzyme. However, a small amount of PG (about 1%) is also present in blood and can be evaluated by measuring serum PG levels. Serum PG levels are generally agreed to reflect the morphological and functional status of the stomach mucosa (Hirschowitz, 1957; Samloff et al., 1982).

In an endoscopic study with Congo red staining, we have shown a strong correlation between an increase in glandular boundary, associated with diagnosed progression of gastric mucosal atrophy, and stepwise reductions in serum PGI levels and the PGI/PGII ratio (**Fig. 1**) (Miki et al., 1987). In other words, by measuring serum PGI and the PGI/II ratio, the progression of CAG, which is involved in GC carcinogenesis, can be objectively evaluated (Ichinose et al., 2001). In addition, during HP infection, serum PGI and PGII increase, and the PG I/II ratio decreases. These findings are improved after eradication treatment (Furuta et al., 1997) and are useful as gastric mucosal inflammatory markers.

Several criteria are used in the serum PG test. As criteria for GC screening, the combination of PGI ≤70 ng/ml and PGI/II ratio ≤3.0, as a reference value by Miki et al., is widely accepted (PG index 1+) (Ichinose et al., 2001; Watanabe et al., 1997). Values lower than this

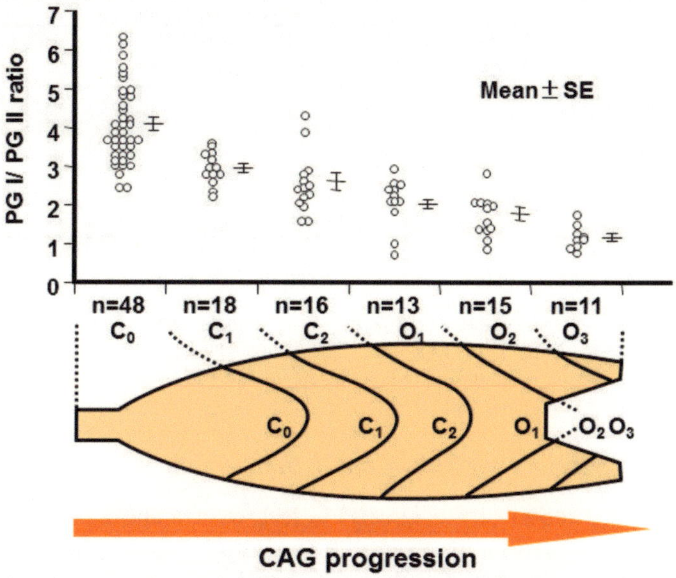

Fig. 1. Relationship between serum pepsinogen (PG)I/PGII ratio and progression of chronic atrophic gastritis (CAG). With atrophic changes in the gastric mucosa progressing from the pyloric glands to more proximally, the serum PGI/II ratio decreases, reflecting an associated loss of PG-producing cells. CAG, chronic atrophic gastritis; SE, standard error.

reference value are considered PG-test positive. In addition to this reference value, to identify more severe CAG progression, criteria of PGI ≤50 ng/ml and PGI/II ratio ≤3.0 (PG index 2+), and PGI ≤30 ng/ml and PGI/II ratio ≤2.0 (PG index 3+) are also used. Since 1992, when PG assay kits became commercially available, a number of screening services provided by workplaces or community health services have adopted this serum test as a filter test (Hattori et al., 1995; Kitahara et al., 1999; Kodoi et al., 1995; Miki et al., 1993; Miki et al., 2003; Ohata et al, 2005; Yoshihara et al., 1997). However, the long-term prognosis of subjects with extensive CAG identified by PG filter test is not fully known.

2.2 Detection accuracy of GC using the serum PG test

We conducted a large-scale cohort study spanning more than 10 years in Wakayama Prefecture, Japan, and identified groups at high risk for GC (Ohata et al., 2004; Yanaoka et al., 2008a; Yanaoka et al., 2008b). Based on the results, accuracy of each criteria of the serum PG test for GC that occurred during the observation period was evaluated (Yanaoka et al, 2008a). Accuracy of the criteria is shown in **Table 1**. For the most favorable criteria (PG index 1+), sensitivity was 58.7%, specificity was 73.4%, and positive predictive value was 2.6%. Compared to a meta-analysis of PG test sensitivity (Dinis-Ribeiro et al., 2004), these results were poor, particularly in terms of sensitivity.

As a reason for these poor results, the presence of GC easy to detect by barium X-ray, and GC easy to detect by the serum PG test, was cited (Ohata et al, 2005). In the above-mentioned meta-analysis, many of the previously reported cases that were reviewed were from studies in populations in which GC screening by conventional barium X-ray had been conducted over a period of many years. In other words, that study reviewed results for GC

	Serum PG test criteria		
	PGI ≤70 and PGI/II ≤3 [PG index 1+]	PGI ≤50 and PGI/II ≤3 [PG index 2+]	PGI ≤30 and PGI/II ≤2 [PG index 3+]
Meta-analysis of reported cases (Dinis-Ribeiro et al., 2004)			
Pooled sensitivity	77.3%	68.4%	51.9%
(95%CI)	(69.8-83.8)	(59.1-76.8)	(40.3-63.5)
Pooled specificity	73.2%	69.3%	84.4%
(95%CI)	(72.8-73.6)	(66.6-70.0)	(83.7-85.0)
Our results (Yanaoka et al., 2008a)			
Sensitivity	58.7%	49.2%	27.0%
(95%CI)	(45.6-70.8)	(36.5-62.0)	(16.9-39.9)
Specificity	73.4%	80.5%	92.0%
(95%CI)	(72.1-74.6)	(79.4-81.6%)	(91.3-92.8)

PG, pepsinogen.
CI, confidential interval.

Table 1. Comparison of accuracy for each criterion in the serum PG test.

detection just after introduction of the serum PG test, over a short period, and targeting a population in whom GC was difficult to detect by barium X-ray, i.e., those in whom GC was easy to detect by the serum PG test. On the other hand, GC cases just after introduction of the serum PG test were excluded from our study, and observation was over a long period of 10 years. Accordingly, results for the detection of GC occurring during the observation period were more rigorously evaluated, and thus more correctly reflective of the accuracy for detecting GC by the serum PG test. Based on the above results, using the serum PG test alone for GC screening has limitations. A more elaborate system must therefore be developed, including for GC screening in PG test-negative cases.

2.3 GC risk in a serum PG test-positive group

Previous studies have examined the accuracy of the serum PG test as a filter test for endoscopy. Recently, as part of an investigation into the natural history of GC occurrence, we evaluated GC risk in populations identified by each criteria for the serum PG test (Yanaoka et al, 2008a). In a population of middle-aged healthy men, in an atrophy-negative group, the annual incidence of GC was 0.07%. In contrast, annual incidence was 0.28% in the PG index 1+ group, 0.32% in the PG index 2+ group, and 0.42% in the PG index 3 +group, showing significant stepwise increases in GC incidence with CAG progression (**Fig. 2**) Based on these results, PG test-positive groups, as assumed, are high-risk groups for GC. In other words, an individual who is serum PG test-positive, even if GC is not currently detectable, still has a high possibility of developing GC in the future. Careful monitoring with detailed testing is clearly indicated in such subjects. This again demonstrates the usefulness of the PG test as a marker of high risk for GC.

2.4 Natural history of HP-related chronic gastritis and GC risk

In addition to the serum PG test, the natural history of HP-related chronic gastritis and associations with GC risk have been examined by evaluating HP infection, as the major cause of onset and progression of chronic gastritis in Japan (Ohata et al, 2004; Yanaoka et al, 2008b). HP infection is diagnosed using anti-HP antibody titers, which, like the serum PG test, is a blood test that is easy to perform. The stages of HP-related chronic gastritis, from

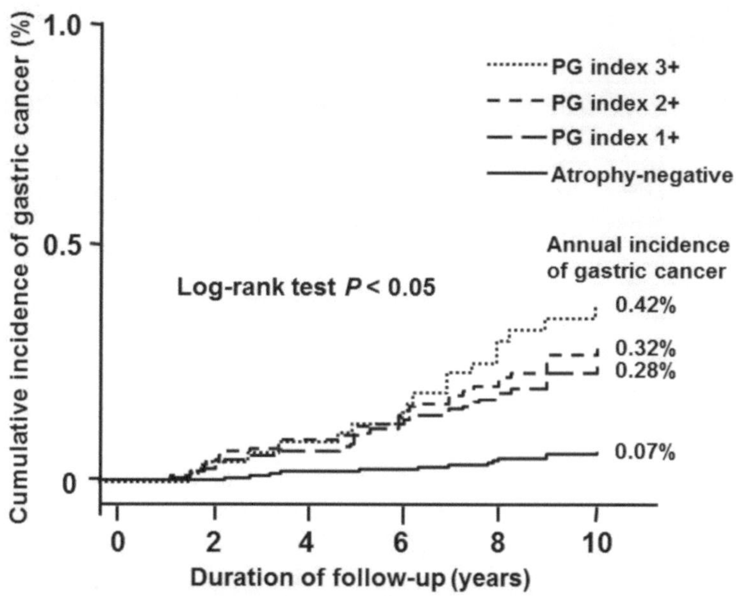

Fig. 2. Kaplan-Meier analysis of gastric cancer development in subjects classified using the criteria of the serum pepsinogen (PG) test. Among middle-aged healthy men, annual incidence of gastric cancer is shown for each population identified using various criteria for the serum PG test. Progression of chronic atrophic gastritis showed a significant stepwise increase in the incidence of gastric cancer.

the onset of HP infection to development of atrophic gastritis, can be classified based on a combination of both serum blood tests: Group A [HP(-), PG(-)], Group B [HP(+), PG(-)], Group C [HP(+), PG(+)], and Group D [HP(-), PG(+)]. Group A comprised HP non-infected healthy subjects. Group B showed established HP infection, but without extensive CAG. Group C had extensive CAG. Group D had severe intestinal metaplasia due to progression of CAG, but HP had been spontaneously eliminated, representing so-called metaplastic gastritis.

The natural history of HP-related chronic gastritis from the onset of HP infection can be shown to progress from each stage: A→B→C→D. Based on a follow-up study, the annual incidence of GC for each group using this stage classification was: 0% for Group A (no occurrence of GC during 10 years in this group); 0.11% for Group B (GC in 1 per 1000 patients per year); 0.24% for Group C (GC in 1 per 400 patients per year); and 1.31% for Group D (GC in about 1 per 80 patients per year). Based on these data, with progression in stage of HP-related chronic gastritis, a stepwise increase is seen for GC incidence (**Fig. 3**). Similar results were reported by Watabe et al. (Watabe et al., 2005). During the 10-year follow-up study, all patients who developed GC were HP infection-positive. These results showed that in Japan, almost all cases of GC are associated with HP-related chronic gastritis. Theoretically, based on this fact, not only a GC high-risk group, but also a GC low-risk group (group A), can be identified. This is expected to contribute greatly to suitable and more intensive GC screening.

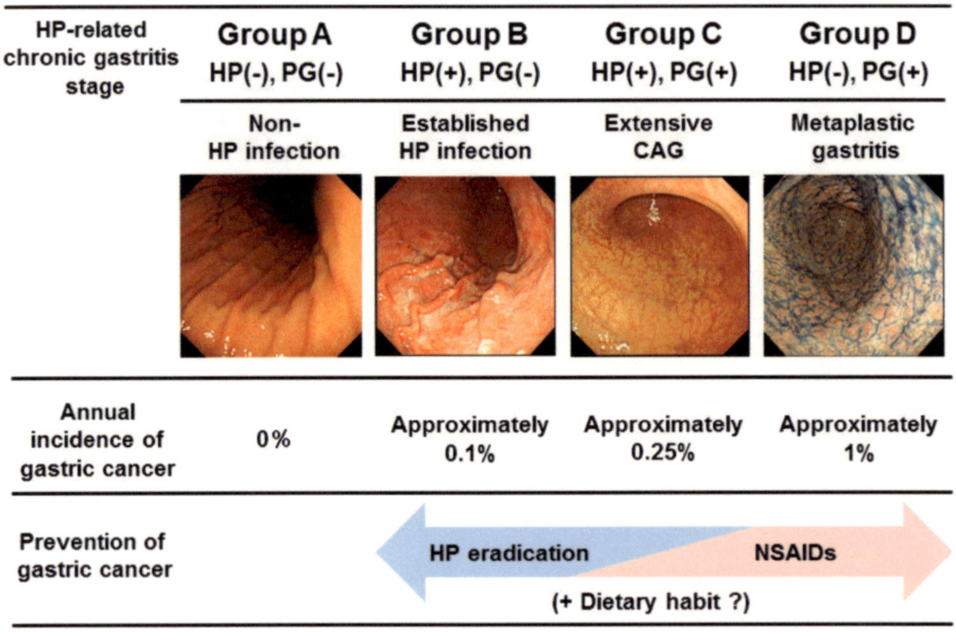

Fig. 3. Gastric cancer risk and prevention of gastric cancer based on *Helicobacter pylori* (HP)-related chronic gastritis stage. This shows the stage classification for HP-related chronic gastritis based on the serum pepsinogen (PG) test and HP antibodies. Among middle-aged healthy men, the annual incidence of gastric cancer showed a significant stepwise increase from Group A to Group D according to stage progression. Regarding gastric cancer prevention based on stage, in Group B, with mild atrophy, prevention of gastric cancer mainly by HP eradication can be expected. In Group D, with progression of atrophy and metaplastic gastritis, prevention of gastric cancer mainly by administration of non-steroidal anti-inflammatory drugs (e.g., cyclooxygenase 2 inhibitors) can be expected. In addition, prevention of gastric cancer may be possible with dietary habits.

2.5 Points in the diagnosis of GC risk using the serum PG test

The serum PG test is clearly a highly useful test for a GC risk marker. However, the occurrence of GC (particularly diffuse-type GC) in PG test-negative groups (group B in the stage classification for HP-related chronic gastritis) cannot be ignored. In our study, even when using the PG test criteria considered as the most balanced in terms of test accuracy (PG index 1+), the fact remains that about 40% of GC cases are PG test-negative. When diagnosing GC risk using the serum PG test, this fact must be carefully considered.

We therefore carefully investigated GC occurrence in a PG test-negative group. Specifically, to evaluate GC incidence, we subdivided the PG test-negative group into 3 groups: α group (serum PGI ≤70 ng/ml and PGI/II >3); β group (serum PGI >70 ng/ml and PGI/II >3), and γ group (serum PGI >70 ng/ml and PGI/II ≤3). The results identified a new group at high risk of GC, with GC incidence in the γ group (high serum PGII levels and severe inflammation of the gastric mucosa) reaching 0.2%, predominantly involving undifferentiated GC (Yanaoka et al, 2008a). This rate in the γ group, although not necessarily high among the PG test-negative group, still indicates a subgroup that deserves particular attention. In addition, a group with high HP antibody titer (a marker that, like serum PGII level, reflects severity of inflammation) showed higher incidence of GC compared to a low-titer group (Yanaoka et al, 2008b).

Among PG test-negative groups, in group A of the stage classification for HP-related chronic gastritis (PG test-negative and HP-negative), we observed no occurrence of GC over a 10-year follow-up period. However, some cautionary points must be considered in a confirmatory diagnosis of Group A status. First, with HP antibody assay kits showing low sensitivity, antibody titers may be negative despite prior HP infection. Second, in HP-negative cases after eradication therapy, it should be kept in mind that "although HP is negative, the risk of GC is not zero." Third, risk assessment by the serum PG test cannot be applied in subjects with post-gastrectomy ,with renal insufficiency, using proton pump inhibitors, or showing an acute gastric mucosal lesion (AGML). In addition, we have reported that in subjects with a PGI/II ratio ≤3.0, serum PGI ≤30 ng/ml, or serum PGII >30 ng/ml, the risk of GC is significantly higher (Yanaoka et al, 2008b). Based on these data, even among group A patients, if the PGI/II ratio is ≤3.0 or serum PGI is ≤30 ng/ml, endoscopy should be performed once to evaluate the possible presence of CAG.

3. Prevention of GC based on the natural history of HP-related chronic gastritis

The evaluation of HP-related chronic gastritis is especially important in the analysis of GC prevention. However, previous studies have not assessed the extent of coexisting CAG or have assessed it only with endoscopic findings and/or histopathology on endoscopic biopsy. In this section, we discuss the strategy of GC prevention according to the evaluation of HP-related chronic gastritis based on the serum PG test.

3.1 Prevention of GC by HP eradication

Many previous studies have been conducted on the inhibition of GC by eradication therapy for HP, a major factor in gastric carcinogenesis. HP eradication therapy has recently been shown to prevent metachronous cancer after endoscopic resection of early GC (Fukase et al., 2008). However, in several reports to date, the effects on prevention of GC have not been as clear-cut as the effects of HP eradication on prevention of peptic ulcers. The studies that found inhibitory effects on gastric carcinogenesis were often non-randomized studies with a short observation period of ≤5 years (Fuccio et al., 2007). Moreover, results have been mixed. For example, in studies of GC occurrence after HP eradication in groups with or without precancerous lesions (CAG or intestinal metaplasia), significant inhibition of GC in the without-precancerous-lesion group was reported (Take et al., 2007; Wong et al., 2004). On the other hand, absence of inhibition of GC, regardless of the presence or absence of precancerous lesions, has also been reported (You et al., 2006). In contrast, in an animal study using HP-infected Mongolian gerbils, inhibition of gastric carcinogenesis by HP eradication was clearly demonstrated (Tatematsu et al., 2007).

These study results suggest several points. First, inhibition of gastric carcinogenesis by HP eradication is not complete, and even after eradication, more than a few GC cases have been observed. Second, the earlier during infection that eradication therapy is started, the greater the inhibitory effect on GC. Third, after a duration has elapsed, irreversible changes due to HP infection develop, representing a "point of no return". This suggests an attenuated eradication effect. Fourth, HP infection promotes the proliferation and growth of cancer cells that have already developed (promoter effect). During long-term observation, clear-cut inhibition of gastric carcinogenesis by HP eradication is not seen, but eradication groups with shorter observation periods may display apparent inhibition of GC, with slower growth rates, and without growth of cancer that can be clinically diagnosed. Fifth, besides promoter effects on GC, HP infection, as previously described in detail, is also involved in gastric carcinogenesis mediated through the development and progression of CAG and intestinal metaplasia. To achieve a reduction in GC risk by eradication, in addition to HP elimination, improvement of CAG and intestinal metaplasia is necessary.

Based on these points, when evaluating the prevention of GC by HP eradication, evaluation of the equivalence of GC risk in the eradication group and non-eradication group (control) is necessary. With regard to this point, in almost all previous studies, either evaluation of CAG progression has been lacking, or even if evaluated, endoscopic or histopathologic findings, with strong subjective elements, were used. We therefore conducted a 10-year follow-up study in middle-aged healthy adults in whom progression of atrophic gastritis was monitored by serum PG (Yanaoka et al., 2009). In that study, although non-randomized, both the HP eradication and control groups showed equivalence with regard to CAG progression (an important risk factor), in addition to major risk factors for GC such as age, gender, and smoking. In this study, no significant inhibition of GC was observed even with HP eradication. However, with assessment by the PG test, evaluation in the PG test-positive (extensive CAG) and PG test-negative (non-extensive CAG) groups showed that HP eradication in the PG test-positive group did not prevent GC, whereas HP eradication in the PG test-negative group only achieved significant inhibition of GC (**Fig. 4**). These results confirm the

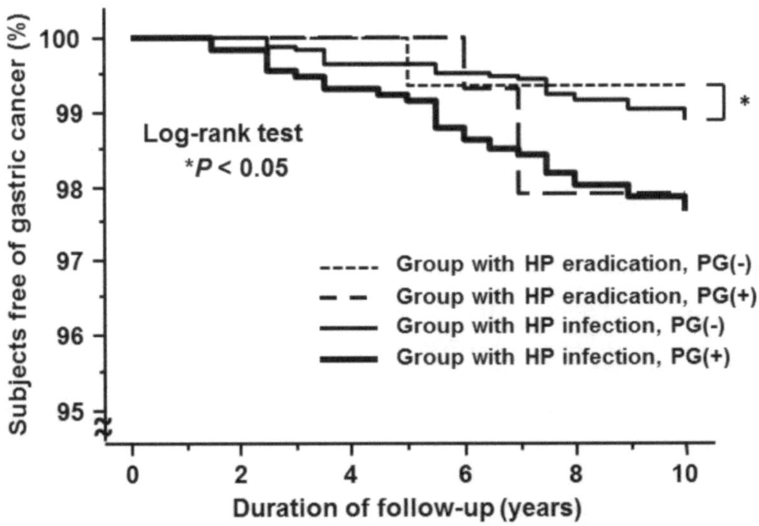

Fig. 4. Kaplan-Meier analysis of the proportion of subjects free of gastric cancer in the serum pepsinogen (PG) test-positive group and the PG test-negative group according to *Helicobacter pylori* (HP) infection status. In the serum PG test-positive group (extensive chronic atrophic gastritis (CAG)), no reduction in gastric cancer incidence was observed with HP eradication. Only the PG test- negative group (non-extensive CAG) showed a reduction in gastric cancer incidence with HP eradication.

previously mentioned results that assumed that no significant prevention of GC by HP eradication was achieved due to advanced CAG. This strongly suggests that in the majority of PG test-positive subjects, the stomach is past the "point of no return." The significance of HP eradication thus lies in achieving: 1) a decrease in GC proliferation and growth rates by inhibiting the GC-promoting effects of HP; 2) inhibition of carcinogenesis by halting progression of CAG; and 3) inhibition of inflammation-based gastric carcinogenesis (particularly diffuse-type GC) by healing chronic active gastritis. In fact, our study also showed that diffuse-type GC can be significantly inhibited by HP eradication.

3.2 Chemoprevention of GC by NSAIDs

Although prevention of GC by HP eradication can be expected, from a more realistic perspective, the effectiveness may be somewhat limited. In particular, among patients with advanced CAG, the chemopreventive effects of HP eradication therapy alone are unlikely to be sufficient. In populations where inhibition of gastric carcinogenesis cannot be achieved by HP eradication therapy alone, chemoprevention with the use of non-steroidal anti-inflammatory drugs (NSAIDs) is promising as a treatment strategy. Cyclooxygenase (COX) is a rate-limiting enzyme of prostaglandin synthesis in the arachidonic acid cascade. Among COX isozymes, attention has been focused on inducible COX-2, which is expressed in inflammatory responses and cancer proliferation (Kujubu et al., 1991). COX-2 expression has been reported in many gastrointestinal cancers, including colorectal cancer (Eberhart et al., 1994), and research has been undertaken into the prevention of carcinogenesis by COX-2 regulation (Giardiello et al., 1993; Kawamori et al., 1998; Kune et al., 1988; Thun et al., 1991).
With regard to COX-2 expression in the gastric mucosa, not only a high rate of COX-2 expression in GC cells, but also COX-2 expression in precancerous lesions such as CAG, intestinal metaplasia, and dysplasia has been reported (Sung et al., 2000). In a study of GC tissue types, a high rate of COX-2 expression was found in intestinal-type GC (Saukkonen et al., 2001). In a study of GC according to site, cancers of the gastric cardia showed decreased COX-2 expression compared to cancers of other gastric areas (Ratnasinghe et al., 1999). In epidemiologic and animal studies, long-term use of aspirin or other NSAIDs has been reported to decrease GC risk in a dose-dependent manner (Duan et al., 2008; Hu et al., 2004; Wang et al., 2003).
In a Mongolian gerbil model of chronic active gastritis, which closely resembles HP-related chronic gastritis in humans, we evaluated the effects of etodolac, a selective COX-2 inhibitor, after initiation with a low dose of N-methyl-N-nitrosourea, a chemical carcinogen (Magari et al., 2005). The results confirmed that treatment with etodolac early in HP infection completely inhibited gastric carcinogenesis, which usually occurs at a high rate. In this model, we confirmed that proliferation of gastric mucosal epithelial tissue was significantly inhibited by etodolac, and that the development of intestinal metaplasia, thought to be a precancerous lesion, was significantly inhibited. In addition, we conducted a clinical study of GC chemoprevention using a COX-2 inhibitor in patients with metaplastic gastritis (Yanaoka et al., 2010). This study, although non-randomized, included patients who had undergone endoscopic resection of intestinal-type GC with a background of metaplastic gastritis. The incidence of metachronous cancer was evaluated in etodolac and non-treatment groups during a mean observation period of 4.2 years. The diagnosis of metaplastic gastritis was based on serum testing, as previously described. Regarding HP-related chronic gastritis stage, these patients were classified as Group D [HP(-), PG(+)]. In this study, long-term treatment with etodolac as a selective COX-2 inhibitor effectively inhibited metachronous cancer development in curatively treated, early GC patients with

metaplastic gastritis. These results are in line with the results of our previous animal experiment using HP-infected Mongolian gerbils, indicating that etodolac can prevent stomach carcinogenesis involving the CAG-metaplasia-dysplasia-cancer sequence. Serious cardiovascular events, depending on the drug, have been reported with long-term administration of COX-2 inhibitors. Whether etodolac is the best choice requires further investigation. However, particularly among patients with extensive CAG, in addition to HP eradication therapy, aggressive chemoprevention using NSAIDs such as selective COX-2 inhibitors may effectively inhibit gastric carcinogenesis (Fig. 3).

3.3 Possible GC prevention by dietary habits

On the other hand, HP eradication therapy and chemoprevention using NSAIDs were not carried out in all subjects, as problems exist with adverse effects of HP eradication or chemoprevention, drug-resistant bacteria, and medical economics. Research into HP-related chronic gastritis and promoters and inhibitors of gastric carcinogenesis, and studies of alternative therapies, primarily in the form of functional foods, has thus been conducted. In the progression of HP-related chronic gastritis, besides HP virulence factors such as VacA and CagA (Hatakeyama, 2004), and host factors such as cytokine polymorphisms (El-Omar et al., 2000), environmental factors such as lifestyle and dietary habits have been shown to be involved. In particular, dietary factors have been highly implicated as the factors to which the gastric mucosa is most frequently and directly exposed. For example, high sodium intake increases gastric mucosal inflammation and the risk of gastric cancer (Nozaki et al., 2002; Shikata et al., 2006) and cigarette smoking is considered to be deeply involved in the transition of CAG to intestinal metaplasia and dysplasia (Kneller et al., 1992; Tredaniel et al., 1997), which are precancerous conditions, in a model of gastric carcinogenesis postulated by Correa (Correa and Houghton, 2007). On the other hand, epidemiologic and animal studies have found that vegetables, fruits, and green tea can inhibit gastritis and reduce gastric carcinogenesis (Kobayashi et al., 2002; Yu et al., 1995).

The Japanese apricot (JA) (*ume* in Japanese; *Prunus mume* Siebold et Zucc.), in extracted or pickled form, has long been empirically used in Japan as a folk remedy for gastrointestinal infections such as gastroenteritis. In an in vitro study, Fujita et al. reported that JA extract displayed bactericidal activity against HP (Fujita et al., 2002). In addition, in an animal study using Mongolian gerbils, Otsuka et al. showed in vivo anti-HP effects of JA extract, demonstrating inhibition of chronic gastritis in HP-infected Mongolian gerbils (Otsuka et al., 2005). Based on these reports, because of the presumably potent anti-HP effects of JA, we conducted a study on associations between regular consumption of JA and HP-related chronic gastritis (Enomoto et al., 2010b; Jones, 2010). As a result, we found that consumption of JA is effective in inhibiting HP-related active inflammation of the stomach and CAG progression, and that development of GC may be inhibited by JA intake. Of course, because dietary habits are greatly influenced by other lifestyle factors, depending on the population being studied, the effectiveness achieved in preventing GC may differ. However, promoting dietary habits that protect against GC, including JA intake, may be an ideal alternative strategy for GC prevention (Fig. 3).

4. Conclusion

In conclusion, based on the natural history of HP-related chronic gastritis from blood test data, including the serum PG test and HP antibodies, specific prediction of the risk of GC in each individual is now possible. With this information, more effective strategies to prevent GC are becoming possible. These are anticipated to have clinical applications such as in more effective GC screening, and in establishing appropriate GC prevention.

5. References

Blaser, MJ.; Perez-Perez, GI.; Kleanthous, H.; Cover, TL.; Peek, RM.; Chyou, PH.; Stemmermann, GN. & Nomura, A. (1995). Infection with Helicobacter pylori strains possessing cagA is associated with an increased risk of developing adenocarcinoma of the stomach. *Cancer Res*, Vol.55, No.10, (May 1995), pp. 2111-2115, ISSN 0008-5472

Correa, P. (1992). Human gastric carcinogenesis: a multistep and multifactorial process-First American Cancer Society Award Lecture on Cancer Epidemiology and Prevention. *Cancer Res*, Vol.52, No.24, (Dec 1992), pp. 6735-6740, ISSN 0008-5472

Correa, P. & Houghton, J. (2007). Carcinogenesis of *Helicobacter pylori*. *Gastroenterology*, Vol.133, No.2, (Aug 2007), pp. 659-672, ISSN 0016-5085

Dinis-Ribeiro, M.; Yamaki, G.; Miki, K.; Costa-Pereira, A.; Matsukawa, M. & Kurihara, M. (2004). Meta-analysis on the validity of pepsinogen test for gastric carcinoma, dysplasia or chronic atrophic gastritis screening. *J Med Screen*, Vol.11, No.3, (Dec 2004), pp. 141-147, ISSN 0969-1413

Dooley, CP.; Cohen, H.; Fitzgibbons, PL.; Bauer, M.; Appleman, MD.; Perez-Perez, GI. & Blaser, MJ. (1989). Prevalence of *Helicobacter pylori* infection and histologic gastritis in asymptomatic persons. *N Engl J Med*, Vol.321, No.23, (Dec 1989), pp. 1562-1566, ISSN 0028-4793

Duan, L.; Wu, AH.; Sullivan-Halley, J. & Bernstein, L. (2008). Nonsteroidal anti-inflammatory drugs and risk of esophageal and gastric adenocarcinomas in Los Angeles County. *Cancer Epidemiol Biomarkers Prev*, Vol.17, No.1, (Jan 2008), pp. 126-134, ISSN 1055-9965

Eberhart, CE.; Coffey, RJ.; Radhika, A.; Giardiello, FM.; Ferrenbach, S. & DuBois, RN. (1994). Up-regulation of cyclooxygenase 2 gene expression in human colorectal adenomas and adenocarcinomas. *Gastroenterology*, Vol.107, No.4, (Oct 1994), pp. 1183-1188, ISSN 0016-5085

El-Omar, EM.; Carrington, M.; Chow, WH.; McColl, KE.; Bream, JH.; Young, HA.; Herrera, J.; Lissowska, J.; Yuan, CC.; Rothman, N.; Lanyon, G.; Martin, M.; Fraumeni, JF, Jr.. & Rabkin, CS. (2000). Interleukin-1 polymorphisms associated with increased risk of gastric cancer. *Nature*, Vol.404, No.6776, (Mar 2000), pp. 398-402, ISSN 0028-0836

Enomoto, S.; Maekita, T.; Ohata, H.; Yanaoka, K.; Oka, M. & Ichinose, M. (2010a). Novel risk markers for gastric cancer screening: Present status and future prospects. *World J Gastrointest Endosc*, Vol.2, No.12, (Dec 2010), pp. 381-387, ISSN 1948-5190

Enomoto, S.; Yanaoka, K.; Utsunomiya, H.; Niwa, T.; Inada, K.; Deguchi, H.; Ueda, K.; Mukoubayashi, C.; Inoue, I.; Maekita, T.; Nakazawa, K.; Iguchi, M.; Arii, K.; Tamai, H.; Yoshimura, N.; Fujishiro, M.; Oka, M. & Ichinose, M. (2010b). Inhibitory effects of Japanese apricot (Prunus mume Siebold et Zucc.; Ume) on *Helicobacter pylori*-related chronic gastritis. *Eur J Clin Nutr*, Vol.64, No.7, (Jul 2010), pp. 714-719, ISSN 1476-5640

EUROGAST Study Group. (1993). An international association between *Helicobacter pylori* infection and gastric cancer. *Lancet*, Vol.341, No.8857, (May 1993), pp. 1359-1362, ISSN 0140-6736

Forman, D.; Newell, DG.; Fullerton, F.; Yarnell, JW.; Stacey, AR.; Wald, N. & Sitas, F. (1991). Association between infection with *Helicobacter pylori* and risk of gastric cancer: evidence from a prospective investigation. *BMJ*, Vol.302, No.6788, (Jun 1991), pp. 1302-1305, ISSN 0959-8138

Fuccio, L.; Zagari, RM.; Minardi, ME. & Bazzoli, F. (2007). Systematic review: *Helicobacter pylori* eradication for the prevention of gastric cancer. *Aliment Pharmacol Ther*, Vol.25, No.2, (Jan 2007), pp. 133-141, ISSN 0269-2813

Fujita, K.; Hasegawa, M.; Fujita, M.; Kobayashi, I.; Ozasa, K. & Watanabe, Y. (2002). Anti-Helicobacter pylori effects of Bainiku-ekisu (concentrate of Japanese apricot juice). *Nippon Shokakibyo Gakkai Zasshi*, Vol.99, No.4, (Apr 2002), pp. 379-385, ISSN 0446-6586

Fukase, K.; Kato, M.; Kikuchi, S.; Inoue, K.; Uemura, N.; Okamoto, S.; Terao, S.; Amagai, K.; Hayashi, S. & Asaka, M. (2008). Effect of eradication of *Helicobacter pylori* on incidence of metachronous gastric carcinoma after endoscopic resection of early gastric cancer: an open-label, randomised controlled trial. *Lancet*, Vol.372, No.9636, (Aug 2008), pp. 392-397, ISSN 1474-547X

Furuta, T.; Kaneko, E.; Baba, S.; Arai, H. & Futami, H. (1997). Percentage changes in serum pepsinogens are useful as indices of eradication of Helicobacter pylori. *Am J Gastroenterol*, Vol.92, No.1, (Jan 1997), pp. 84-88, ISSN 0002-9270

Giardiello, FM.; Hamilton, SR.; Krush, AJ.; Piantadosi, S.; Hylind, LM.; Celano, P.; Booker, SV.; Robinson, CR. & Offerhaus, GJ. (1993). Treatment of colonic and rectal adenomas with sulindac in familial adenomatous polyposis. *N Engl J Med*, Vol.328, No.18, (May 1993), pp. 1313-1316, ISSN 0028-4793

Gotoda, T. (2007). Endoscopic resection of early gastric cancer. *Gastric Cancer*, Vol.10, No.1, (Feb 2007), pp. 1-11, ISSN 1436-3291

Guarner, J.; Herrera-Goepfert, R.; Mohar, A.; Sanchez, L.; Halperin, D.; Ley, C. & Parsonnet, J. (1999). Interobserver variability in application of the revised Sydney classification for gastritis. *Hum Pathol*, Vol.30, No.12, (Dec 1999), pp. 1431-1434, ISSN 0046-8177

Hatakeyama, M. (2004). Oncogenic mechanisms of the *Helicobacter pylori* CagA protein. *Nat Rev Cancer*, Vol.4, No.9, (Sep 2004), pp. 688-694, ISSN 1474-175X

Hattori, Y.; Tashiro, H.; Kawamoto, T. & Kodama, Y. (1995). Sensitivity and specificity of mass screening for gastric cancer using the measurment of serum pepsinogens. *Jpn J Cancer Res*, Vol.86, No.12, (Dec 1995), pp. 1210-1215, ISSN 0910-5050

Hirayama, F.; Takagi, S.; Iwao, E.; Yokoyama, Y.; Haga, K. & Hanada, S. (1999). Development of poorly differentiated adenocarcinoma and carcinoid due to long-term *Helicobacter pylori* colonization in Mongolian gerbils. *J Gastroenterol*, Vol.34, No.4, (Aug 1999), pp. 450-454, ISSN 0944-1174

Hirschowitz, BI. (1957). Pepsinogen: its origins, secretion and excretion. *Physiol Rev*, Vol.37, No.4, (Oct 1957), pp. 475-511, ISSN 0031-9333

Honda, S.; Fujioka, T.; Tokieda, M.; Satoh, R.; Nishizono, A. & Nasu, M. (1998). Development of *Helicobacter pylori*-induced gastric carcinoma in Mongolian gerbils. *Cancer Res*, Vol.58, No.19, (Oct 1998), pp. 4255-4259, ISSN 0008-5472

Hu, PJ.; Yu, J.; Zeng, ZR.; Leung, WK.; Lin, HL.; Tang, BD.; Bai, AH. & Sung, JJ. (2004). Chemoprevention of gastric cancer by celecoxib in rats. *Gut*, Vol.53, No.2, (Feb 2004), pp. 195-200, ISSN 0017-5749

Huang, JQ.; Sridhar, S.; Chen, Y. & Hunt, RH. (1998). Meta-analysis of the relationship between *Helicobacter pylori* seropositivity and gastric cancer. *Gastroenterology*, Vol.114, No.6, (Jun 1998), pp. 1169-1179, ISSN 0016-5085

Ichinose, M.; Yahagi, N.; Oka, M.; Ikeda, H.; Miki, K. & Omata, M. (2001). Screening for gastric cancer in Japan, In: *Cancer Screening*, Wu GY, Aziz K, editors, pp. 255−268, Humana Press, ISBN 0896038653, Totowa, New Jersey

International Agency for Research on Cancer (IARC). (1994). Schistosomes,liver flukes, and *Helicobacter pylori* Working group on the evaluation of carcinogenic risks to humans. *IARC Monogr Eval Carcinog Risks Hum*, Vol.61, (June 1994), pp. 177-241

Jones, R. (2010). Japanese apricots reported to inhibit inflammation and gastritis progression related to *Helicobacter pylori* infection. *Nat Rev Gastroenterol Hepatol*, Vol.7, No.9, (Sep 2010), pp. 478

Kageyama, T. & Ichinose, M. (2003). Diversity of structure and function of pepsinogens and pepsins *Rescent Research Developments and Biophysics and Biochemistry*, Vol.3, (2003), pp. 159-178

Kakushima, N. & Fujishiro, M. (2008). Endoscopic submucosal dissection for gastrointestinal neoplasms. *World J Gastroenterol*, Vol.14, No.19, (May 2008), pp. 2962-2967, ISSN 1007-9327

Kawamori, T.; Rao, CV.; Seibert, K. & Reddy, BS. (1998). Chemopreventive activity of celecoxib, a specific cyclooxygenase-2 inhibitor, against colon carcinogenesis. *Cancer Res*, Vol.58, No.3, (Feb 1998), pp. 409-412, ISSN 0008-5472

Kimura, K. (1972). Chronological transition of the fundic-pyloric border determined by stepwise biopsy of the lesser and greater curvatures of the stomach. *Gastroenterology*, Vol.63, No.4, (Oct 1972), pp. 584-592, ISSN 0016-5085

Kitahara, F.; Kobayashi, K.; Sato, T.; Kojima, Y.; Araki, T. & Fujino, MA. (1999). Accuracy of screening for gastric cancer using serum pepsinogen concentrations. *Gut*, Vol.44, No.5, (May 1999), pp. 693-697, ISSN 0017-5749

Kneller, RW.; You, WC.; Chang, YS.; Liu, WD.; Zhang, L.; Zhao, L.; Xu, GW.; Fraumeni, JF, Jr.. & Blot, WJ. (1992). Cigarette smoking and other risk factors for progression of precancerous stomach lesions. *J Natl Cancer Inst*, Vol.84, No.16, (Aug 1992), pp. 1261-1266, ISSN 0027-8874

Kobayashi, M.; Tsubono, Y.; Sasazuki, S.; Sasaki, S. & Tsugane, S. (2002). Vegetables, fruit and risk of gastric cancer in Japan: a 10-year follow-up of the JPHC Study Cohort I. *Int J Cancer*, Vol.102, No.1, (Nov 2002), pp. 39-44, ISSN 0020-7136

Kodoi, A.; Yoshihara, M.; Sumii, K.; Haruma, K. & Kajiyama, G. (1995). Serum pepsinogen in screening for gastric cancer. *J Gastroenterol*, Vol.30, No.4, (Aug 1995), pp. 452-460, ISSN 0944-1174

Kujubu, DA.; Fletcher, BS.; Varnum, BC.; Lim, RW. & Herschman, HR. (1991). TIS10, a phorbol ester tumor promoter-inducible mRNA from Swiss 3T3 cells, encodes a novel prostaglandin synthase/cyclooxygenase homologue. *J Biol Chem*, Vol.266, No.20, (Jul 1991), pp. 12866-12872, ISSN 0021-9258

Kune, GA.; Kune, S. & Watson, LF. (1988). Colorectal cancer risk, chronic illnesses, operations, and medications: case control results from the Melbourne Colorectal Cancer Study. *Cancer Res*, Vol.48, No.15, (Aug 1988), pp. 4399-4404, ISSN 0008-5472

Magari, H.; Shimizu, Y.; Inada, K.; Enomoto, S.; Tomeki, T.; Yanaoka, K.; Tamai, H.; Arii, K.; Nakata, H.; Oka, M.; Utsunomiya, H.; Tsutsumi, Y.; Tsukamoto, T.; Tatematsu, M. & Ichinose, M. (2005). Inhibitory effect of etodolac, a selective cyclooxygenase-2 inhibitor, on stomach carcinogenesis in *Helicobacter pylori*-infected Mongolian gerbils. *Biochem Biophys Res Commun*, Vol.334, No.2, (Aug 2005), pp. 606-612, ISSN 0006-291X

Marshall, BJ. & Warren, JR. (1984). Unidentified curved bacilli in the stomach of patients with gastritis and peptic ulceration. *Lancet*, Vol.1, No.8390, (Jun 1984), pp. 1311-1315, ISSN 0140-6736

Meister, H.; Holubarsch, C.; Haferkamp, O.; Schlag, P. & Herfarth, C. (1979). Gastritis, intestinal metaplasia and dysplasia versus benign ulcer in stomach and duodenum and gastric carcinoma -- a histotopographical study. *Pathol Res Pract*, Vol.164, No.3, (Jan 1979), pp. 259-269, ISSN 0344-0338

Miki, K.; Ichinose, M.; Shimizu, A.; Huang, SC.; Oka, H.; Furihata, C.; Matsushima, T. & Takahashi, K. (1987). Serum pepsinogens as a screening test of extensive chronic gastritis. *Gastroenterol Jpn*, Vol.22, No.2, (Apr 1987), pp. 133-141, ISSN 0435-1339

Miki, K.; Ichinose, M.; Ishikawa, KB.; Yahagi, N.; Matsushima, M.; Kakei, N.; Tsukada, S.; Kido, M.; Ishihama, S.; Shimizu, Y.; Suzuki, T. & Kurokawa, K. (1993). Clinical application of serum pepsinogen I and II levels for mass screening to detect gastric cancer. *Jpn J Cancer Res*, Vol.84, No.10, (Oct 1993), pp. 1086-1090, ISSN 0910-5050

Miki, K.; Morita, M.; Sasajima, M.; Hoshina, R.; Kanda, E. & Urita, Y. (2003). Usefulness of gastric cancer screening using the serum pepsinogen test method. *Am J Gastroenterol*, Vol.98, No.4, (Apr 2003), pp. 735-739, ISSN 0002-9270

Mukoubayashi, C.; Yanaoka, K.; Ohata, H.; Arii, K.; Tamai, H.; Oka, M. & Ichinose, M. (2007). Serum pepsinogen and gastric cancer screening. *Intern Med*, Vol.46, No.6, (Mar 2007), pp. 261-266, ISSN 1349-7235

Nakajima, T.; Oda, I.; Gotoda, T.; Hamanaka, H.; Eguchi, T.; Yokoi, C. & Saito, D. (2006). Metachronous gastric cancers after endoscopic resection: how effective is annual endoscopic surveillance? *Gastric Cancer*, Vol.9, No.2, (May 2006), pp. 93-98, ISSN 1436-3291

Nomura, A.; Stemmermann, GN.; Chyou, PH.; Kato, I.; Perez-Perez, GI. & Blaser, MJ. (1991). *Helicobacter pylori* infection and gastric carcinoma among Japanese Americans in Hawaii. *N Engl J Med*, Vol.325, No.16, (Oct 1991), pp. 1132-1136, ISSN 0028-4793

Nozaki, K.; Shimizu, N.; Inada, K.; Tsukamoto, T.; Inoue, M.; Kumagai, T.; Sugiyama, A.; Mizoshita, T.; Kaminishi, M. & Tatematsu, M. (2002). Synergistic promoting effects of *Helicobacter pylori* infection and high-salt diet on gastric carcinogenesis in Mongolian gerbils. *Jpn J Cancer Res*, Vol.93, No.10, (Oct 2002), pp. 1083-1089, ISSN 0910-5050

Ohata, H.; Kitauchi, S.; Yoshimura, N.; Mugitani, K.; Iwane, M.; Nakamura, H.; Yoshikawa, A.; Yanaoka, K.; Arii, K.; Tamai, H.; Shimizu, Y.; Takeshita, T.; Mohara, O. & Ichinose, M. (2004). Progression of chronic atrophic gastritis associated with *Helicobacter pylori* infection increases risk of gastric cancer. *Int J Cancer*, Vol.109, No.1, (Mar 2004), pp. 138-143, ISSN 0020-7136

Ohata, H.; Oka, M.; Yanaoka, K.; Shimizu, Y.; Mukoubayashi, C.; Mugitani, K.; Iwane, M.; Nakamura, H.; Tamai, H.; Arii, K.; Nakata, H.; Yoshimura, N.; Takeshita, T.; Miki, K.; Mohara, O. & Ichinose, M. (2005). Gastric cancer screening of a high-risk population in Japan using serum pepsinogen and barium digital radiography. *Cancer Sci*, Vol.96, No.10, (Oct 2005), pp. 713-720, ISSN 1347-9032

Otsuka, T.; Tsukamoto, T.; Tanaka, H.; Inada, K.; Utsunomiya, H.; Mizoshita, T.; Kumagai, T.; Katsuyama, T.; Miki, K. & Tatematsu, M. (2005). Supressive effect of fruits-juice concentrate of *Prunus Mume* Sieb. et Zucc. (Japanese apricot, Ume) on *Helicobacter pylori*-induced glandular stoach lesion in Mongolian gerbils *Asian Pacific J Cancer Prev*, Vol.6, (Jul-Sep 2005), pp. 337-341

Parsonnet, J.; Friedman, GD.; Vandersteen, DP.; Chang, Y.; Vogelman, JH.; Orentreich, N. & Sibley, RK. (1991). *Helicobacter pylori* infection and the risk of gastric carcinoma. *N Engl J Med*, Vol.325, No.16, (Oct 17 1991), pp. 1127-1131, ISSN 0028-4793

Plummer, M.; Buiatti, E.; Lopez, G.; Peraza, S.; Vivas, J.; Oliver, W. & Munoz, N. (1997). Histological diagnosis of precancerous lesions of the stomach: a reliability study. *Int J Epidemiol*, Vol.26, No.4, (Aug 1997), pp. 716-720, ISSN 0300-5771

Ratnasinghe, D.; Tangrea, JA.; Roth, MJ.; Dawsey, SM.; Anver, M.; Kasprzak, BA.; Hu, N.; Wang, QH. & Taylor, PR. (1999). Expression of cyclooxygenase-2 in human adenocarcinomas of the gastric cardia and corpus. *Oncol Rep*, Vol.6, No.5, (Sep-Oct 1999), pp. 965-968, ISSN 1021-335X

Samloff, IM.; Varis, K.; Ihamaki, T.; Siurala, M. & Rotter, JI. (1982). Relationships among serum pepsinogen I, serum pepsinogen II, and gastric mucosal histology. A study in relatives of patients with pernicious anemia. *Gastroenterology*, Vol.83, No.1 Pt 2, (Jul 1982), pp. 204-209, ISSN 0016-5085

Saukkonen, K.; Nieminen, O.; van Rees, B.; Vilkki, S.; Harkonen, M.; Juhola, M.; Mecklin, JP.; Sipponen, P. & Ristimaki, A. (2001). Expression of cyclooxygenase-2 in dysplasia of the stomach and in intestinal-type gastric adenocarcinoma. *Clin Cancer Res*, Vol.7, No.7, (Jul 2001), pp. 1923-1931, ISSN 1078-0432

Shikata, K.; Kiyohara, Y.; Kubo, M.; Yonemoto, K.; Ninomiya, T.; Shirota, T.; Tanizaki, Y.; Doi, Y.; Tanaka, K.; Oishi, Y.; Matsumoto, T. & Iida, M. (2006). A prospective study of dietary salt intake and gastric cancer incidence in a defined Japanese population: the Hisayama study. *Int J Cancer*, Vol.119, No.1, (Jul 2006), pp. 196-201, ISSN 0020-7136

Shimizu, N.; Inada, K.; Nakanishi, H.; Tsukamoto, T.; Ikehara, Y.; Kaminishi, M.; Kuramoto, S.; Sugiyama, A.; Katsuyama, T. & Tatematsu, M. (1999). *Helicobacter pylori* infection enhances glandular stomach carcinogenesis in Mongolian gerbils treated with chemical carcinogens. *Carcinogenesis*, Vol.20, No.4, (Apr 1999), pp. 669-676, ISSN 0143-3334

Sipponen, P.; Kekki, M.; Haapakoski, J.; Ihamaki, T. & Siurala, M. (1985). Gastric cancer risk in chronic atrophic gastritis: statistical calculations of cross-sectional data. *Int J Cancer*, Vol.35, No.2, (Feb 15 1985), pp. 173-177, ISSN 0020-7136

Sipponen, P.; Kosunen, TU.; Valle, J.; Riihela, M. & Seppala, K. (1992). *Helicobacter pylori* infection and chronic gastritis in gastric cancer. *J Clin Pathol*, Vol.45, No.4, (Apr 1992), pp. 319-323, ISSN 0021-9746

Siurala, M.; Varis, K. & Wiljasalo, M. (1966). Studies of patients with atrophic gastritis: a 10-15-year follow-up. *Scand J Gastroenterol*, Vol.1, No.1, (1966), pp. 40-48, ISSN 0036-5521

Sugiyama, A.; Maruta, F.; Ikeno, T.; Ishida, K.; Kawasaki, S.; Katsuyama, T.; Shimizu, N. & Tatematsu, M. (1998). *Helicobacter pylori* infection enhances N-methyl-N-nitrosourea-induced stomach carcinogenesis in the Mongolian gerbil. *Cancer Res*, Vol.58, No.10, (May 1998), pp. 2067-2069, ISSN 0008-5472

Sung, JJ.; Leung, WK.; Go, MY.; To, KF.; Cheng, AS.; Ng, EK. & Chan, FK. (2000). Cyclooxygenase-2 expression in *Helicobacter pylori*-associated premalignant and malignant gastric lesions. *Am J Pathol*, Vol.157, No.3, (Sep 2000), pp. 729-735, ISSN 0002-9440

Take, S.; Mizuno, M.; Ishiki, K.; Nagahara, Y.; Yoshida, T.; Yokota, K. & Oguma, K. (2007). Baseline gastric mucosal atrophy is a risk factor associated with the development of gastric cancer after *Helicobacter pylori* eradication therapy in patients with peptic ulcer diseases. *J Gastroenterol*, Vol.42 Suppl 17, (Jan 2007), pp. 21-27, ISSN 0944-1174

Talley, NJ.; Zinsmeister, AR.; Weaver, A.; DiMagno, EP.; Carpenter, HA.; Perez-Perez, GI. & Blaser, MJ. (1991). Gastric adenocarcinoma and *Helicobacter pylori* infection. *J Natl Cancer Inst*, Vol.83, No.23, (Dec 1991), pp. 1734-1739, ISSN 0027-8874

Tatematsu, M.; Tsukamoto, T. & Toyoda, T. (2007). Effects of eradication of *Helicobacter pylori* on gastric carcinogenesis in experimental models. *J Gastroenterol*, Vol.42 Suppl 17, (Jan 2007), pp. 7-9, ISSN 0944-1174

Tatsuta, M.; Saegusa, T. & Okuda, S. (1973). Studies on Gastritis in the Upper Portion of Stomach by Endoscopic Congo Red Test *Endoscopy*, Vol.5, (Feb 1973), pp. 61-69

Tatsuta, M.; Iishi, H.; Nakaizumi, A.; Okuda, S.; Taniguchi, H.; Hiyama, T.; Tsukuma, H. & Oshima, A. (1993). Fundal atrophic gastritis as a risk factor for gastric cancer. *Int J Cancer*, Vol.53, No.1, (Jan 1993), pp. 70-74, ISSN 0020-7136

Testoni, PA.; Masci, E.; Marchi, R.; Guslandi, M.; Ronchi, G. & Tittobello, A. (1987). Gastric cancer in chronic atrophic gastritis. Associated gastric ulcer adds no further risk. *J Clin Gastroenterol*, Vol.9, No.3, (Jun 1987), pp. 298-302, ISSN 0192-0790

Thun, MJ.; Namboodiri, MM. & Heath, CW, Jr. (1991). Aspirin use and reduced risk of fatal colon cancer. *N Engl J Med*, Vol.325, No.23, (Dec 1991), pp. 1593-1596, ISSN 0028-4793

Tokieda, M.; Honda, S.; Fujioka, T. & Nasu, M. (1999). Effect of *Helicobacter pylori* infection on the N-methyl-N'-nitro-N-nitrosoguanidine-induced gastric carcinogenesis in mongolian gerbils. *Carcinogenesis*, Vol.20, No.7, (Jul 1999), pp. 1261-1266, ISSN 0143-3334

Tredaniel, J.; Boffetta, P.; Buiatti, E.; Saracci, R. & Hirsch, A. (1997). Tobacco smoking and gastric cancer: review and meta-analysis. *Int J Cancer*, Vol.72, No.4, (Aug 1997), pp. 565-573, ISSN 0020-7136

Uemura, N.; Okamoto, S.; Yamamoto, S.; Matsumura, N.; Yamaguchi, S.; Yamakido, M.; Taniyama, K.; Sasaki, N. & Schlemper, RJ. (2001). *Helicobacter pylori* infection and the development of gastric cancer. *N Engl J Med*, Vol.345, No.11, (Sep 2001), pp. 784-789, ISSN 0028-4793

Wang, WH.; Huang, JQ.; Zheng, GF.; Lam, SK.; Karlberg, J. & Wong, BC. (2003). Non-steroidal anti-inflammatory drug use and the risk of gastric cancer: a systematic review and meta-analysis. *J Natl Cancer Inst*, Vol.95, No.23, (Dec 2003), pp. 1784-1791, ISSN 1460-2105

Watabe, H.; Mitsushima, T.; Yamaji, Y.; Okamoto, M.; Wada, R.; Kokubo, T.; Doi, H.; Yoshida, H.; Kawabe, T. & Omata, M. (2005). Predicting the development of gastric cancer from combining *Helicobacter pylori* antibodies and serum pepsinogen status: a prospective endoscopic cohort study. *Gut*, Vol.54, No.6, (Jun 2005), pp. 764-768, ISSN 0017-5749

Watanabe, T.; Tada, M.; Nagai, H.; Sasaki, S. & Nakao, M. (1998). *Helicobacter pylori* infection induces gastric cancer in mongolian gerbils. *Gastroenterology*, Vol.115, No.3, (Sep 1998), pp. 642-648, ISSN 0016-5085

Watanabe, Y.; Kurata, JH.; Mizuno, S.; Mukai, M.; Inokuchi, H.; Miki, K.; Ozasa, K. & Kawai, K. (1997). *Helicobacter pylori* infection and gastric cancer. A nested case-control study in a rural area of Japan. *Dig Dis Sci*, Vol.42, No.7, (Jul 1997), pp. 1383-1387, ISSN 0163-2116

Wong, BC.; Lam, SK.; Wong, WM.; Chen, JS.; Zheng, TT.; Feng, RE.; Lai, KC.; Hu, WH.; Yuen, ST.; Leung, SY.; Fong, DY.; Ho, J. & Ching, CK. (2004). *Helicobacter pylori* eradication to prevent gastric cancer in a high-risk region of China: a randomized controlled trial. *JAMA*, Vol.291, No.2, (Jan 2004), pp. 187-194, ISSN 1538-3598

Yanaoka, K.; Oka, M.; Mukoubayashi, C.; Yoshimura, N.; Enomoto, S.; Iguchi, M.; Magari, H.; Utsunomiya, H.; Tamai, H.; Arii, K.; Ohata, H.; Fujishiro, M.; Takeshita, T.; Mohara, O. & Ichinose, M. (2008a). Cancer high-risk subjects identified by serum pepsinogen tests: outcomes after 10-year follow-up in asymptomatic middle-aged males. *Cancer Epidemiol Biomarkers Prev*, Vol.17, No.4, (Apr 2008), pp. 838-845, ISSN 1055-9965

Yanaoka, K.; Oka, M.; Yoshimura, N.; Mukoubayashi, C.; Enomoto, S.; Iguchi, M.; Magari, H.; Utsunomiya, H.; Tamai, H.; Arii, K.; Yamamichi, N.; Fujishiro, M.; Takeshita, T.; Mohara, O. & Ichinose, M. (2008b). Risk of gastric cancer in asymptomatic, middle-aged Japanese subjects based on serum pepsinogen and *Helicobacter pylori* antibody levels. *Int J Cancer*, Vol.123, No.4, (Aug 2008), pp. 917-926, ISSN 1097-0215

Yanaoka, K.; Oka, M.; Ohata, H.; Yoshimura, N.; Deguchi, H.; Mukoubayashi, C.; Enomoto, S.; Inoue, I.; Iguchi, M.; Maekita, T.; Ueda, K.; Utsunomiya, H.; Tamai, H.; Fujishiro, M.; Iwane, M.; Takeshita, T.; Mohara, O. & Ichinose, M. (2009). Eradication of *Helicobacter pylori* prevents cancer development in subjects with mild gastric atrophy identified by serum pepsinogen levels. *Int J Cancer*, Vol.125, No.11, (Dec 2009), pp. 2697-2703, ISSN 1097-0215

Yanaoka, K.; Oka, M.; Yoshimura, N.; Deguchi, H.; Mukoubayashi, C.; Enomoto, S.; Maekita, T.; Inoue, I.; Ueda, K.; Utsunomiya, H.; Iguchi, M.; Tamai, H.; Fujishiro, M.; Nakamura, Y.; Tsukamoto, T.; Inada, K.; Takeshita, T. & Ichinose, M. (2010). Preventive effects of etodolac, a selective cyclooxygenase-2 inhibitor, on cancer development in extensive metaplastic gastritis, a *Helicobacter pylori*-negative precancerous lesion. *Int J Cancer*, Vol.126, No.6, (Mar 2010), pp. 1467-1473, ISSN 1097-0215

Yoshihara, M.; Sumii, K.; Haruma, K.; Kiyohira, K.; Hattori, N.; Tanaka, S.; Kajiyama, G. & Shigenobu, T. (1997). The usefulness of gastric mass screening using serum pepsinogen levels compared with photofluorography. *Hiroshima J Med Sci*, Vol.46, No.2, (Jun 1997), pp. 81-86, ISSN 0018-2052

You, WC.; Brown, LM.; Zhang, L.; Li, JY.; Jin, ML.; Chang, YS.; Ma, JL.; Pan, KF.; Liu, WD.; Hu, Y.; Crystal-Mansour, S.; Pee, D.; Blot, WJ.; Fraumeni, JF, Jr..; Xu, GW. & Gail, MH. (2006). Randomized double-blind factorial trial of three treatments to reduce the prevalence of precancerous gastric lesions. *J Natl Cancer Inst*, Vol.98, No.14, (Jul 2006), pp. 974-983, ISSN 1460-2105

Yu, GP.; Hsieh, CC.; Wang, LY.; Yu, SZ.; Li, XL. & Jin, TH. (1995). Green-tea consumption and risk of stomach cancer: a population-based case-control study in Shanghai, China. *Cancer Causes Control*, Vol.6, No.6, (Nov 1995), pp. 532-538, ISSN 0957-5243

Zheng, Q.; Chen, XY.; Shi, Y. & Xiao, SD. (2004). Development of gastric adenocarcinoma in Mongolian gerbils after long-term infection with Helicobacter pylori. *J Gastroenterol Hepatol*, Vol.19, No.10, (Oct 2004), pp. 1192-1198, ISSN 0815-9319

11

Role of Genetic and Environmental Risk Factors in Gastric Carcinogenesis Pathway

Bárbara Peleteiro and Nuno Lunet
Department of Clinical Epidemiology, Predictive Medicine and Public Health, University of Porto Medical School
Institute of Public Health – University of Porto (ISPUP)
Portugal

1. Introduction

Gastric carcinoma has been considered an aetiologically heterogeneous entity, with the role of its potential determinants differing with tumour location (Cavaleiro-Pinto et al., 2011; Helicobacter and Cancer Collaborative Group, 2001; Huang et al., 1998; Huang et al., 2003; Ladeiras-Lopes et al., 2008; Larsson et al., 2006; Lunet et al., 2007; Tredaniel et al., 1997; World Cancer Research Fund & American Institute for Cancer Research, 2007) and histological type (Helicobacter and Cancer Collaborative Group, 2001; Huang et al., 1998; Ladeiras-Lopes et al., 2008; Larsson et al., 2006; Lunet et al., 2007; World Cancer Research Fund & American Institute for Cancer Research, 2007). Regarding the latter, Laurén proposed an histo-clinical classification (Laurén, 1965) comprising two main histological types – diffuse and intestinal – with different frequency and distribution across populations (Muñoz & Asvall, 1971; Muñoz & Connelly, 1971). Most gastric carcinomas belong to the intestinal type, representing between 52% and 82% of all gastric cancers (Kaneko & Yoshimura, 2001; Laurén & Nevalainen, 1993; Wu et al., 2009). A higher incidence of intestinal type tumours was observed in males, blacks and older subjects, while the diffuse type had a similar incidence in both genders and was more frequent in younger individuals (Correa et al., 1973; Ekström et al., 2000). Also, there was a wide geographical variation in the frequency of intestinal type tumours, whereas the occurrence of diffuse adenocarcinomas was more uniform across regions (Laurén & Nevalainen, 1993). In addition, the decrease in cancer incidence among migrants from high- to low-risk areas was observed predominantly for tumours of the intestinal type (Correa et al., 1973). These findings were taken as evidence of a relatively greater impact of environmental factors in the aetiology of intestinal type carcinomas, while the diffuse type was considered more dependent on the genetic profile of the individuals (Tahara, 2004). Pelayo Correa (Correa et al., 1975) proposed a model for the development of the intestinal type tumours, according to which the precancerous lesions occur in sequential steps: chronic atrophic gastritis, intestinal metaplasia, and dysplasia. It provided a framework for understanding the role of different environmental and constitutional factors in gastric carcinogenesis, which has evolved with the epidemiologic findings on this topic.

2. Gastric carcinogenesis models

In his initial model (Correa et al., 1975), Correa postulated that both deleterious and protective exposures could modulate the progression towards intestinal type cancers, by acting in different stages of the pathway. With the rediscovery of *Helicobacter pylori* in 1984 (Marshall & Warren, 1984) and the gradual recognition of its role as a carcinogen, the model was redefined to accommodate the causal relation between *H. pylori* infection and gastric cancer (Correa, 1992), assuming that its effects were exerted at the early phases of gastric carcinogenesis (Figure 1).

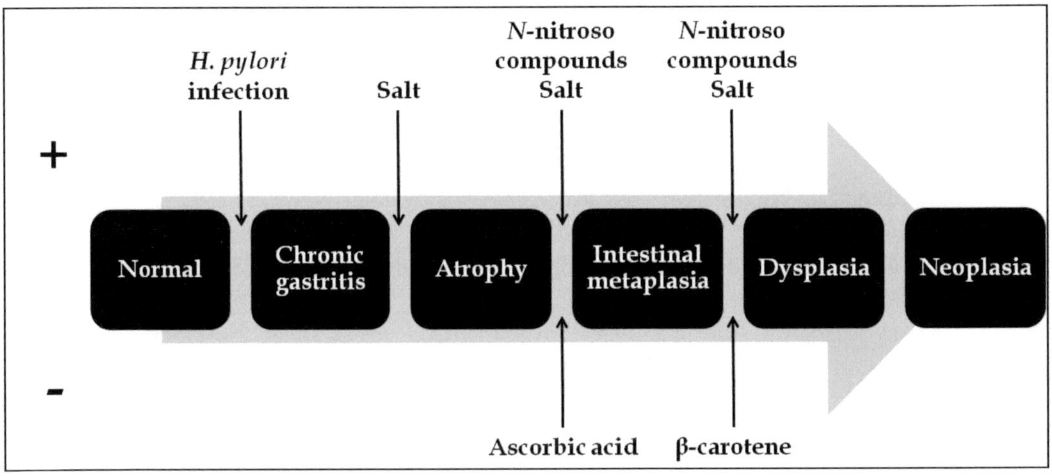

+ positive associations (increase the risk of gastric cancer); – negative associations (decrease the risk of gastric cancer).

Fig. 1. Gastric carcinogenesis model for the carcinomas of Laurén intestinal type, according to the proposed by Pelayo Correa (Correa, 1992)

The models proposed by Pelayo Correa more than 15 years ago still provide the essential framework for research on gastric carcinogenesis. The understanding of potentially alternative pathways, the more accurate definition of the endpoints for research, and the identification of the carcinogenesis steps where each of the gastric cancer causal components may act will contribute for a better understanding of cancer aetiology and support the development of preventive strategies.

2.1 The effect of risk factors for gastric cancer across the carcinogenesis pathway

The research on the determinants of gastric cancer precursors has been less extensive than for the cancer endpoints. In Table 1 we present a summary of the systematic reviews and meta-analyses of research conducted to assess the determinants of the lesions that precede the cancer. The contribution of these findings for improvement of the currently accepted gastric carcinogenesis model will be discussed in the following sections of this chapter.

Author, year (ref)	Exposure	Outcome	Databases searched	Number of studies included	Main results
Adamu, 2010 (Adamu et al., 2010)	*H. pylori* infection	CAG incidence	MEDLINE, EMBASE	14	<u>*H. pylori*-infected *vs.* uninfected</u> RR=5.0 (95%CI: 3.1-8.3) Includes studies with follow-up periods ranging from 5 to 32 years
Peleteiro, 2010 (Peleteiro et al., 2010b)	*IL1RN* VNTR *IL1B-511* *TNFA-308*	CAG prevalence IM prevalence	PubMed	15	<u>*IL1RN* VNTR (22 *vs.* LL)</u> CAG and IM: OR=2.27 (95%CI: 1.40-3.70) CAG: OR=1.65 (95%CI: 1.02-2.66) IM: OR=2.27 (95%CI: 1.14-4.51) <u>*IL1B-511* (TT *vs.* CC)</u> CAG and IM: OR=1.34 (95%CI: 0.87-2.07) CAG: OR=1.20 (95%CI: 0.70-2.05) IM: OR=1.94 (95%CI: 1.14-3.31) <u>*TNFA-308* (AA *vs.* GG)</u> CAG and IM: OR=0.93 (95%CI: 0.35-2.43)
Dias-Neto, 2010 (Dias-Neto et al., 2010)	Salt intake	IM prevalence	PubMed	17	<u>Salted/salty meat intake (highest *vs.* lowest exposure)</u> OR=1.68 (95%CI: 0.98-2.90) <u>Preference for salted/salty foods or use of table salt (highest *vs.* lowest exposure)</u> OR=1.53 (95%CI: 0.72-3.24)
Weck, 2008 (Weck & Brenner, 2008)	*H. pylori* infection	CAG prevalence evaluated by: - gastroscopy with biopsy - PG I only - PG I/PG II ratio	MEDLINE	66	<u>*H. pylori*-infected *vs.* uninfected</u> Gastroscopy with biopsy: OR=6.4 (95%CI: 4.0-10.1) PG I only *: OR=0.9 (95%CI: 0.7-1.2) PG I/PG II ratio: OR=7.2 (95%CI: 3.1-16.8) Combination of PG I and PG I/PG II ratio: OR=5.7 (95%CI: 4.4-7.4)

Author, year (ref)	Exposure	Outcome	Databases searched	Number of studies included	Main results
		- combination of PG I and PG I/PG II ratio			All methods: OR=4.7 (95%CI: 3.7-6.0) All methods, except PG I only: OR=6.1 (95%CI: 4.8-7.7)
Peleteiro, 2008 (Peleteiro et al., 2008)	*H. pylori* infection Smoking	IM prevalence	PubMed	22	Systematic review for identification of estimates for IM prevalence among *H. pylori*-infected subjects in different populations and ecological analysis of the association with smoking Pearson correlation coefficient = 0.45 (p=0.02)
Rokkas, 2007 (Rokkas et al., 2007)	*H. pylori* eradication	CAG incidence IM incidence	MEDLINE	8	<u>*H. pylori*-eradicated *vs.* placebo</u> CAG in the antrum: OR=0.554 (95%CI: 0.372-0.825) CAG in the corpus: OR=0.209 (95%CI: 0.081-0.538) IM in the antrum: OR=0.795 (95%CI: 0.587-1.078) IM in the corpus: OR=0.891 (95%CI: 0.633-1.253) Includes studies with follow-up periods ranging from 10 to 137 months

CAG – chronic atrophic gastritis; RR – relative risk; VNTR – variable number tandem repeat; IM – intestinal metaplasia; OR – odds ratio; PG – pepsinogen.

* the magnitude of the association depends on the method used to assess atrophy; previous studies showed that PG I alone had a low sensitivity for serological definition of chronic atrophic gastritis (Miki, 2006).

† systematic reviews and meta-analyses were identified through PubMed search, from its inception to December 2010, under the following expression *(gastritis OR chronic OR atroph* OR intestinal metaplasia OR dysplasia) AND (gastric OR stomach) AND (helicobacter pylori OR gene OR polymorphism OR SNPs OR smoking OR tobacco OR cigarette OR salt OR antioxidant OR diet OR lifestyle OR environmental OR behaviour) AND (meta-analysis OR "systematic review").*

Table 1. Summary of systematic reviews and meta-analyses † addressing the role of genetic and environmental factors on the occurrence of gastric precancerous lesions

2.1.1 The role of *Helicobacter pylori* infection

The association between *H. pylori* infection and gastric cancer is well established, with several meta-analyses reporting an odds ratio of approximately 2 (Figure 2). The prevalence of *H. pylori* infection is high (74% in developing and 58% in developed countries, on average) and nearly two-thirds of all gastric cancers occurring worldwide are attributed to it (Parkin, 2006). Pelayo Correa proposed that *H. pylori* infection acted at the early phases of the carcinogenesis based on the fact that the inflammatory reaction could disappear after clearance of the bacteria with antibiotic treatment (Correa, 1992), and this has received support from several lines of evidence. On the one hand, the longer the lag between the assessment of *H. pylori* infection status and the diagnosis of gastric cancer, the stronger is the association between infection and cancer (Helicobacter and Cancer Collaborative Group, 2001; Huang et al., 1998), as *H. pylori* clearance tends to occur with the progression to the cancer endpoint (Gao et al., 2009; Kokkola et al., 2003). Case-control designs tend to underestimate the relation between infection and gastric cancer, but studies that used more sensitive methods to detect past infection or restricted the analysis to less advanced cases yielded stronger relative risk estimates (Brenner et al., 2004; Ekstrom et al., 2001; Mitchell et al., 2008; Peleteiro et al., 2010a). On the other hand, this is also in accordance with the stronger associations observed between *H. pylori* and precancerous lesions (Table 1) than with gastric cancer, as depicted in Figure 2.

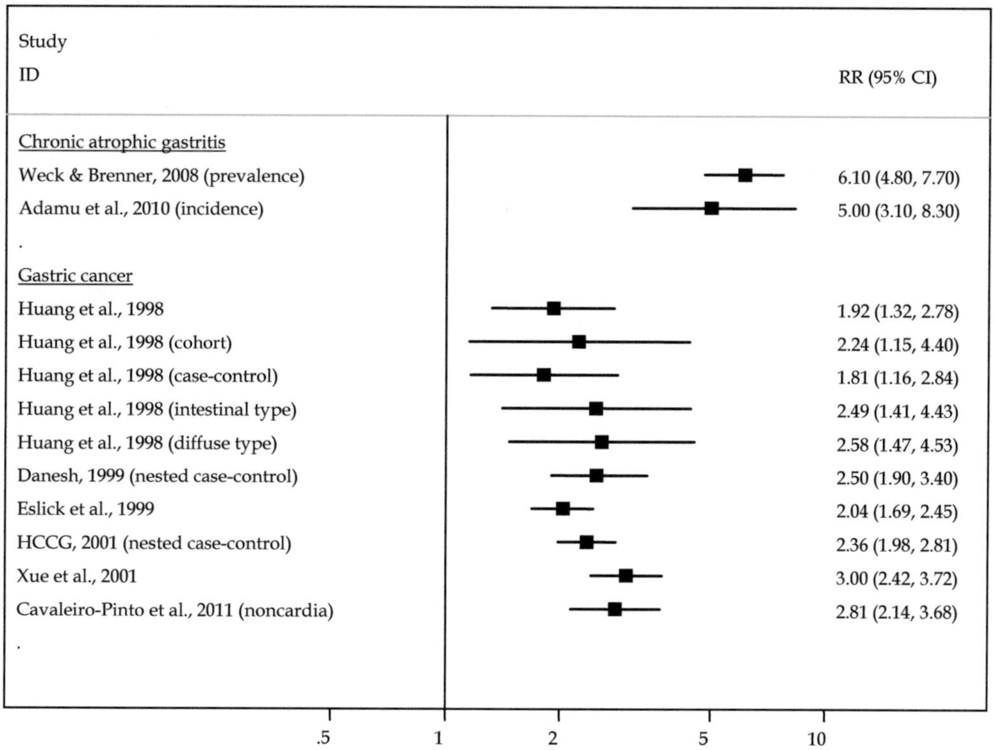

Fig. 2. Meta-analyses on the association between *Helicobacter pylori* infection and chronic atrophic gastritis, and gastric cancer (Adamu et al., 2010; Cavaleiro-Pinto et al., 2011; Danesh, 1999; Eslick et al., 1999; Helicobacter and Cancer Collaborative Group, 2001; Huang et al., 1998; Weck & Brenner, 2008; Xue et al., 2001).

A direct correlation between *H. pylori* prevalence and gastric cancer rates is not observed when countries with different patterns of infection and gastric cancer risk are considered, namely because some of them present low gastric cancer incidences despite the high prevalences of infection, the so-called African and Asian enigmas (Holcombe, 1992; Miwa et al., 2002). In the latter settings, the cancer precursor lesions, especially intestinal metaplasia, are also less frequent than expected given the high prevalence of infection (Campbell et al., 2001; Carrilho et al., 2009; Kalebi et al., 2007; Kidd et al., 1999; Oluwasola & Ogunbiyi, 2004), supporting the hypothesis that *H. pylori* infection acts before their development (in earlier steps of the carcinogenesis) and that other genetic and/or environmental exposures modulate the progression towards cancer (Campbell et al., 2001; Louw et al., 2001; Lunet & Barros, 2003; Mitchell et al., 2002).

2.1.1.1 The impact of *Helicobacter pylori* eradication

Since the recognition of the causal link between *H. pylori* and gastric cancer, research has focused on the potential of eradication of the infection as preventive tool. Some clinical trials concluded that *H. pylori* eradication reduces gastric cancer risk (Fuccio et al., 2009; Ito et al., 2009) (Figure 3). However, one of the trials (Wong et al., 2004) analysed separately the subjects with and without precancerous lesions, and eradication of *H. pylori* infection was significantly associated with a decreased risk of developing gastric cancer only among the

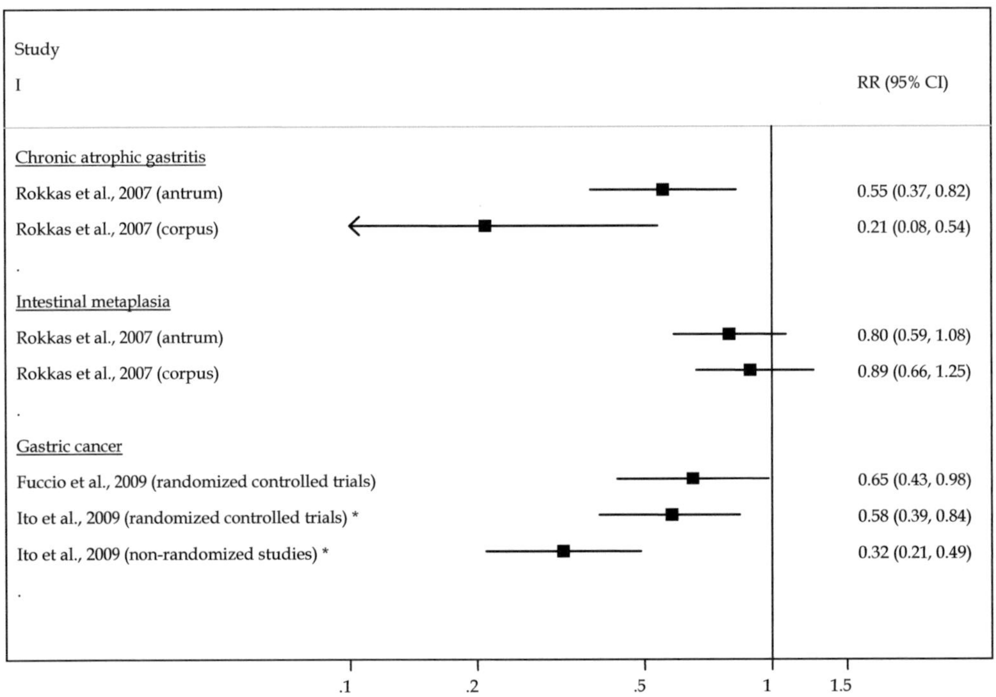

* this report refers to a systematic review but does not include a meta-analysis, and summary estimates were computed by the authors of this chapter based on the results presented for each individual study.

Fig. 3. Meta-analyses on the association between *Helicobacter pylori* eradication and incidence of chronic atrophic gastritis, intestinal metaplasia, and gastric cancer (Fuccio et al., 2009; Ito et al., 2009; Rokkas et al., 2007).

latter, supporting the hypothesis of the effects of infection in the early stages of gastric carcinogenesis. This is also in accordance with the lack of association between eradication and cancer in a trial conducted in Colombia, which only included subjects with gastric precancerous lesions at baseline evaluation (Correa et al., 2000; Mera et al., 2005).

Also, a meta-analysis from Rokkas *et al.* (Rokkas et al., 2007) estimated the long-term impact of *H. pylori* eradication on the incidence of gastric precancerous lesions (Table 1), with significant reduction in chronic atrophic gastritis risk but not for intestinal metaplasia (Figure 3).

Taken together, these results support the irreversibility of intestinal metaplasia, since *H. pylori* eradication must occur before a point of no return in order to be effective. This represents one more piece of evidence of an early role for *H. pylori* infection in the gastric carcinogenesis, as it leads to intestinal metaplasia but must be complemented with other factors for progression towards cancer.

2.1.2 The role of lifestyle factors

Although *H. pylori* infection is the most important gastric cancer determinant, only a small proportion of infected subjects will reach this endpoint (Hsu et al., 2007; Uemura et al., 2001), and several other potential causal components have to be considered.

2.1.2.1 Smoking

Stomach cancer is now considered a tobacco-related cancer, with 17% of cases among men and 11% among women being attributed to it in the more developed countries (IARC Working Group on the Evaluation of Carcinogenic Risks to Humans, 2004). Compared to never-smokers, current smokers have a 20% (among women) to 62% (among men) higher risk of gastric cancer, while gastric cancer is 16% (among women) to 34% (among men) more frequent in former smokers (Ladeiras-Lopes et al., 2008). This shows that the interruption of the exposure to tobacco contributes to a reduction in gastric cancer risk, supporting that its effects are exerted at the later steps of carcinogenesis. Furthermore, the risk of cancer was higher in subjects quitting smoking more recently (summary RR for studies with a mean/median follow-up time < 10 *vs.* ≥ 10 years: 1.39, 95%CI: 1.30-1.49 *vs.* 1.09, 95%CI: 0.95-1.25, among men) (Ladeiras-Lopes et al., 2008), in accordance with the hypothesis that smoking acts predominantly by promoting the progression from the more advanced precursor lesions to cancer.

Among lifestyle exposures, the relation between smoking and precancerous lesions, especially intestinal metaplasia, has been the more extensively studied, but no systematic reviews of studies quantifying this association are available. The individual reports that have been published yielded relative risk estimates ranging from 1.42 to 4.91 (Kim et al., 2008; Mesquita et al., 2006). An ecological analysis showed a strong correlation between apparent tobacco consumption and the frequency of intestinal metaplasia among *H. pylori*-infected subjects (Peleteiro et al., 2008), suggesting that the low cigarette consumption observed in developing countries may be a contributory factor for the disruption of the carcinogenesis pathway, precluding the progression to the more advanced lesions. This was also supported by another ecological analysis that showed lower gastric cancer incidence rates in settings with high prevalence of infection and low apparent tobacco consumption than in those where smoking was more frequent (Lunet & Barros, 2003).

Taken together, these results are indicative of a role for smoking in the stages closer to cancer.

2.1.2.2 Salt

The proposed mechanisms by which salt can cause gastric cancer are either the direct damage of the gastric mucosa causing excessive cell replication or an indirect effect by increasing of the mutagenic potential of *N*-nitroso compounds, which is compatible with the action of salt intake at the initial and late stages of gastric carcinogenesis, respectively (Correa, 1992). More recently, it was shown that the damage caused by salt may also increase gastric *H. pylori* colonization (Fox et al., 1999; Nozaki et al., 2002), which is also supportive of an early role in the pathway.
Many methodological limitations preclude valid measurements of salt consumption (Chen et al., 1990), and the excretion of sodium in urine over a 24-h period is the method that reflects more accurately the sodium ingested from different sources (World Cancer Research Fund & American Institute for Cancer Research, 2007). The latter, however, was used only in an ecological study assessing the association between salt and intestinal metaplasia (ECP-EURONUT, 1994).
The summary estimates for the relation between total salt use and gastric cancer obtained in the World Cancer Research Fund meta-analysis correspond to a relative risk of approximately 2 (Figure 4). However, only 17 of the 71 studies identified trough systematic review were included in the meta-analysis, due to the large heterogeneity in the presentation of results (World Cancer Research Fund & American Institute for Cancer Research, 2007).

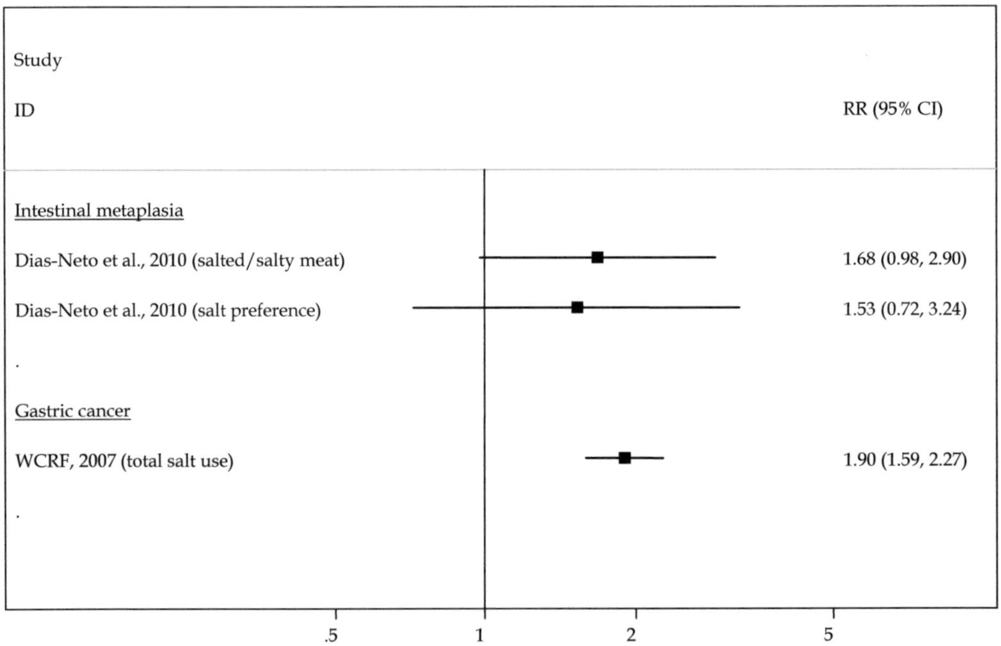

Fig. 4. Meta-analyses on the association between salt intake and intestinal metaplasia, and gastric cancer (Dias-Neto et al., 2010; World Cancer Research Fund & American Institute for Cancer Research, 2007).

In the meta-analysis conducted by Dias-Neto *et al.* (Dias-Neto et al., 2010), salted/salty meat intake and preference for salted/salty foods or use of table salt were associated with an approximately 60% increased risk of intestinal metaplasia (Figure 4), but the authors concluded that the large methodological heterogeneity and in the presentation of the results did not allow a more comprehensive quantitative synthesis or a conclusive overall interpretation of the findings.

The evidence currently available on this topic precludes definite conclusions on the magnitude of the effects of salt consumption, overall and in different steps of carcinogenesis.

2.1.2.3 Antioxidants

Based on the inverse association between ingestion of fresh fruits and vegetables and gastric cancer observed in epidemiological studies, antioxidants such as ascorbic acid and beta-carotene were postulated to play a protective role in the stages closer to cancer by acting as free-radical scavengers (Correa, 1992). This protective effect of fruits and vegetables, however, seems to be weaker than initially expected. The summary estimates from several meta-analyses on this topic are closer to 1 when derived from cohort studies, ranging from 0.89 to 0.95 for fruits intake and from 0.89 to 0.98 for vegetables consumption (Figure 5).

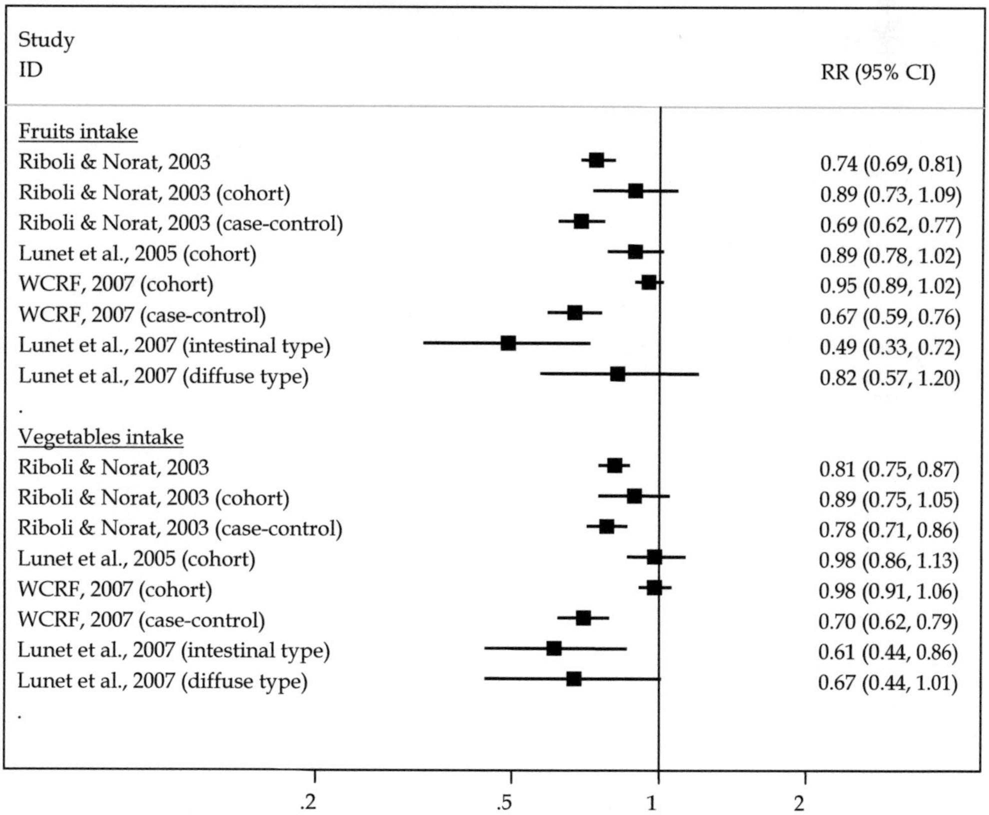

Fig. 5. Meta-analyses on the association between fruits and vegetables intake and gastric cancer (Lunet et al., 2005; Lunet et al., 2007; Riboli & Norat, 2003; World Cancer Research Fund & American Institute for Cancer Research, 2007).

However, a stronger protective effect was observed in studies with a follow-up of 10 or more years (OR=0.66, 95%CI: 0.52-0.83 for fruits and OR=0.71, 95%CI: 0.53-0.94 for vegetables in incidence studies) (Lunet et al., 2005), which may be seen as evidence of a relatively early effect of these factors in the gastric carcinogenesis pathway. Research on this topic having cancer precursor lesions as the outcome has seldom been conducted, with few studies reporting conflicting results regarding chronic atrophic gastritis and intestinal metaplasia (Jedrychowski et al., 1999; Kato et al., 2004; Kuwahara et al., 2000; Sierra et al., 2008).

Chemoprevention trials have found no evidence of a beneficial effect for antioxidant supplementation on gastric cancer prevention (Bjelakovic et al., 2004; Druesne-Pecollo et al., 2010).

Although it is plausible that naturally occurring antioxidants may inhibit the carcinogenesis progression, there is limited evidence on the specific steps where these factors may act.

2.1.2.4 *N*-nitroso compounds

N-nitroso compounds were hypothesized to act in gastric carcinogenesis by promoting the synthesis of carcinogens via nitrosation reactions (Correa, 1992). Processed meat is often an important source of exposure to carcinogenic *N*-nitroso compounds, and a meta-analysis of studies that quantified the association between processed meat consumption and stomach cancer found stronger associations for case-control studies (case-control *vs.* cohort: OR=1.63, 95%CI: 1.31-2.01 *vs.* OR=1.24, 95%CI: 0.98-1.56) (Larsson et al., 2006). The relation between these exposures and cancer precursor lesions has seldom been addressed (Sobala et al., 1991; You et al., 1996) and the effect of these compounds in the gastric carcinogenesis pathway remains to be fully understood.

2.1.3 The role of genetic factors

The genetic profile of the individuals was not included in the first versions of the model proposed by Correa (Correa, 1992; Correa et al., 1975) but, along with the advent of new technologies and their use in epidemiological research, several studies addressing the association between genetic polymorphisms and gastric cancer have been conducted. In the aetiological model of gastric cancer, individual genetic susceptibility may be critical in a variety of processes relevant to gastric carcinogenesis, namely mucosal protection, inflammatory response, carcinogen detoxification, antioxidant protection, DNA repair and oncogenes and tumour suppressor genes expression. The most widely studied polymorphisms, and for which more promising results have been achieved, are those related to proinflammatory cytokines, namely within interleukin-1 (*IL1*) and tumour necrosis factor α (*TNFA*) gene clusters.

2.1.3.1 Cytokine gene polymorphisms

H. pylori infection induces both interleukin-1β (IL-1β) and tumour necrosis factor-α (TNF-α) production, and these cytokines inhibit gastric acid secretion, leading to the development of gastric precancerous lesions and cancer (El-Omar et al., 2000; Hwang et al., 2002). The *IL1B* gene codes for the IL-1β and the *IL1RN* gene for an anti-inflammatory cytokine, interleukin-1 receptor antagonist (IL-1ra). Polymorphisms within the *IL1B* gene increase IL-1β expression and IL-1ra binds to the IL-1 receptors, modulating the pro-inflammatory effects of IL-1β. Regarding the *IL1RN* gene, a variable number tandem repeat (VNTR) polymorphism has been detected within intron 2, and five allelic variants have been identified in the number of repeats varying from 2 to 6 (El-Omar, 2001; Gonzalez et al., 2002). The ability of *H. pylori* to infect and remain in the human stomach induces a chronic inflammatory response, which may be of variable magnitude depending on the genetic make-up of the host. Most of the single nucleotide polymorphisms (SNPs) studied are situated in the gene promoter region and play important roles in modulating gene expression and thus the inflammatory response.

Previous meta-analyses have shown an increased gastric cancer risk associated with polymorphisms in *IL1RN*, *IL1B-511* and *TNFA-308* (Figure 6). The *IL1RN**22 genotype increases the risk of gastric precancerous lesions, suggesting a role for this polymorphism in the early stages of gastric carcinogenesis, while positive associations between *IL1B-511* TT genotype and gastric precancerous lesions only became apparent when studies addressing intestinal metaplasia as the outcome were considered (Figure 6). These associations were

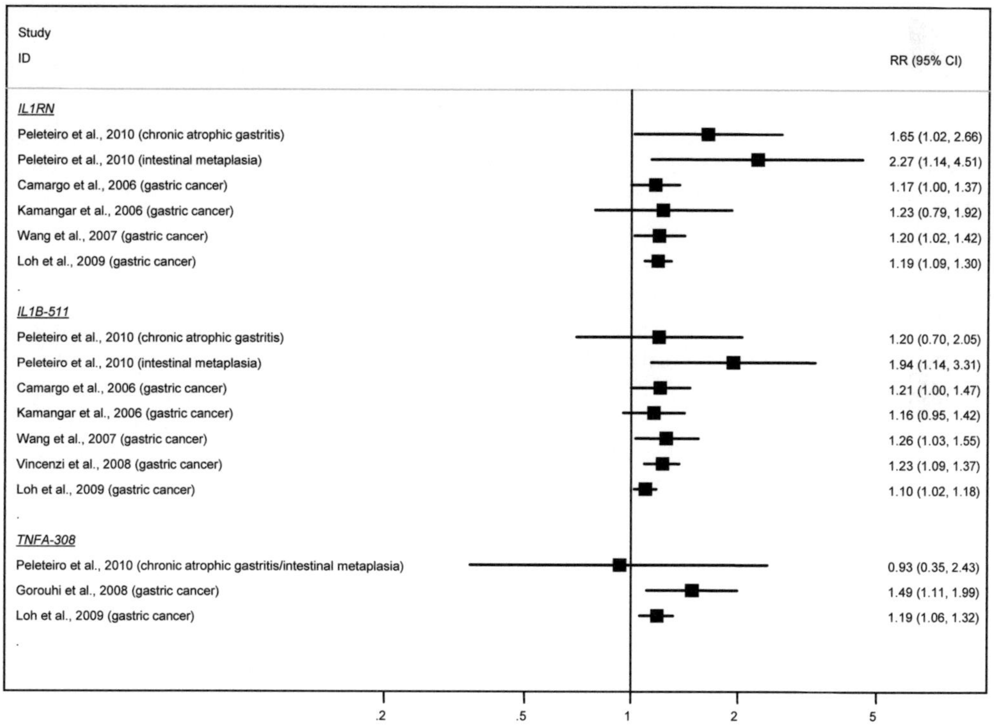

Fig. 6. Meta-analyses on the association between cytokine gene polymorphisms and chronic atrophic gastritis, intestinal metaplasia, and gastric cancer (Camargo et al., 2006; Gorouhi et al., 2008; Kamangar et al., 2006; Loh et al., 2009; Peleteiro et al., 2010b; Vincenzi et al., 2008; Wang et al., 2007).

stronger among studies conducted in samples with high *H. pylori* prevalence, in accordance to what is known about the gene function and its potential interaction with infection. No overall association was found for *TNFA-308* AA genotype (Figure 6).

2.2 Other markers of gastric cancer development

The currently available evidence shows no substantial aetiological differences between the main Laurén subtypes, despite the relatively small number of studies addressing the effect of environmental exposures on the risk of gastric cancer according to histological subtypes (Figures 2 and 5). This may partially reflect misclassification of the histological type, due to inter-observer variability, the type of specimen available for diagnosis, and the proportion of tumours classified as unknown (Carneiro et al., 2007).

An additional concern is the ability for the classification proposed by Laurén to define aetiologically homogeneous subgroups of gastric cancer cases. The cascade of events that involve intestinal differentiation is mediated by CDX1 and/or CDX2 (Guo et al., 2004), and may result in the development of both intestinal and diffuse gastric carcinoma (Almeida et al., 2003). In particular, CDX2 expression is regarded as a marker of the intestinal epithelial phenotype, and the transdifferentiation of normal epithelia has been experimentally induced by changes in local environment (Marchetti et al., 2003), which supports the hypothesis that environmental exposures may modulate the CDX2 expression. This may be seen as an early marker of intestinal differentiation, that may be used as an endpoint occurring in the gastric carcinogenesis pathway even earlier than chronic atrophic gastritis or intestinal metaplasia. Research relying on these tools to define the outcomes is still scarce (Yuasa et al., 2009; Yuasa et al., 2005), but may be important to understand the aetiological heterogeneity of gastric cancer.

Histopathological and histochemical studies allowed the identification of two main types of intestinal metaplasia. The complete, also designated type I, and the incomplete, comprising types II and III (Filipe & Jass, 1986). In the classical multistep model of the gastric precancerous process, incomplete follows complete intestinal metaplasia sequentially (Correa, 1992). However, according to the patterns of mucin expression observed within each intestinal metaplasia type, it has been hypothesised that the complete and incomplete types of intestinal metaplasia may represent two alternative pathways, rather than successive steps; or that type II may represent a first step in the pathway, which may evolve to type I or to type III (Reis et al., 1999). The evaluation of specific risk factors for these endpoints may clarify the gastric carcinogenesis pathways and the role of environmental exposures in the aetiology of cancer (Peleteiro et al., 2007; Pintalhao et al., 2010).

3. Conclusion

The accumulated evidence so far led to the gradual acceptance and better understanding of the role of *H. pylori* infection and smoking in gastric carcinogenesis. For other exposures, however, there is much less robust evidence on the magnitude of the associations or their role throughout carcinogenesis. This allows an update of the model proposed by Correa, that still provides the best framework for gastric cancer etiological research, taking into account the evidence generated in the last two decades (Figure 7).

Research relying on more accurate tools to define specific gastric cancer subtypes and the evaluation of specific risk factors for early endpoints in the gastric carcinogenesis pathway may further contribute to the understanding of gastric cancer aetiology.

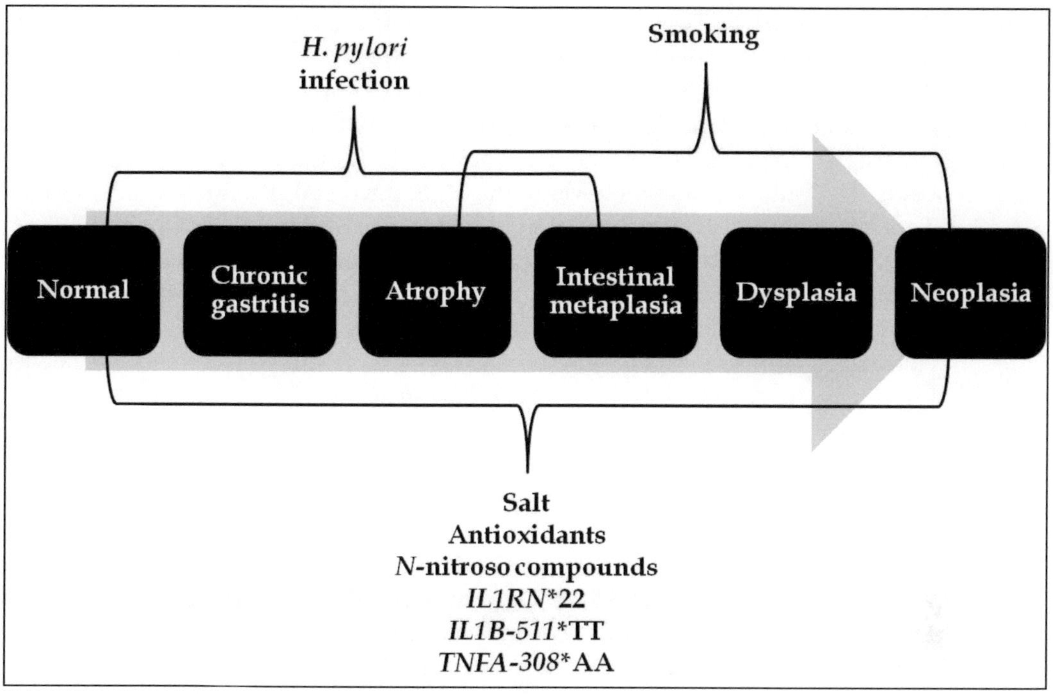

Fig. 7. Framework for the carcinogenesis pathway leading to gastric cancer, taking into account the model proposed by Correa (Correa, 1992) and the more robust evidence gathered up to 2010.

4. References

Adamu, M. A., Weck, M. N., Gao, L., & Brenner, H. (2010). Incidence of chronic atrophic gastritis: systematic review and meta-analysis of follow-up studies. *Eur J Epidemiol, 25*, 439-448.

Almeida, R., Silva, E., Santos-Silva, F., Silberg, D. G., Wang, J., De Bolos, C., & David, L. (2003). Expression of intestine-specific transcription factors, CDX1 and CDX2, in intestinal metaplasia and gastric carcinomas. *J Pathol, 199*, 36-40.

Bjelakovic, G., Nikolova, D., Simonetti, R. G., & Gluud, C. (2004). Antioxidant supplements for prevention of gastrointestinal cancers: a systematic review and meta-analysis. *Lancet, 364*, 1219-1228.

Brenner, H., Arndt, V., Stegmaier, C., Ziegler, H., & Rothenbacher, D. (2004). Is Helicobacter pylori infection a necessary condition for noncardia gastric cancer? *Am J Epidemiol, 159*, 252-258.

Camargo, M. C., Mera, R., Correa, P., Peek, R. M., Jr., Fontham, E. T., Goodman, K. J., Piazuelo, M. B., Sicinschi, L., Zabaleta, J., & Schneider, B. G. (2006). Interleukin-1beta and interleukin-1 receptor antagonist gene polymorphisms and gastric cancer: a meta-analysis. *Cancer Epidemiol Biomarkers Prev, 15*, 1674-1687.

Campbell, D. I., Warren, B. F., Thomas, J. E., Figura, N., Telford, J. L., & Sullivan, P. B. (2001). The African enigma: low prevalence of gastric atrophy, high prevalence of chronic inflammation in West African adults and children. *Helicobacter, 6*, 263-267.

Carneiro, F., Moutinho, C., Pera, G., Caldas, C., Fenger, C., Offerhaus, J., Save, V., Stenling, R., Nesi, G., Mahlke, U., Blaker, H., Torrado, J., Roukos, D. H., Sabourin, J. C., Boeing, H., Palli, D., Bueno-de-Mesquita, H. B., Overvad, K., Bingham, S., Clavel-Chapelon, F., Lund, E., Trichopoulou, A., Manjer, J., Riboli, E., & Gonzalez, C. A. (2007). Pathology findings and validation of gastric and esophageal cancer cases in a European cohort (EPIC/EUR-GAST). *Scand J Gastroenterol, 42*, 618-627.

Carrilho, C., Modcoicar, P., Cunha, L., Ismail, M., Guisseve, A., Lorenzoni, C., Fernandes, F., Peleteiro, B., Almeida, R., Figueiredo, C., David, L., & Lunet, N. (2009). Prevalence of Helicobacter pylori infection, chronic gastritis, and intestinal metaplasia in Mozambican dyspeptic patients. *Virchows Arch, 454*, 153-160.

Cavaleiro-Pinto, M., Peleteiro, B., Lunet, N., & Barros, H. (2011). Helicobacter pylori infection and gastric cardia cancer: systematic review and meta-analysis. *Cancer Causes Control, 22*, 375-387.

Chen, V. W., Abu-Elyazeed, R. R., Zavala, D. E., Ktsanes, V. K., Haenszel, W., Cuello, C., Montes, G., & Correa, P. (1990). Risk factors of gastric precancerous lesions in a high-risk Colombian population. I. Salt. *Nutr Cancer, 13*, 59-65.

Correa, P. (1992). Human gastric carcinogenesis: a multistep and multifactorial process--First American Cancer Society Award Lecture on Cancer Epidemiology and Prevention. *Cancer Res, 52*, 6735-6740.

Correa, P., Fontham, E. T., Bravo, J. C., Bravo, L. E., Ruiz, B., Zarama, G., Realpe, J. L., Malcom, G. T., Li, D., Johnson, W. D., & Mera, R. (2000). Chemoprevention of gastric dysplasia: randomized trial of antioxidant supplements and anti-helicobacter pylori therapy. *J Natl Cancer Inst, 92*, 1881-1888.

Correa, P., Haenszel, W., Cuello, C., Tannenbaum, S., & Archer, M. (1975). A model for gastric cancer epidemiology. *Lancet, 2*, 58-60.

Correa, P., Sasano, N., Stemmermann, G. N., & Haenszel, W. (1973). Pathology of gastric carcinoma in Japanese populations: comparisons between Miyagi prefecture, Japan, and Hawaii. *J Natl Cancer Inst, 51*, 1449-1459.

Danesh, J. (1999). Helicobacter pylori infection and gastric cancer: systematic review of the epidemiological studies. *Aliment Pharmacol Ther, 13*, 851-856.

Dias-Neto, M., Pintalhao, M., Ferreira, M., & Lunet, N. (2010). Salt intake and risk of gastric intestinal metaplasia: systematic review and meta-analysis. *Nutr Cancer, 62*, 133-147.

Druesne-Pecollo, N., Latino-Martel, P., Norat, T., Barrandon, E., Bertrais, S., Galan, P., & Hercberg, S. (2010). Beta-carotene supplementation and cancer risk: a systematic review and metaanalysis of randomized controlled trials. *Int J Cancer, 127*, 172-184.

ECP-EURONUT. (1994). ECP-EURONUT-Intestinal Metaplasia Study: urinary and gastric juice analyses. *Eur J Cancer Prev, 3*, 413-418.

Ekström, A. M., Hansson, L. E., Signorello, L. B., Lindgren, A., Bergstrom, R., & Nyren, O. (2000). Decreasing incidence of both major histologic subtypes of gastric adenocarcinoma--a population-based study in Sweden. *Br J Cancer, 83*, 391-396.

Ekstrom, A. M., Held, M., Hansson, L. E., Engstrand, L., & Nyren, O. (2001). Helicobacter pylori in gastric cancer established by CagA immunoblot as a marker of past infection. *Gastroenterology, 121*, 784-791.

El-Omar, E. M. (2001). The importance of interleukin 1beta in Helicobacter pylori associated disease. *Gut, 48*, 743-747.

El-Omar, E. M., Carrington, M., Chow, W. H., McColl, K. E., Bream, J. H., Young, H. A., Herrera, J., Lissowska, J., Yuan, C. C., Rothman, N., Lanyon, G., Martin, M., Fraumeni, J. F., Jr., & Rabkin, C. S. (2000). Interleukin-1 polymorphisms associated with increased risk of gastric cancer. *Nature, 404*, 398-402.

Eslick, G. D., Lim, L. L., Byles, J. E., Xia, H. H., & Talley, N. J. (1999). Association of Helicobacter pylori infection with gastric carcinoma: a meta-analysis. *Am J Gastroenterol, 94*, 2373-2379.

Filipe, M. I., & Jass, J. R. (1986). Intestinal metaplasia subtypes and cancer risk. In M. I. Filipe & J. R. Jass (Eds.), *Gastric carcinoma* (pp. 87-115). London: Churchill Livingstone.

Fox, J. G., Dangler, C. A., Taylor, N. S., King, A., Koh, T. J., & Wang, T. C. (1999). High-salt diet induces gastric epithelial hyperplasia and parietal cell loss, and enhances Helicobacter pylori colonization in C57BL/6 mice. *Cancer Res, 59*, 4823-4828.

Fuccio, L., Zagari, R. M., Eusebi, L. H., Laterza, L., Cennamo, V., Ceroni, L., Grilli, D., & Bazzoli, F. (2009). Meta-analysis: can Helicobacter pylori eradication treatment reduce the risk for gastric cancer? *Ann Intern Med, 151*, 121-128.

Gao, L., Weck, M. N., Nieters, A., & Brenner, H. (2009). Inverse association between a pro-inflammatory genetic profile and Helicobacter pylori seropositivity among patients with chronic atrophic gastritis: enhanced elimination of the infection during disease progression? *Eur J Cancer, 45*, 2860-2866.

Gonzalez, C. A., Sala, N., & Capella, G. (2002). Genetic susceptibility and gastric cancer risk. *Int J Cancer, 100*, 249-260.

Gorouhi, F., Islami, F., Bahrami, H., & Kamangar, F. (2008). Tumour-necrosis factor-A polymorphisms and gastric cancer risk: a meta-analysis. *Br J Cancer, 98*, 1443-1451.

Guo, R. J., Suh, E. R., & Lynch, J. P. (2004). The role of Cdx proteins in intestinal development and cancer. *Cancer Biol Ther, 3*, 593-601.

Helicobacter and Cancer Collaborative Group. (2001). Gastric cancer and Helicobacter pylori: a combined analysis of 12 case control studies nested within prospective cohorts. *Gut, 49*, 347-353.

Holcombe, C. (1992). Helicobacter pylori: the African enigma. *Gut, 33*, 429-431.

Hsu, P. I., Lai, K. H., Hsu, P. N., Lo, G. H., Yu, H. C., Chen, W. C., Tsay, F. W., Lin, H. C., Tseng, H. H., Ger, L. P., & Chen, H. C. (2007). Helicobacter pylori infection and the risk of gastric malignancy. *Am J Gastroenterol, 102*, 725-730.

Huang, J. Q., Sridhar, S., Chen, Y., & Hunt, R. H. (1998). Meta-analysis of the relationship between Helicobacter pylori seropositivity and gastric cancer. *Gastroenterology, 114*, 1169-1179.

Huang, J. Q., Zheng, G. F., Sumanac, K., Irvine, E. J., & Hunt, R. H. (2003). Meta-analysis of the relationship between cagA seropositivity and gastric cancer. *Gastroenterology, 125*, 1636-1644.

Hwang, I. R., Kodama, T., Kikuchi, S., Sakai, K., Peterson, L. E., Graham, D. Y., & Yamaoka, Y. (2002). Effect of interleukin 1 polymorphisms on gastric mucosal interleukin 1beta production in Helicobacter pylori infection. *Gastroenterology, 123*, 1793-1803.

IARC Working Group on the Evaluation of Carcinogenic Risks to Humans. (2004). Tobacco smoke and involuntary smoking. *IARC Monogr Eval Carcinog Risks Hum, 83*, 1-1438.

Ito, M., Takata, S., Tatsugami, M., Wada, Y., Imagawa, S., Matsumoto, Y., Takamura, A., Kitamura, S., Matsuo, T., Tanaka, S., Haruma, K., & Chayama, K. (2009). Clinical prevention of gastric cancer by Helicobacter pylori eradication therapy: a systematic review. *J Gastroenterol, 44*, 365-371.

Jedrychowski, W., Popiela, T., Drews, M., Gabryelewicz, A., Marlicz, K., Misiunia, P., Wajda, Z., Matyja, A., Nowak, K., Ramroth, H., & Wahrendorf, J. (1999). Effect of Helicobacter pylori infection, smoking and dietary habits on the occurrence of antrum intestinal metaplasia. Clinico-epidemiological study in Poland. *Pol J Pathol, 50*, 289-295.

Kalebi, A., Rana, F., Mwanda, W., Lule, G., & Hale, M. (2007). Histopathological profile of gastritis in adult patients seen at a referral hospital in Kenya. *World J Gastroenterol, 13*, 4117-4121.

Kamangar, F., Cheng, C., Abnet, C. C., & Rabkin, C. S. (2006). Interleukin-1B polymorphisms and gastric cancer risk--a meta-analysis. *Cancer Epidemiol Biomarkers Prev, 15*, 1920-1928.

Kaneko, S., & Yoshimura, T. (2001). Time trend analysis of gastric cancer incidence in Japan by histological types, 1975-1989. *Br J Cancer, 84*, 400-405.

Kato, I., Vivas, J., Plummer, M., Lopez, G., Peraza, S., Castro, D., Sanchez, V., Cano, E., Andrade, O., Garcia, R., Franceschi, S., Oliver, W., & Munoz, N. (2004). Environmental factors in Helicobacter pylori-related gastric precancerous lesions in Venezuela. *Cancer Epidemiol Biomarkers Prev, 13*, 468-476.

Kidd, M., Louw, J. A., & Marks, I. N. (1999). Helicobacter pylori in Africa: observations on an 'enigma within an enigma'. *J Gastroenterol Hepatol, 14*, 851-858.

Kim, N., Park, Y. S., Cho, S. I., Lee, H. S., Choe, G., Kim, I. W., Won, Y. D., Park, J. H., Kim, J. S., Jung, H. C., & Song, I. S. (2008). Prevalence and risk factors of atrophic gastritis and intestinal metaplasia in a Korean population without significant gastroduodenal disease. *Helicobacter, 13*, 245-255.

Kokkola, A., Kosunen, T. U., Puolakkainen, P., Sipponen, P., Harkonen, M., Laxen, F., Virtamo, J., Haapiainen, R., & Rautelin, H. (2003). Spontaneous disappearance of Helicobacter pylori antibodies in patients with advanced atrophic corpus gastritis. *APMIS, 111*, 619-624.

Kuwahara, Y., Kono, S., Eguchi, H., Hamada, H., Shinchi, K., & Imanishi, K. (2000). Relationship between serologically diagnosed chronic atrophic gastritis, Helicobacter pylori, and environmental factors in Japanese men. *Scand J Gastroenterol, 35*, 476-481.

Ladeiras-Lopes, R., Pereira, A. K., Nogueira, A., Pinheiro-Torres, T., Pinto, I., Santos-Pereira, R., & Lunet, N. (2008). Smoking and gastric cancer: systematic review and meta-analysis of cohort studies. *Cancer Causes Control, 19*, 689-701.

Larsson, S. C., Orsini, N., & Wolk, A. (2006). Processed meat consumption and stomach cancer risk: a meta-analysis. *J Natl Cancer Inst, 98*, 1078-1087.

Laurén, P. A. (1965). The two histological main types of gastric carcinoma: diffuse and so-called intestinal-type carcinoma. An attempt at a histo-clinical classification. *Acta Pathol Microbiol Scand, 64*, 31-49.

Laurén, P. A., & Nevalainen, T. J. (1993). Epidemiology of intestinal and diffuse types of gastric carcinoma. A time-trend study in Finland with comparison between studies from high- and low-risk areas. *Cancer, 71*, 2926-2933.

Loh, M., Koh, K. X., Yeo, B. H., Song, C. M., Chia, K. S., Zhu, F., Yeoh, K. G., Hill, J., Iacopetta, B., & Soong, R. (2009). Meta-analysis of genetic polymorphisms and gastric cancer risk: variability in associations according to race. *Eur J Cancer, 45*, 2562-2568.

Louw, J. A., Kidd, M. S., Kummer, A. F., Taylor, K., Kotze, U., & Hanslo, D. (2001). The relationship between Helicobacter pylori infection, the virulence genotypes of the infecting strain and gastric cancer in the African setting. *Helicobacter, 6*, 268-273.

Lunet, N., & Barros, H. (2003). Helicobacter pylori infection and gastric cancer: facing the enigmas. *Int J Cancer, 106*, 953-960.

Lunet, N., Lacerda-Vieira, A., & Barros, H. (2005). Fruit and vegetables consumption and gastric cancer: a systematic review and meta-analysis of cohort studies. *Nutr Cancer, 53*, 1-10.

Lunet, N., Valbuena, C., Vieira, A. L., Lopes, C., David, L., Carneiro, F., & Barros, H. (2007). Fruit and vegetable consumption and gastric cancer by location and histological type: case-control and meta-analysis. *Eur J Cancer Prev, 16*, 312-327.

Marchetti, M., Caliot, E., & Pringault, E. (2003). Chronic acid exposure leads to activation of the cdx2 intestinal homeobox gene in a long-term culture of mouse esophageal keratinocytes. *J Cell Sci, 116*, 1429-1436.

Marshall, B. J., & Warren, J. R. (1984). Unidentified curved bacilli in the stomach of patients with gastritis and peptic ulceration. *Lancet, 1*, 1311-1315.

Mera, R., Fontham, E. T., Bravo, L. E., Bravo, J. C., Piazuelo, M. B., Camargo, M. C., & Correa, P. (2005). Long term follow up of patients treated for Helicobacter pylori infection. *Gut, 54*, 1536-1540.

Mesquita, P., Raquel, A., Nuno, L., Reis, C. A., Silva, L. F., Serpa, J., Van Seuningen, I., Barros, H., & David, L. (2006). Metaplasia--a transdifferentiation process that facilitates cancer development: the model of gastric intestinal metaplasia. *Crit Rev Oncog, 12*, 3-26.

Miki, K. (2006). Gastric cancer screening using the serum pepsinogen test method. *Gastric Cancer, 9*, 245-253.

Mitchell, H., English, D. R., Elliott, F., Gengos, M., Barrett, J. H., Giles, G. G., & Forman, D. (2008). Immunoblotting using multiple antigens is essential to demonstrate the true risk of Helicobacter pylori infection for gastric cancer. *Aliment Pharmacol Ther, 28*, 903-910.

Mitchell, H. M., Ally, R., Wadee, A., Wiseman, M., & Segal, I. (2002). Major differences in the IgG subclass response to Helicobacter pylori in the first and third worlds. *Scand J Gastroenterol, 37*, 517-522.

Miwa, H., Go, M. F., & Sato, N. (2002). H. pylori and gastric cancer: the Asian enigma. *Am J Gastroenterol, 97*, 1106-1112.

Muñoz, N., & Asvall, J. (1971). Time trends of intestinal and diffuse types of gastric cancer in Norway. *Int J Cancer, 8*, 144-157.

Muñoz, N., & Connelly, R. (1971). Time trends of intestinal and diffuse types of gastric cancer in the United States. *Int J Cancer, 8*, 158-164.

Nozaki, K., Shimizu, N., Inada, K., Tsukamoto, T., Inoue, M., Kumagai, T., Sugiyama, A., Mizoshita, T., Kaminishi, M., & Tatematsu, M. (2002). Synergistic promoting effects of Helicobacter pylori infection and high-salt diet on gastric carcinogenesis in Mongolian gerbils. *Jpn J Cancer Res, 93*, 1083-1089.

Oluwasola, A. O., & Ogunbiyi, J. O. (2004). Chronic gastritis and Helicobacter pylori infection in University College Hospital Ibadan, Nigeria--a study of 85 fibre optic gastric biopsies. *Niger J Med, 13*, 372-378.

Parkin, D. M. (2006). The global health burden of infection-associated cancers in the year 2002. *Int J Cancer, 118*, 3030-3044.

Peleteiro, B., Bastos, J., Barros, H., & Lunet, N. (2008). Systematic review of the prevalence of gastric intestinal metaplasia and its area-level association with smoking. *Gac Sanit, 22*, 236-247.

Peleteiro, B., Lunet, N., Barros, R., La Vecchia, C., & Barros, H. (2010a). Factors contributing to the underestimation of Helicobacter pylori-associated gastric cancer risk in a high-prevalence population. *Cancer Causes Control, 21*, 1257-1264.

Peleteiro, B., Lunet, N., Carrilho, C., Duraes, C., Machado, J. C., La Vecchia, C., & Barros, H. (2010b). Association between cytokine gene polymorphisms and gastric precancerous lesions: systematic review and meta-analysis. *Cancer Epidemiol Biomarkers Prev, 19*, 762-776.

Peleteiro, B., Lunet, N., Figueiredo, C., Carneiro, F., David, L., & Barros, H. (2007). Smoking, Helicobacter pylori virulence, and type of intestinal metaplasia in Portuguese males. *Cancer Epidemiol Biomarkers Prev, 16*, 322-326.

Pintalhao, M., Dias-Neto, M., Peleteiro, B., Lopes, C., Figueiredo, C., David, L., & Lunet, N. (2010). Salt intake and type of intestinal metaplasia in Helicobacter pylori-infected Portuguese men. *Nutr Cancer, 62*, 1153-1160.

Reis, C. A., David, L., Correa, P., Carneiro, F., de Bolos, C., Garcia, E., Mandel, U., Clausen, H., & Sobrinho-Simoes, M. (1999). Intestinal metaplasia of human stomach displays distinct patterns of mucin (MUC1, MUC2, MUC5AC, and MUC6) expression. *Cancer Res, 59*, 1003-1007.

Riboli, E., & Norat, T. (2003). Epidemiologic evidence of the protective effect of fruit and vegetables on cancer risk. *Am J Clin Nutr, 78*, 559S-569S.

Rokkas, T., Pistiolas, D., Sechopoulos, P., Robotis, I., & Margantinis, G. (2007). The long-term impact of Helicobacter pylori eradication on gastric histology: a systematic review and meta-analysis. *Helicobacter, 12 Suppl 2*, 32-38.

Sierra, R., Une, C., Ramirez, V., Alpizar-Alpizar, W., Gonzalez, M. I., Ramirez, J. A., De Mascarel, A., Cuenca, P., Perez-Perez, G., & Megraud, F. (2008). Relation of atrophic gastritis with Helicobacter pylori-CagA(+) and interleukin-1 gene polymorphisms. *World J Gastroenterol, 14*, 6481-6487.

Sobala, G. M., Pignatelli, B., Schorah, C. J., Bartsch, H., Sanderson, M., Dixon, M. F., Shires, S., King, R. F., & Axon, A. T. (1991). Levels of nitrite, nitrate, N-nitroso compounds, ascorbic acid and total bile acids in gastric juice of patients with and without precancerous conditions of the stomach. *Carcinogenesis, 12*, 193-198.

Tahara, E. (2004). Genetic pathways of two types of gastric cancer. *IARC Sci Publ*, 327-349.

Tredaniel, J., Boffetta, P., Buiatti, E., Saracci, R., & Hirsch, A. (1997). Tobacco smoking and gastric cancer: review and meta-analysis. *Int J Cancer, 72*, 565-573.

Uemura, N., Okamoto, S., Yamamoto, S., Matsumura, N., Yamaguchi, S., Yamakido, M., Taniyama, K., Sasaki, N., & Schlemper, R. J. (2001). Helicobacter pylori infection and the development of gastric cancer. *N Engl J Med, 345*, 784-789.

Vincenzi, B., Patti, G., Galluzzo, S., Pantano, F., Venditti, O., Santini, D., Ruzzo, A., Schiavon, G., Caraglia, M., Marra, M., Graziano, F., & Tonini, G. (2008). Interleukin 1beta-511T gene (IL1beta) polymorphism is correlated with gastric cancer in the Caucasian population: results from a meta-analysis. *Oncol Rep, 20*, 1213-1220.

Wang, P., Xia, H. H., Zhang, J. Y., Dai, L. P., Xu, X. Q., & Wang, K. J. (2007). Association of interleukin-1 gene polymorphisms with gastric cancer: a meta-analysis. *Int J Cancer, 120*, 552-562.

Weck, M. N., & Brenner, H. (2008). Association of Helicobacter pylori infection with chronic atrophic gastritis: Meta-analyses according to type of disease definition. *Int J Cancer, 123*, 874-881.

Wong, B. C., Lam, S. K., Wong, W. M., Chen, J. S., Zheng, T. T., Feng, R. E., Lai, K. C., Hu, W. H., Yuen, S. T., Leung, S. Y., Fong, D. Y., Ho, J., & Ching, C. K. (2004). Helicobacter pylori eradication to prevent gastric cancer in a high-risk region of China: a randomized controlled trial. *JAMA, 291*, 187-194.

World Cancer Research Fund, & American Institute for Cancer Research. (2007). Food, Nutrition, Physical Activity, and the Prevention of Cancer: a Global Perspective. In. Washington DC: AICR.

Wu, H., Rusiecki, J. A., Zhu, K., Potter, J., & Devesa, S. S. (2009). Stomach carcinoma incidence patterns in the United States by histologic type and anatomic site. *Cancer Epidemiol Biomarkers Prev, 18*, 1945-1952.

Xue, F. B., Xu, Y. Y., Wan, Y., Pan, B. R., Ren, J., & Fan, D. M. (2001). Association of H. pylori infection with gastric carcinoma: a Meta analysis. *World J Gastroenterol, 7*, 801-804.

You, W. C., Zhang, L., Yang, C. S., Chang, Y. S., Issaq, H., Fox, S. D., Utermahlen, W. E., Zhao, L., Keefer, L., Liu, W. D., Chow, W. H., Ma, J. L., Kneller, R., Ho, M. Y., Fraumeni, J. F., Jr., Xu, G. W., & Blot, W. J. (1996). Nitrite, N-nitroso compounds, and other analytes in physiological fluids in relation to precancerous gastric lesions. *Cancer Epidemiol Biomarkers Prev, 5*, 47-52.

Yuasa, Y., Nagasaki, H., Akiyama, Y., Hashimoto, Y., Takizawa, T., Kojima, K., Kawano, T., Sugihara, K., Imai, K., & Nakachi, K. (2009). DNA methylation status is inversely correlated with green tea intake and physical activity in gastric cancer patients. *Int J Cancer, 124*, 2677-2682.

Yuasa, Y., Nagasaki, H., Akiyama, Y., Sakai, H., Nakajima, T., Ohkura, Y., Takizawa, T., Koike, M., Tani, M., Iwai, T., Sugihara, K., Imai, K., & Nakachi, K. (2005). Relationship between CDX2 gene methylation and dietary factors in gastric cancer patients. *Carcinogenesis, 26*, 193-200.

12

Effects of *Helicobacter pylori* Infection on the Histology, Cellular Phenotype, K-*ras* Mutations, and Cell Kinetics in Gastric Intestinal Metaplasia in Patients with Chronic Gastritis and Gastric Cancer

Jiro Watari et al.*
[1]*Division of Upper Gastroenterology, Department of Internal Medicine, Hyogo College of Medicine, Nishinomiya, Japan*

1. Introduction

Helicobacter pylori (*H. pylori*) infection is a main risk factor for the development of gastric cancer (Correa et al., 1990; Sipponen & Hyvarinen, 1993; International Agency for Research on Cancer [IARC], 1994; Graham, 2000; Uemura et al., 2001). It has been postulated that *H. pylori* infection causes chronic gastritis, gastric atrophy, usually with gastric intestinal mataplasia (GIM) and dysplasia, and gastric cancer. The stepwise fashion of this infection, which usually continues over decades, has been defined as a sequence of histological events that confer an increasing risk of malignant transformation as described in Correa's hypothesis (Correa & Shiao, 1994). Although it is fairly well accepted that *H. pylori* infection plays a significant role in causing gastric cancer, the exact mechanisms involved in the pathogenesis remain obscure. In general, GIM is believed to be a preneoplastic lesion of the stomach (Correa, 1995), which increases the risk of gastric adenocarcinoma, especially intestinal type (Correa & Shiao, 1994; Correa, 1988). It remains unclear, however, as to whether or not GIM is a precancerous lesion or a marker for an increased risk of malignancy (Filipe et al., 1994; Miehlke et al., 1998).

Although there are many reports regarding the histological changes including metaplasia and dysplasia following eradication of *H. pylori,* the results have been conflicting (Table 1).

* Hiroki Tanabe[2], Kentaro Moriichi[2], Mikihiro Fujiya[2], Peter S. Amenta[3], Hiroto Miwa[1], Yutaka Kohgo[2] and Kiron M. Das[3]
[1]*Division of Upper Gastroenterology, Department of Internal Medicine, Hyogo College of Medicine, Nishinomiya, Japan;*
[2]*Division of Gastroenterology and Hematology/Oncology, Department of Medicine, Asahikawa Medical University, Asahikawa, Japan;*
[3]*Crohn's and Colitis Center of New Jersey, Division of Gastroenterology and Hepatology, Department of Medicine and Pathology, UMDNJ-Robert Wood Johnson Medical School, New Brunswick, NJ, USA*

Study	Materials	Follow-up period
Improvement		
Genta RM, et al.	Peptic ulcer (n=8) and others (n=3)	1 yr
Uemura N, et al.	Gastric cancer (n=65)	6 mo
Nardone G, et al.	Dyspepsia (n=45)	1 yr
Sung JJ, et al.	Volunteer (n=226)	1 yr
Ohkusa T, et al.	Dyspepsia (n=115)	12-15 mo
Kokkola A, et al.	Atrophic corpus gastritis (n=22)	2.5 yr
Correa P, et al.	Volunteer (n=226)	72 mo
Ley C, et al.	Volunteer (n=248)	1 yr
Mera R, et al.	Volunteer (n=394)	12 yr
You WC, et al.	Volunteer (n=3365)	7 yr
Unchanged		
Witteman EM, et al.	Dyspepsia (n=23)	1 yr
Forbes GM, et al.	Duodenal ulcer (n=32)	85 mo
van der Hulst RW, et al.	Dyspepsia & Peptic ulcer (n=106)	1 yr
Hibi K et al.	Gastric ulcer (n=16) Duodenal ulcer (n=9)	6 mo
Satoh K, et al.	Atrophic gastritis (n=20)	12-33 mo
Tucci A, et al.	Fundic atrophic gastritis (n=20)	3 yr
Tepes B, et al.	Duodenal ulcer (n=63)	4 yr
El-Omar EM, et al.	Cancer patients' relatives (n=40)	1 yr
Kim N, et al.	Gastric ulcer (n=41) Duodenal ulcer (n=72)	2 yr
Kuipers EJ, et al.	Reflux esophagitis (n=231)	2 yr
Tanaka A, et al.	Atrophic gastritis (n=39) Early gastric cancer (n=25)	1 yr

Table 1. Summary of studies on changes of GIM scores after successful *H. pylori* eradication

Some reported that the histologic grade of GIM had improved after eradication (Genta et al., 1993; Uemura et al., 1997; Nardone et al., 1999; Sung et al., 2000; Ohkusa et al., 2001; Kokkola et al., 2002; Correa et al., 2000; Ley et al., 2004; Mera et al., 2005; You et al., 2006) but the others did not find any change (Witteman et al., 1995; Forbes et al., 1996; van der Hulst et al., 1997; Hibi et al., 1997; Satoh et al., 1998; Tucci A et al., 1998; Tepes et al., 1999; El-Omar et al., 2000 ; Kim et al., 2000 ; Kuipers et al., 2004 ; Tanaka et al., 2006). Some of the reasons for these discrepancies may be ethnic variations, completeness of eradication of the disease and the stage of the disease when treatment is initiated and short follow-up (most studies up to 1 year) (Kokkola et al., 2002; Forbes et al., 1996; Tucci A et al., 1998; Tepes et al., 1999; Kim et al., 2000; Tanaka et al., 2006). Uemura et al (Uemura et al, 1997) studied the changes of GIM after treatment of *H. pylori* in the patients with intramucosal gastric cancer who underwent endoscopic mucosal resection (EMR). In this study, they showed that GIM score regressed at 6 months after *H. pylori* eradication. To our knowledge, however, there are no studies about the long-term effects after *H. pylori* eradication on the difference of histologic changes of GIM between the patients with and without gastric neoplasms.

We developed a monoclonal antibody (mAb), Das-1 (formerly known as $7E_{12}H_{12}$, IgM isotype), that specifically reacts with colonic epithelium (Das et al. 1987). Using both immunoperoxidase and immunofluorescence assays, we and others have demonstrated that the antibody specifically reacts with colonic epithelium (both goblet and non-goblet absorptive cells), but not with enterocytes (including goblet cells) from jejunum or ileum and normal epithelium from the stomach and esophagus (Das et al. 1987; Halstensen et al., 1993). However, mAb Das-1 reacts sensitively (95%) and specifically (100%) to Barrett's epithelium (BE), a pre-neoplastic condition of the esophagus, and adenocarcinoma of the esophagus (Das et al. 1994; Griffel et al., 2000). These data support that BE is a "colonic" or "incomplete" type of intestinal metaplasia (Das et al. 1994). Although normal small intestinal epithelium does not react with mAb Das-1, small intestinal adenoma and adenocarcinoma strongly react with the antibody, suggesting a phenotypic change in the pre-cancerous state and in carcinoma (Onuma et al., 2001). We also reported that GIM of colonic phenotype, such as type II or type III (incomplete type) detected by the mucin histochemistry (Filipe & Jass, 1986) and detected by mAb Das-1, is strongly associated with gastric cancer (Mirza et al., 2002). Ninety-three percent of GIM as well as gastric cancer from the same patients at a different area reacted with mAb Das-1, whereas GIM from patients without gastric cancer reacted less frequently (35%) with the antibody ($p<0.0001$) (Mirza et al., 2002).

More recently, during screening a complimentary DNA library prepared from a human colon cancer cell line, T84, we isolated and cloned a novel human tropomyosin (hTM) isoform, termed TC22 (Lin et al. 2002). The amino acid sequence analysis of TC22 demonstrated that it is identical to normal colon epithelial tropomyosin isoform 5 (hTM5) except the C-terminal peptide aminoacids 222-247 coding exon 9. Using this C terminal peptide, we developed a mAb, termed TC22-4, which is specific to TC22 (Lin et al. 2002). The expression of TC22, identified by the TC22-4 mAb, progressively increased in benign adenomatous polyp of colon (35%) and polyps with mild (57%) and severe dysplasia (100%) and in colon cancer (100%) (Lin et al., 2002). hTMs are microfilament-associated proteins present in all eukaryotic cells with organ-specific isoforms and distinct functions (Lees-Miller & Helfman, 1991; Pittenger & Helfman, 1992; Lin et al, 1997), and at least 8 isoforms of hTM are detected in human (Lin et al, 1997; Novy et al. 1993). hTM isoform 5 (hTM5) is the predominant isoform in normal colon epithelium and it acts as an autoantigen in ulcerative colitis (UC) (Das et al., 1993; Geng et al. 1998). We and others have shown that patients with UC demonstrate both humoral and cellular immune responses against hTM, particularly against isoform 5 (hTM5) (Das et al., 1993; Geng et al. 1998; Onuma et al., 2000; Biancone et al., 1995 ; Sakamaki et al., 2000 ; Taniguchi et al., 2001).

A K-*ras* mutation occurs relatively early in human carcinogenesis (Vogelstein et al., 1988), and it is detected in various types of human malignancies (Soh et al., 1993; Cooper 1995). Mutations of K-*ras* gene are found in ~10% of intestinal-type gastric cancer but they are rarely detected in the diffuse type (Tahara, 1993; Arber et al., 2000; Hiyama et al., 2002). Furthermore, a K-*ras* mutation has been detected in preneoplastic lesions, such as mucous cell hyperplasia of the pancreas, which current term is pancreatic intraepithelial neoplasia, grade 1, suffering from chronic inflammation and regenerative or dysplastic epithelia of ulcerative colitis (Yanagisawa et al., 1993; Chaubert et al. 1994). However, there have been only a few reports of this oncogene in *H. pylori*-associated chronic gastritis and GIM either with or without gastric cancer (Hiyama et al., 2002; Gong et al., 1999). Moreover, changes in K-*ras* mutations in GIM after *H. pylori* eradication have not yet been investigated.

In addition to genetic alterations, one of the pathways by which *H. pylori* is linked to gastric carcinogenesis may be related to the disruption in the balance between gastric epithelial cell proliferation and apoptosis as some investigators have reported (Moss et al., 1996; Wagner et al. 1997; Jones et al., 1997; Hoshi et al., 1999; Leung et al. 2001). However, such previous studies on the cell kinetics before and after *H. pylori* eradication have yielded conflicting results.

Epidemiological studies indicate that Asian countries have a high prevalence of *H. pylori* infection, with a correspondingly high incidence of gastric cancer. The annual incidence rate of gastric cancer per 100,000 population in various Asian countries, as reported by Parkin et al (Parkin et al., 1997), is very high in the northern parts of Asia, especially in Japan. In this paragraph, we illustrated around our previous studies (Watari et al., 2007; Watari et al., 2008) in the Japanese population, (i) if the eradication of *H. pylori* affects subsequent (over the course of up to 4 years) histological grade of GIM, (ii) if mAb Das-1 reactivity that identifies colonic phenotype of GIM associated with gastric carcinogenesis changes after eradication of *H. pylori*, and (iii) to assess the expression of the novel tropomyosin isoform TC22 in GIM before and after *H. pylori* treatment. p53 expression was also examined, in parallel. Additionally, we investigated (iv) if *H. pylori* eradication affects K-*ras* mutations and cell kinetics including cell proliferation and apoptosis in GIM.

2. Patients and methods

2.1 Study 1

Gastric biopsy samples (during 288 endoscopic procedures) from 96 *H. pylori*-positive Japanese patients were obtained prior to introduction of therapy, and, subsequently, over a follow-up period of up to 4 years. In all patients, biopsy specimens were taken to assess *H. pylori* infection, two from the greater curvature of the antrum and two from the greater curvature of the corpus of the stomach. *H. pylori* status was analyzed in each patient by two methods: Wartin-Starry staining and *H. pylori* culture. A patient was regarded as positive for *H. pylori* if at least one is positive, and the patient received anti-*H. pylori* therapy. All of the patients underwent upper endoscopy again after 2 to 3 months post-therapy to ensure successful eradication of *H. pylori*, and then were followed-up with yearly endoscopy, up to 4 years (mean 2.6 yrs, range; 1 to 4). At each endoscopy, successful eradication was documented by the above methods. None of the patients showed positive for *H. pylori* during the follow-up period.

2.1.1 Histology and patient classification

GIM was defined as replacement of the gastric epithelium by intestinal type epithelium, and was composed of two types; the presence of absorptive enterocytes with brush border along with goblet cells, or columnar cells with foamy cytoplasm, lacking brush border (Filipe et al., 1994).

In this study, the patients with chronic gastritis with gastric ulcers or gastroduodenal ulcers were included. Almost half of the patients (53.9%) had gastric ulcers and the remainder had both gastric as well as duodenal ulcers (Take et al. 2005). The patients with duodenal ulcer only were excluded because most duodenal ulcers were categorized as antral predominat gastritis (Uemura et al., 2001) or non-atrophic gastritis (Mera et al. 2005), which has a low risk for gastric cancer and difference from gastric and gastroduodenal ulcers in pathophysiology (Uemura et al., 2001; Take et al. 2005).

The 96 *H. pylori*-positive patients were divided into 3 groups on the basis of history and initial histology by a single experienced pathologist (P.S.A.). Group CG (n=36) had histologically chronic gastritis, but no GIM. This group was considered to correspond to non-metaplastic multifocal atrophic gastritis according to the global diagnosis by Mera et al (Mera et al. 2005). Thirty of the 36 patients had peptic ulcers, comprising 34 gastric ulcers and 2 gastroduodenal ulcers, and 6 patients had chronic gastritis without ulcer. Group IM consisted of patients with chronic gastritis with GIM (n=33). Twenty-six patients had gastric ulcers and 7 patients had gastroduedenal ulcers. Group DYS consisted of patients with dysplasia (n=27). This comprised low-grade dysplasia (n=13), high grade-dysplasia (n=13), and cancer with microinvasion to the submucosa (n=1). All patients in Group DYS underwent EMR for dysplasia, and then received treatment for *H. pylori*.

Serial sections (4 μm) were made and consecutive sections were used for histologic examination by H&E staining, mucin stainings by alcian blue and high iron diamine, pH2.5 (AB/HID), and for immunohistochemistry, as described below. All slides were sent from Japan to NJ, USA, and evaluated and scored for GIM according to the updated Sydney system (Dixon et al., 1996; Rugge et al., 2000) by a single pathologist (P.S.A.) in NJ, who was unaware of the patient groups and treatment status. Scores were given numerically as follows: 0 for absence, and 1, 2, 3 for mild, moderate, or severe GIM. The GIM score was assessed in the samples obtained from the antrum, including patients with dysplasia at a different site of the stomach (Group DYS).

2.1.2 Alcian blue (pH2.5)/High iron diamine (AB/HID) staining

Serial sections were stained with AB/HID to identify neutral mucins, sialomucins, and sulphomucins using the standard method (Filipe et al., 1994). Briefly, slides were immersed in HID solution for 24 hours at room temperature. Slides were rinsed with distilled water, and then stained with 1% Alcian blue (pH 2.5) for 30 minutes. Three phenotypes of GIM were classified as described by Filipe and Jass (Filipe & Jass, 1986) namely type I (complete or small intestinal type), types II & III (incomplete or colonic type). When more than one type of GIM coexisted in a given sample, the case was classified according to the dominant type present in the section.

2.1.3 Immnoperoxidase assays with mAb Das-1, TC22-4, and anti-p53

Serial sections were stained with mAb Das-1 (mouse IgM mAb highly specific against Barrett's epithelium), TC22-4 (mouse IgG1 mAb against a novel tropomyosin isoform, TC22, specific for colon cancer) and anti-p53 monoclonal antibody, DO7 (mouse IgG 2b, Dako, Carpenteria, CA) using sensitive immnoperoxidase assays as described previously (Das et al., 1994; Mirza et al., 2003; Lin et al., 2002). Briefly, after deparaffinization and rehydration, free aldehydes were reduced with 0.05% sodium borohydride for 20 min at 4°C. The tissue sections were treated with the antigen-retrieval technique for TC22 and p53 staining. They were then sequentially incubated with mAb Das-1, mAb TC22-4 and DO7 for 45 min at room temperature (for DO7), overnight at 4°C (for mAb Das-1), and 5 hr at 4°C (for mAb TC22-4), followed by biotinylated rabbit antimouse IgM or IgG (Dako), 3% hydrogen peroxide, and streptoavidin peroxidase (Dako). Subsequently, the slides were treated with diaminobenzidine-H_2O_2 solution for 20 min at room temperature. Each experiment included positive controls for mAb Das-1, normal colon section, and colon cancer tissue sections as positive controls for mAb TC22-4 and anti-p53 immunostainings. As negative controls, jejunum (for mAb Das-1) and normal colon (for TC22-4 and p53) were used.

2.2 Study 2

We enrolled 64 patients with successful *H. pylori* treatment who had atrophic gastritis (n=39) and intestinal-type mucosal gastric cancer after EMR (n=25). Following successful eradication, all patients were followed up by endoscopy for 1 year. All these patients histologically showed GIM in gastric biopsy samples both before and after *H. pylori* eradication. In order to improve the accuracy regarding the genetic alterations, the number of samples was increased. Twenty-eight intestinal-type early gastric cancer cases that had undergone a surgical resection were randomly selected from the histopathology files of Asahikawa Medical University Hospital during the same period and thus were added to this study.

Finally, the patients in this study included, Group IM (n=39): chronic gastritis cases with GIM, and Group DYS (n=53): intestinal-type early gastric cancer, further divided into Group DYS-1 (n=25): EMR cases diagnosed as mucosal cancer and Group DYS-2 (n=28): surgical resection cases, consisting of 10 mucosal cancers and 18 submucosal invasive cancers. All patients in Group DYS-1 underwent EMR for their mucosal cancer lesions, and thereafter received treatment for *H. pylori*.

2.2.1 DNA preparation and detection of K-*ras* mutations

Four tissue sections, each measuring 10 µm in thickness, were serially cut from paraffin embedded tissue blocks. DNA was extracted from only GIM (Fig. 1). In this procedure of DNA extraction, the tissue specimens were precisely microdissected under microscopic visualization, using a PixCell laser capture microdissection system (Arcturus Engineering, Mountain View, CA) to avoid any DNA contamination of inflammatory or stromal cell nuclei. DNA was then extracted from the microdissected tissue specimen by proteinase K treatment, followed by phenol-chloroform extraction.

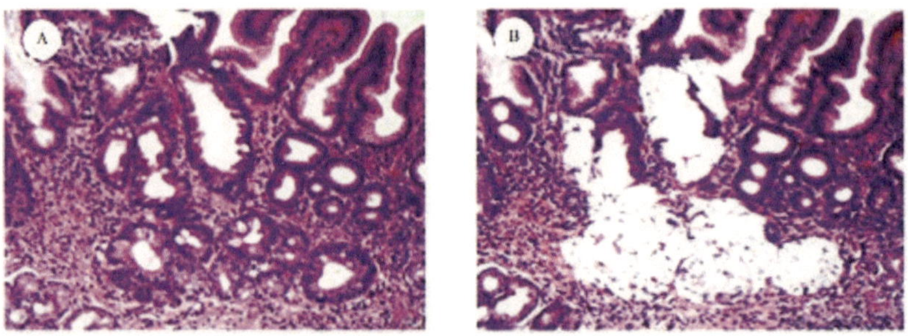

Fig. 1. Metaplastic glands were isolated by a laser capture microdissection. (A) H&E stained section, (B) The same section, after the removal of metaplastic glands.

The detection of point mutations in codon 12 of the K-*ras* gene was performed by enriched polymerase chain reaction-restriction fragment length polymorphism (PCR-RFLP) as previously described with minor modifications (Levi et al., 1991; Sanger et al., 1997). The DNA from the K-*ras* sequence of exon 1 was amplified by a first PCR using the mismatched primers as previously described (Levi et al., 1991). After restriction enzyme digestion using *MvaI* (Toyobo Company, Tokyo, Japan), PCR was performed in a 20µl reaction mixture using Ampli-Taq Gold DNA polymerase (Perkin Elmer Applied Biosystems Division, Foster City, CA) according to the manufacturer's manual. In a second PCR and after another round of *MvaI* digestion, wild type fragments were cleaved to yield 29 and 106 base pair (bp) products, whereas mutant fragments yielded 135 bp. Electrophoresis of the digested sample on 3% agarose gel confirmed the mutation band. SW480, a colon cancer cell line, and HT29 were used as a positive and negative control for K-*ras* codon 12, respectively (Fig. 2).

2.2.2 Sequencing analysis

The mutant fragments identified by enriched PCR-RFLP were confirmed by direct sequencing. The sequence of codon 12 was determined by automated fluorescent DNA sequencing using the dideoxy chain termination method (Sanger et al., 1997). PCR products were used for the cycle sequencing. The products were purified using Centricon-100 (Amicon Inc, Beverly, MA) following the manufacturer's protocol and then were sequenced using the Dye Terminator Cycle Sequencing Ready Reaction (Perkin Elmer Applied Biosystems Division, Foster City, CA) according to the manufacturer's instructions as reported previously (Watari et al., 2002). The sequencing reaction products were analyzed on ABI PRISM Geluxe™ (Perkin Elmer) on an ABI PRISM 310 DNA sequencer (Perkin Elmer).

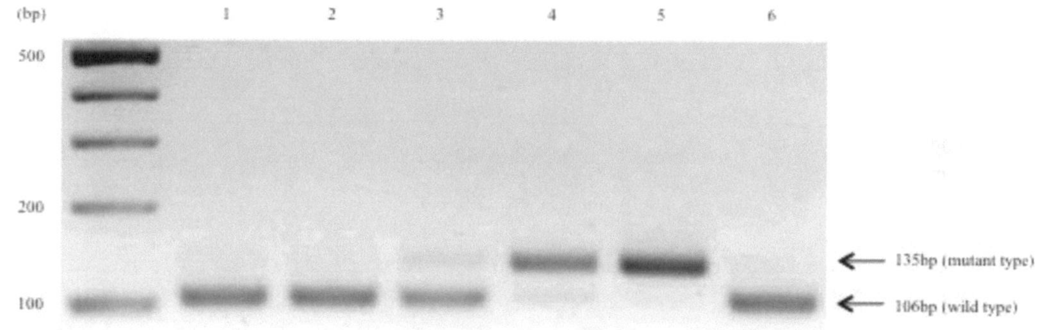

Fig. 2. A K-*ras* mutation in codon 12 was detected by enriched PCR-restriction fragment length polymorphism in gastric intestinal metaplasia (GIM) from patients with and without gastric cancer. The arrows indicate the positions of the mutant (135bp) and wild-type (106bp) bands. Lane 1: GIM from patient with gastric cancer; lanes 2-4: GIM from patients without gastric cancer; lane 5: SW480 as positive control; lane 6: HT29 as negative control.

2.2.3 Detection of proliferation and apoptosis

Dewaxed paraffin sections were examined by the avidin-biotin peroxidase complex (ABC, Vector Laboratories, Burlingame, CA) method using the primary antibody for Ki-67 antigen of proliferating cells (mouse IgG, Invitrogen, Calsbad, CA, USA). The slides were treated with the antigen-retrieval technique based on microwave oven heating.

Apoptotic cells *in situ* were detected by the terminal deoxynucleotidyl transferase-mediated dUTP nick-end labeling (TUNEL) method as previously described (Gavrieli et al., 1992). The slides were dewaxed and rehydrated through a graded alcohol series. The tissue specimens were digested with 20 µg/ml proteinase K (Boehringer, Mannheim, Germany) for 30 min at 37°C. After treating with a 2% H_2O_2 solution, the sections were preincubated with 100 mM potassium cacodylate, 2 mM cobalt chloride, 0.2 mM dithiothreitol, pH 7.2 for 3 min, and then were incubated with the same buffer containing 0.3U/µl terminal deoxynucleotidyl transferase (TdT, GIBCO BRL Gaithersburg, MD) and 0.04 nmol/µl biotinylated dUTP (Boehringer, Mannheim, Germany) in a humid chamber at 37°C for 1 hr. The slides were rinsed in 30mM sodium citrate, 300 mM sodium chloride for 30 minutes at RT, and washed in phosphate-buffered saline (PBS). After blocking with 10% rabbit serum for 10 min and rinsing briefly in PBS, sections were incubated with ABC for 30 min at RT. Labeled cells were visualized with diaminobenzidine. The sections were then counterstained with hematoxylin. In GIM in each case, a minimum of 300 cells from some fields randomly selected were counted and the fractions (%) of cells that showed positive nuclear staining for Ki-67 antigen (Fig. 3A) and TUNEL (Fig. 3B) were considered to be the proliferative indices (PI) and the apoptotic indices (AI), respectively. The PI and AI were determined independently by a single physician (J.W.).

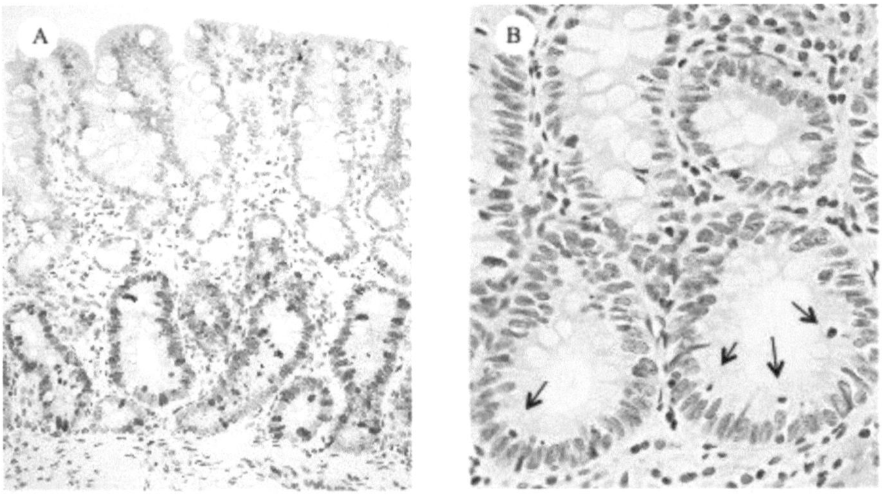

Fig. 3. Ki-67 staining and TUNEL in a representative case of gastric intestinal metaplasia (GIM). (A) Proliferating cells were found predominantly in the lower portion of GIM. (B) Apoptotic cells (arrows), detected by the TUNEL method were seen.

2.3 Consent and ethical approval

Regarding the above studied, written informed consent was obtained from the patients, and the Ethics Committee of Asahikawa Medical University gave their approval for this study.

2.4 Statistical analysis

All data are presented as means ± SEM. Statistical analyses were assessed by the Student *t* test, by Mann-Whitney *U* test, by the Kruskal-Wallis test, by chi-square test and by Fisher's exact test. The Wilcoxon signed-rank test was used in the comparison of parameters before and after treatment in the same patient. Statistical significance was defined as $p<0.05$.

3. Results

3.1 Study 1

3.1.1 Histologic score at initial diagnosis

Patients in Group CG had evidence of chronic gastritis, but did not have GIM. At the initial diagnosis, GIM scores in Group DYS were significantly higher than those in Group IM ($p<0.05$) and Group CG ($p<0.0001$) (Fig. 4).

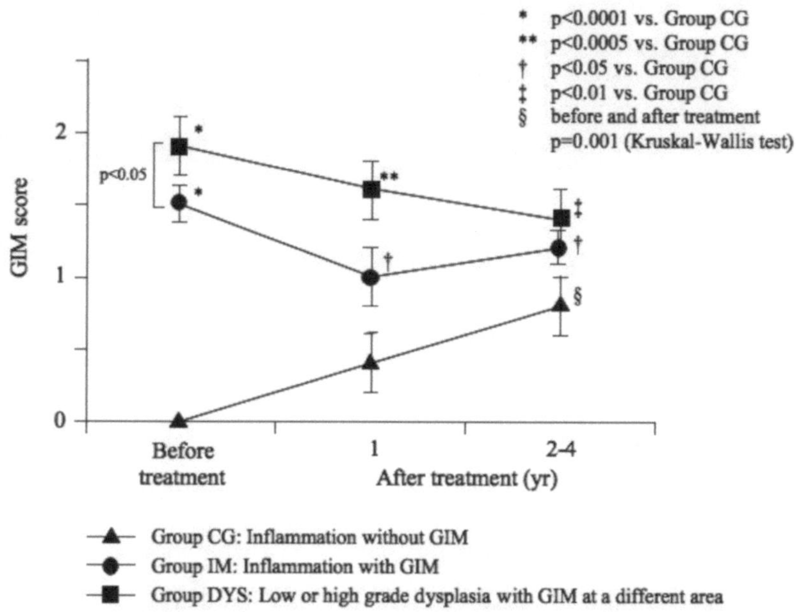

Fig. 4. Initial histologic GIM scores and changes in the score in patients followed up over 4 years after *H. pylori* eradication. GIM scores were significantly higher in Group DYS than in Group IM before eradication ($p<0.05$). At initial stage, none of the patients in Group CG had GIM, although all had gastritis. GIM scores in Groups IM and DYS were higher than those in Group CG at 1 year after treatment ($p<0.05$ and $p<0.0005$, respectively), as well as at 2 to 4 years. After eradication of *H. pylori* in both Groups IM and DYS there were slow minor declines of GIM scores that were not statistically significant. However, GIM score in patients from Group CG increased even if *H. pylori* was eliminated, and this difference was statistically significant ($p=0.001$, Kruskal-Wallis test). The GIM score in Group CG was significantly lower than in Groups IM and DYS at the 1-year follow-up evaluation, as well as at the end of 4 years.

3.1.2 Reactivity against mAb Das-1, TC22-4 and anti-p53 before treatment

In Group CG, with chronic gastritis without GIM, there was no immunoreactivity with any of the gastric mucosal samples against mAb Das-1, TC22-4 and anti-p53 (Fig. 5). In Group IM patients, the immunoreactivity against mAb Das-1 was 39% (13 of 33) and against TC22-4 it was 36% (12 of 33). The reactivity against anti-p53 was 3% (1 of 33). The reactivity of mAb Das-1 is diffuse cytoplasmic with higher intensity at the periphery of cells and is present in both goblet cells and non-goblet cells in the GIM areas (Fig. 6E). The TC22 reactivity is seen as intracellular cytoplasmic dot-like staining in a punctate manner (Fig. 6F), and p53 staining is detected in scattered cells mainly in the nuclei of the glands (Fig. 6N). In patients from Group DYS, the reactivity of mAb Das-1, TC22-4 and anti-53 in GIM areas away from dysplastic areas was 63% (17 of 27), 48% (13 of 27) and 15% (4 of 27), respectively. Twenty-four of 27 (89%) of patients showed positive reactivity with mAb Das-1 at the dysplastic areas (Fig. 5). If the dysplastic area is positive with mAb Das-1, GIM areas away from the dysplastic areas of the same patients were also positive. Of the 13 patients who were positive with TC22-4 in the GIM areas, 11 of these 13 (85%) patients' dysplastic areas also showed reactivity to TC22-4. The mAb Das-1 reactivity showed progressive increase between Group IM and Group DYS (Fig. 5). TC22 expression, although numerically higher in Group DYS than in Group IM (48% vs. 36%), was not statistically significant. However, in the same patients following eradication, as described below, there was a significant decline of immunoreactivity. p53 expression in the GIM areas in the 2 groups (IM and DYS) were 3% vs. 15% respectively. Anti-p53 reactivity was much higher in the dysplastic areas in Group DYS (59%, 16 of 27) (Fig. 5).

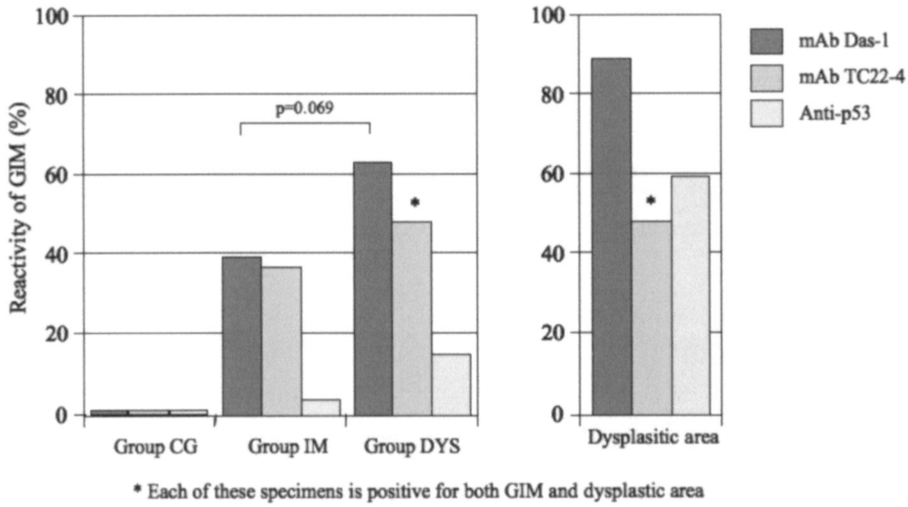

Fig. 5. Reactivity of GIM to mAb Das-1, TC22-4 and anti-p53 in patients from Groups CG, IM, and DYS before treatment. In Group CG, no reactivity to mAb Das-1, TC22-4 and anti-p53 was found in the normal mucosa or in gastritis area without GIM. The immunoreactivity of mAb Das-1 to GIM from Group C was higher (63%) than Group IM (39%) (p=0.069). In the GIM areas from Group DYS, mAb TC22-4 reactivity (48%) was higher than that from Group IM (36%). However, in the dysplastic areas of Group DYS, the mAb Das-1 reactivity was the highest (89%). Each of the dysplastic areas and GIM mucosa away from this mucosal cancer area from the same patients reacted with mAb Das-1. Anti-p53 reactivity was absent in normal and inflamed mucosa as well as in GIM areas from Groups CG and IM (3%), except in Group DYS where 4 of 27 (15%) showed reactivity at the GIM areas. However, 59% of dysplastic areas reacted with anti-p53.

3.1.3 Changes of the GIM score after eradication of *H. pylori* during prospective follow-ups

GIM scores before and after treatment of *H. pylori* in each group are shown in Fig. 4. Although initially none of the patients in Group CG had GIM, during the follow-up period, 8 patients at 1 year and 6 additional patients developed GIM during subsequent 4 years (p=0.001, Kruskal-Wallis test). Furthermore, GIM scores were higher in Group IM and DYS than in Group CG at 1 year after treatment ($p<0.05$ and $p<0.0005$, respectively). At 2-4 years after treatment, GIM scores continued to increase in Group CG and there was a significant difference in GIM score between Group CG and Group IM ($p<0.05$) as well as Group DYS ($p<0.01$) at 4 years. This difference suggests chronicity of the metaplastic process over a long time. Although in Group DYS there was some decline of GIM score over 4 years, it was not significant. The histologic scores in Group IM remained essentially unchanged (Fig. 4).

3.1.4 Changes in the GIM phenotypes on the basis of mucin histochemistry before and after treatment for *H. pylori*

Patients from Group CG did not have GIM before treatment, however, 14 patients (39%) developed GIM during the 4 years of follow-up and GIM in these patients consisted of type I (complete type) in 8 (57%) and type II or III (incomplete type) in 6 (43%) patients (Table 2). In Group IM, type I and type II/III were found in 22 (67%) and in 11 (33%) patients respectively before treatment for eradication of *H. pylori*. On the contrary, in Group DYS, the majority (59%) (16 out of 27) of GIM belonged to type II/III (incomplete type) compared to type I (41%, 11 of 27), prior to treatment. The incidence of incomplete type of GIM was significantly ($p<0.05$) higher in Group DYS than in Group IM. In Group IM, of the 22 patients initially classified as type I GIM, 7 (32%) had "progressed" to type II/III, while in two no GIM was found after treatment and three of the 11 patients initially classified with type II/III had "regressed" to type I GIM. Similarly, in Group DYS, 5 of the 11 patients (46%) with type I GIM changed to type II/III, and in one, no GIM was found following treatment. Three of 16 patients (19%) initially classified as type II/III GIM regressed to type I and one had no GIM after eradication (Table 2).

3.1.5 Reactivity to mAb Das-1, TC22-4 and anti-p53 in GIM during the follow-up period

mAb Das-1 did not react with any of the 36 samples in Group CG who had chronic gastritis without GIM prior to treatment (Fig. 5). Of the 39% of patients in Group CG who developed GIM during the 4 year follow-up period subsequent to the eradication of *H. pylori*, 43% (6 of 14) showed reactivity to mAb Das-1, similar to the incomplete (type II/III) determined by immunohistochemistry. Fig. 6A and 6B are an example from a patient in Group CG showing chronic gastritis in pretreatment biopsy (Fig. 6A) and subsequent development of GIM (Fig. 6B) despite eradication following triple therapy. However, no mAb Das-1 reactivity to GIM was found in this patient (Fig. 6C). The H&E staining, and mAb Das-1 reactivities of serial sections of the biopsy specimen from a patient in Group IM are shown in Fig. 6D and E, respectively. Fig. 6G and H show serial sections from the biopsy specimen from a patient in Group DYS (GIM area) stained by H&E and mAb Das-1 respectively. The mAb Das-1 reactivity is restricted to the glandular epithelium in the GIM areas (Fig. 6E and 6H). Both the non-goblet metaplastic cells and goblet cells reacted with mAb Das-1, and normal gastric mucosa did not react. Fig. 6J and 6K show serial sections from a patient in Group DYS with cancer stained by H&E and mAb Das-1 respectively. Cancer cells invading microscopically into the sub-mucosa can be seen. The reactivity with mAb Das-1 against the dysplastic glands is more diffuse and intense (Fig. 6K).

There were 30 patients (13 in Group IM and 17 in Group DYS) that reacted to mAb Das-1 before treatment. When the immunoreactivity in the biopsy tissue from the same patients were compared before and after treatment, in 40% of the patients the reactivity disappeared ($p<0.0001$) after eradication of *H. pylori* (Table 3, Fig. 6I), despite the presence of GIM. The disappearance of the reactivity was seen in both Group IM and Group DYS.

The reactivity of mAb TC22-4 is restricted to GIM areas both in goblet and non-goblet cells. The reactivity is dense globular dot like staining mainly along the apical areas (Fig. 6F). In Group DYS, the GIM areas and cancer areas also showed similar staining with TC22-4, as in

		Pretreatment		Posteradiucation	
		Types	Number	Types	Number
Group CG	(n=36)	No GIM		I	8
				II/III	6
Total					14
Group IM	(n=33)	I	22	I	13
				II/III	7
Total					20 [a]
		II/III [c]	11	I	3
				II/III	8
Total					11
Group DYS	(n=27)	I	11	I	5
				II/III	5
Total					10 [b]
		II/III	16	I	3
				II/III	12
Total					15 [b]

[a] GIM disappeared in 2 patients after eradication.
[b] GIM disappeared in 2 patients after eradication.
[c] *P*<0.05 in the incidence of type II/III GIM between Group IM and Group DYS in pretreatment.

Table 2. Types of GIM on the basis of mucin histochemistry

	Pretreatment	Posteradiucation		
	Positive	Positive	Negative	*P*
Groups IM + DYS	30 (100%)	17 (57%)	12 (40%)	<0.0001
Group IM	13 (100%)	7 (54%)	5 (38%)	<0.01
Group DYS	17 (100%)	10 (59%)	7 (41%)	<0.007

Table 3. Changes in the immunoreactivity of mAb Das-1-positive GIM after *H. pylori* eradication in the same patients

Figure 6F. Twelve of 33 patients (36%) in Group IM were positive prior to treatment, and following treatment the reactivity declined to 6 of 29 (21%) (Fig. 6M). There was no difference in TC22 reactivity before and after treatment. Seven patients in Group IM and 10 patients in Group DYS were positive for both mAb Das-1 and TC22-4 reactivity. Following eradication of *H. pylori*, the immunoreactivity for both the markers disappeared in 5 of the 7 patients in Group IM (p<0.05). However, in only 3 of 10 patients in Group DYS was the reactivity absent. This was not significant (Table 4).

	Pretreatment	Posteradiucation		
	Positive	Positive	Negative	*P*
Groups IM + DYS	17 (100%)	9 (53%)	8 (40%)	<0.005
Group IM	7 (100%)	2 (29%)	5 (38%)	<0.05
Group DYS	10 (100%)	7 (70%)	3 (41%)	NS

Table 4. Changes in the immunoreactivity of TC22-4-positive GIM after *H. pylori* eradication in the same patients

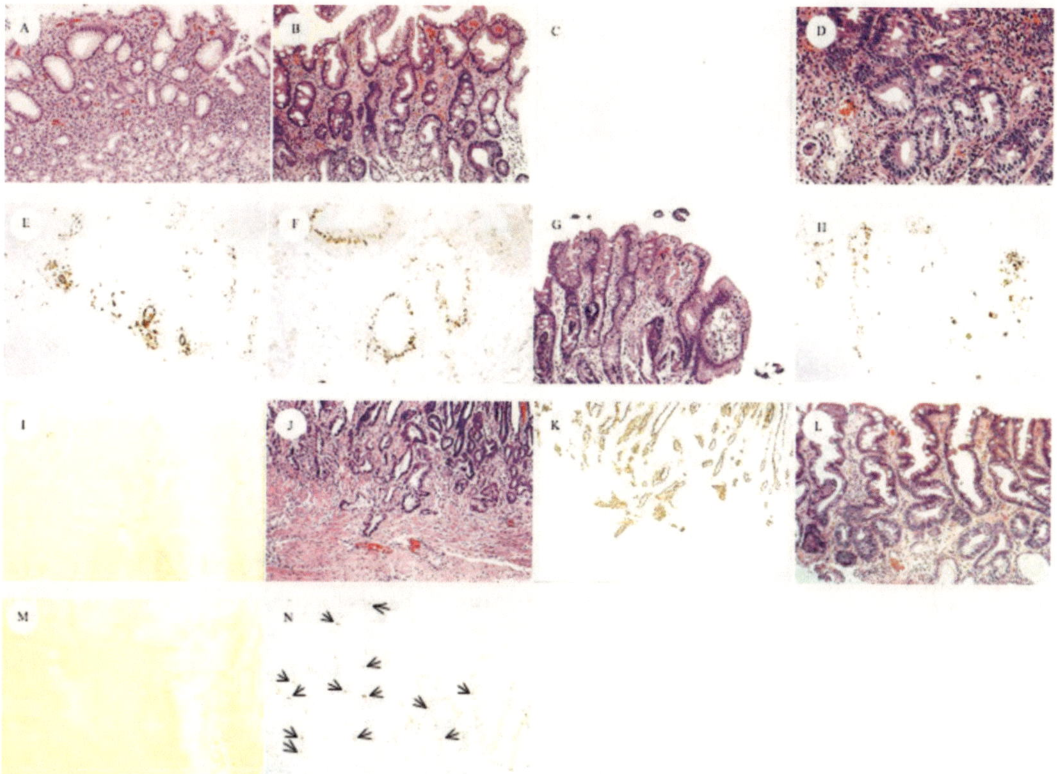

Fig. 6. Representative sections of H&E and immunoperoxidase staining with mAb Das-1, TC22-4, and anti-p53. (A and B) Example of a patient from group CG whose gastric mucosa only had mild gastritis, (A) without any GIM before treatment (magnification, 200X), but (B) GIM clearly developed after eradication (magnification, 200X). (C) However, GIM did not react with mAb Das-1 after treatment (magnification, 200X). In a patient from group IM, serial sections from the initial biopsy specimen before eradication show (D) GIM (H&E magnification, 200X) that reacted with both (E) mAb Das-1 (magnification, 200X) and (F) TC22-4 (magnification, 400X). Serial sections of the biopsy tissue from a patient from group DYS before treatment show (G) GIM (H&E magnification, 200X) and (H) reactivity to mAb Das-1 (magnification, 200X). A serial section of the same tissue also reacted with TC22-4 (figure not shown). (I) The reactivity to mAb Das-1 (magnification, 200X) disappeared in two fifths of the patients from both groups IM and DYS (Table 3) after *H. pylori* treatment (p<0.0001). (J and K) Representative pictures of the serial tissue sections from a patient in the severe dysplasia group (group DYS) stained with (J) H&E and (K) mAb Das-1. (J) Cancerous glands, with microinvasion into the submucosa, seen in H&E staining (magnification, 100X), and all of these tissue strongly reacted with (K) mAb Das-1 (magnification, 100X). (L) GIM in a patient from group IM after eradication of *H. pylori*. (M) TC22 reactivity disappeared in this patient (H&E magnification, 200X). (N) GIM from a patient from group DYS stained with anti-p53. p53 protein staining is shown in scattered cells (arrows), mainly in the nuclei of the glands.

The p53-positive nuclear staining was mainly detected in the dispersed cells mostly at the GIM glands located at the deeper plane (Fig. 6N, arrows). In Group IM, p53 expression was observed in only one of 33 patients before treatment, and its expression was noted in one additional patient during the follow-up period after treatment. In Group DYS, in the GIM areas, 4 of 27 (15%) had p53 expression at initial examination. During the follow-up period, additional patients, 7 of 25 (28%), exhibited p53 expression. However, in the dysplastic areas in Group DYS, p53 expression was high (16 of 27, 59%). The p53 expression did not change in these patients during the follow-up period. All of the patients in Group DYS who were anti-p53 positive, also had mAb Das-1 reactivity and TC22 expression (both GIM and dysplastic areas).

3.2 Study 2

3.2.1 K-*ras* codon 12 mutations in GIM

The mutant K-*ras* in codon 12 was detected in 18 (46.2%) of 39 GIM in Group IM and 1 (1.9%) of 53 GIM areas away from cancer in Group DYS before eradication, and 2 (3.8%) of 53 cancers, respectively. One case who had a K-*ras* mutation in Group DYS belonged to Group DYS-1. One of the 2 cancers which were positive for K-*ras* mutations was also positive in parallel with the GIM areas. Group IM showed a significantly more frequent incidence of K-*ras* codon 12 point mutations than Group DYS ($p<0.005$). Moreover, the incidence (46.2%) of the K-*ras* gene alterations significantly decreased to 12.8% (5 of 39) after treatment in Group IM but not in Group DYS. Of the lesions with K-*ras* mutations in Group IM before treatment, GGT (Gly) showed AGT (Ser) transition in 9 (50.0%), GAT (Asp) transition in 6 (33.3%) and TGT (Cys) transversion in 3 (16.7%). Following treatment, four (75.0%) showed a transition to AGT (Ser) and 1 (25.0%) showed a transition to GAT (Asp). Hence, mutation patterns showed convergence to Ser transformation by *H. pylori* treatment. The mutation pattern in the patient from Group DYS-1 was AGT (Ser). After eradication, the patterns of AGT (Ser) disappeared and one subject who had previously been negative for K-*ras* mutation showed a positive finding for the K-*ras* mutation of GAT (Asp). The cancer showed two patterns: GCT (Ala) in 1 and GTT (Val) in 1 (Table 5).

	Helicobacter pylori eradication			
	Before	n	After	n
Group IM	AGT (Ser)	9	AGT (Ser)	4
	GAT (Asp)	6	GAT (Asp)	1
	TGT (Cys)	3		
Group DYS-1	AGT (Ser)	1	GAT (Asp)	1
Cancer areas	GCT (Ala)	1		
	GTT (Val)	1		

Table 5. Patterns of K-*ras* mutation in gastric intestinal metaplasia

3.2.2 Cell kinetics of GIM

PI and AI in IM before *H. pylori* eradication were 36.71% and 0.27% in Group IM, 45.69% and 0.52% in Group DYS, respectively. PI in Group DYS was significantly higher than that in Group IM ($p<0.05$). AI also showed a similar tendency, but the difference did not reach statistical significance. Regarding the cell kinetics after treatment in each group, PI and AI were 40.43% and 0.47% in Group IM, 42.32% and 0.83% in Group DYS, respectively. Although there were no significant changes in the PI before and after *H. pylori* eradication, the level of AI increased after *H. pylori* eradication in both groups ($p<0.05$ in Group IM) (Table 6).

	PI		AI		AI/PI ratio	
	H. pylori eradication		*H. pylori* eradication		*H. pylori* eradication	
	Before	After	Before	After	Before	After
Group IM	36.71 ± 2.71*	40.43 ± 2.71	0.27 ± 0.07	0.47 ± 0.10	0.020 ± 0.012	0.013 ± 0.004
Group DYS	45.69 ± 2.65*	42.32 ± 3.20	0.52 ± 0.16	0.83 ± 0.30	0.010 ± 0.003	0.021 ± 0.001

* $p<0.05$, Numbers are mean ± standard error. PI, proliferative indices; AI, apoptotic indices; *H. pylori*, *Helicobacter pylori*

Table 6. Comparison of cell kinetics before and after *Helicobacter pylori* eradication

	Neutrophils		Mononucler cells		Intestinal metaplasia	
	H pylori eradication		*H pylori* eradication		*H pylori* eradication	
	Before	After	Before	After	Before	After
Group IM	0.65 ± 0.10 [a]	0.03 ± 0.03 [a]	1.54 ± 0.11 [c,d]	1.03 ± 0.10 [c]	1.4 ± 0.6 [f]	1.3 ± 0.8
Group DYS	0.40 ± 0.13	0.20 ± 0.09	1.15 ± 0.17 [d]	1.00 ± 0.10	2.1 ± 0.9 [f]	1.9 ± 0.9

a,c,d $p<0.0001$, c $p<0.005$, d $p<0.05$, e $p<0.005$, f $p<0.05$, Numbers are mean ± standard error. *H. pylori*, *Helicobacter pylori*

Table 7. Comparison of scores for histological findings before and after *Helicobacter pylori* eradication

3.2.3 Inflammation and GIM scores

The grade of inflammation and GIM before and after treatment was shown in Table 7. All GIMs investigated in the current study were diagnosed as incomplete type without dysplastic glands. At 1 year after successful *H. pylori* eradication, the median score of inflammation such as neutrophils and mononuclear cells significantly improved in Group A ($p<0.0001$ and $p<0.005$, respectively), but it did not change in Group B. The score of mononuclear cells was significantly higher in Group IM than in Group DYS ($p<0.05$), although no significant difference was observed in the neutrophils between the two groups. The GIM scores were also significantly higher in Group DYS than in Group IM before *H. pylori* therapy ($p<0.05$). After 1 yr of follow-up, however, the GIM score remained unchanged in comparison to their pretreatment values in both Groups IM and DYS.

4. Discussion

4.1 Study 1

In this study, we show that *H. pylori* eradication did not significantly improve GIM histologically, but changed the cellular phenotype, as evidenced by the significant reduction of reactivity against monoclonal antibody, mAb Das-1, indicating a reduction of colonic phenotype (incomplete type) of metaplasia over the course of subsequent follow-up, up to 4 years. This was further supported by prospectively following the same patients who were initially positive. We further demonstrate that eradication of *H. pylori* might reverse TC22 expression at the earlier stage (Group IM). However, once dysplasia/cancer has developed in the background mucosa (Group DYS), both cellular phenotype, as detected by mAb Das-1 and neoplastic marker TC22, did not show significant change following *H. pylori* eradication. These data support the conclusion reported by some investigators that at a certain stage of progression of GIM there is a "Point of no return" (Wong et al., 2004; Wright, 1998).

GIM is considered to be a pre-cancerous lesion of the stomach (Uemura et al., 2001; Correa & Shiao, 1994; Wong et al., 2004), especially when it is incomplete or colonic type (type II & type III) metaplasia (Filipe & Jass, 1986; Mirza et al., 2003). There are an equal number of studies showing either improvement or no change in the incidence of gastric cancer following eradication of *H. pylori* (Table 1). However, a large population based study showed decrease in cancer incidence following eradication of *H. pylori* (You et al., 2006; Take et al., 2005; Wong et al., 2004). The reasons for these discrepancies are the limited number of patients in some of the series, short follow-up, and also unawareness of the stage when the treatment was initiated. Our results support the reports that showed that 2 years following *H. pylori* eradication there was no significant histologic improvement in GIM (Forbes et al. 1996; Tucci et al., 1998; Tepes et al., 1999; Kim et al., 2000; Kuipers et al., 2004), although two other reports showed improvement (Kokkola et al., 2002; Correa et al., 2000). It was suggested that effective anti-*H. pylori* treatment might interfere with the pre-cancerous process, mostly by increasing the rate of regression of GIM (Correa et al., 2000). Our study demonstrates that this "regression" may be related to the change of cellular phenotype. Taking into account previous studies and our finding, it, therefore, appears that eradication of the bacteria may not influence the course of the histologic process (Farinati et al., 1998). We further demonstrate that even after eradication of *H. pylori*, in 14 of 36 patients (39%) who at initial diagnosis had gastritis without GIM (Group CG), developed GIM subsequently during the 4 years of follow-up evaluation. However, it appears that these GIMs are mostly of complete type (type I) of metaplasia that have a low risk for gastric carcinoma (Filipe et al. 1986; Mirza et al., 2003; Wong et al., 2004). Wong et al suggested that eradication of *H. pylori* should be done prior to the development of GIM in order to prevent gastric cancer (Wong et al., 2004). Our data further support that once the dysplastic process has occurred, eradication of *H. pylori* may not be helpful in changing the course (Sakaki et al., 2002; Asaka et al., 2002). Some investigators showed that older subjects are more likely to demonstrate progression in GIM in persistent *H. pylori* infection than younger patients (Sung et al., 2000; Sakaki et al., 2002; Asaka et al., 2002). Indeed, the average age of the patients in Group DYS was significantly higher than from Group CG and IM ($p<0.005$ and $p<0.05$, respectively), indicating that GIM in Group DYS was in an advanced stage among the three groups. The mean age of the patients in Group IM was in between the mean ages of Group CG and Group DYS. Furthermore, the GIM score in Group DYS is significantly higher than Group IM ($p<0.05$). Hence, our findings support the postulation that GIM grade ensues sequentially over a period of a decade (Uemura et al., 2001; Correa et al., 1990).

We previously reported a highly significant ($p<0.0001$) reactivity of mAb Das-1 against GIM adjacent to gastric cancer when compared to GIM from non-cancer patients (Mirza et al., 2003). We further reported that the reactivity of mAb Das-1 in other precancerous conditions, such as Barrett's epithelium was highly sensitive and specific (100%) (Das et al., 1994). In the small intestine, although mAb Das-1 does not react with normal epithelium, mAb Das-1 reactivity was evident in most of the small intestinal adenoma and adenocarcinoma (Onuma et al., 2001). All of these studies suggest a colonic or incomplete phenotype of metaplasia in the pre-cancerous conditions of the esophagus, stomach and small intestine. The present study shows that the immunoreactivity to mAb Das-1 was higher in the GIM in patients from Group DYS compared to those from Group IM ($p<0.05$) at the initial diagnosis before *H. pylori* eradication. Furthermore, mAb Das-1 reacted with GIM areas away from the dysplastic areas from each of the patients whose dysplastic areas were positive with mAb Das-1. Twelve out of 30 patients (40%) with GIM from Groups IM and DYS who were positive to mAb Das-1 before treatment, lost the reactivity ($p<0.0001$) after eradication of *H. pylori*, suggesting the reversibility of the process if *H. pylori* is eradicated. Thus, the patients with *H. pylori* infection with GIM that showed the reactivity for mAb Das-1 (incomplete type of metaplasia) may benefit from eradication for future development of cancer. This observation may be clinically useful for surveillance.

TC22 is a neoplastic marker. It is expressed by transformed cells but not by normal epithelial cells (Lin et al., 2002). In the present study, TC22-4 reactivity in GIM did not significantly change after eradication in both Group IM and DYS. Thus, the reactivity of Das-1 against GIM may suggest an early stage of neoplastic process compared with that of TC22-4. In a pilot study, we also observed that the frequency of mAb TC22-4 reactivity in gastric cancer was 86% (19/22) (Das-Bhattacharya et al., 2001). In each of these 19 patients, the GIM area away from the cancer area was also positive for TC22. Therefore, eradication of *H. pylori* at this stage may not be beneficial to avoid cancer development.

Mutation of the tumor suppressor gene p53 has been described in gastric carcinogenesis. Some GIM shows p53 mutations and its overexpression (El-Zimaity et al., 2001; Shiao et al., 1994; Imatani et al., 1996 ; Hamamoto et al., 1997; Jones et al., 1997), and accumulation of p53 is detected in gastric mucosa infected with *H. pylori* (Hibi et al., 1997; Satoh et al., 2001). Of interest, it was reported that p53 overexpression decreased after eradication of *H. pylori* (Hibi et al., 1997; Jones et al., 1997). Some of the discrepancies may be due to various reagents, and in some reports, p53 positivity index was used by calculating p53-positive cells in gastric glands (Hibi et al., 1997; Jones et al., 1997). p53 expression in our patients with GIM was very low, 3% in Group IM, and only 15% in Group DYS, and there was no regression following treatment. In the patients from Group DYS before treatment, the incidence (15%) of p53 expression was significantly lower than that of mAb TC22-4 reactivity in GIM areas (48%). In the paired samples of tissue with dysplasia/cancer, the overexpression of p53 increased from 15% in the GIM areas to 59% in the dysplastic areas. However, TC22 expression was essentially the same. Thus, p53 protein accumulation seems to be a late event, whereas TC22-4 expression is an earlier event, as also reported in colonic neoplasm (Lin et al., 2002).

As many investigators pointed out, it will certainly need a much longer follow-up period, more than 4 yrs., in order to evaluate the effect of eradication for the cancer prevention. However, the end-point of the current study was to assess the changes in the expression of biomarkers in GIM, one associated with cell phenotype and the other associated with epithelial neoplasia, but not the development of gastric cancer after *H. pylori* treatment. Indeed, we recently found that cell kinetics and genetic alterations, i.e. microsatellite instability and K-*ras* mutations in GIM, play a role in the early events leading to gastric carcinogenesis, and *H. pylori* eradication settled these genetic events during only the one-

year post-treatment period (Tanaka et al. 2006; Watari et al. 2008). Thus, we believe that the follow-up period, up to 4 yrs in this study, is enough to investigate the changes in cellular phenotype and neoplastic biomarkers related to carcinogenesis after *H. pylori* eradication. Taking our present and previous data (Tanaka et al. 2006; Watari et al. 2008) together, eradication of *H. pylori* may inhibit this intracellular dysfunction; thereby may inhibit carcinogenesis.
The data presented in the current study based on careful initial stratification of patients by an independent expert pathologist without the knowledge of clinical information, and prospective follow-up for 4 years, provide important information about the cellular changes in the GIM using the two novel biomarkers. Strategies to identify individuals who are at a "high risk" for gastric cancer screening are very much needed. Immunostaining with mAb Das-1 and TC22-4, that can easily be performed along with routine histology, may be clinically useful in this regard.

4.2 Study 2

The mutant K-*ras* was detected in only 3.8% of the cancer, and this finding was consistent with the findings of previous reports (Tahara et al. 1993; Arber et al., 2000; Hiyama et al., 2002). On the other hand, we found a significantly higher frequency of K-*ras* mutations in GIM (46.2%) in patients with chronic gastritis in comparison those with gastric cancer (1.9%) with *H. pylori* infection. Furthermore, we also observed that K-*ras* mutations significantly decreased to 12.8% after *H. pylori* eradication. Regarding the K-*ras* mutation types in Group IM, various patterns such as G to A (Ser and Asp) transitions and G to T (Cys) transversion were seen before treatment. It is interesting to note that after *H. pylori* eradication, most individuals (80.0%, 4 of 5) showed transition to AGT (Ser) while other mutation patterns such as TGT (Cys) and GAT (Asp) disappeared. In our data, since the number of cases that could be investigated based on the changes in the K-*ras* mutation patterns was small, statistical significance could therefore not be applied to them. These results indicate, however, that K-*ras* mutations in GIM with GAT and TGT types may thus be early and unstable in gastric carcinogenesis because they disappeared after *H. pylori* treatment. AGT (Ser) still remained in most cases treated with *H. pylori* in our study. Gong et al. reported the G to A transition (Ser) to be important for the progression of gastric mucosal cells to a more advanced premalignant stage (Gong et al., 1999). Lee et al. also showed a similar result, so that frequent G to A transversions were detected in gastric cancers (Lee et al., 1995). Taking both our results and other data into consideration, mutations with AGT (Ser) were thus considered to more likely be advantageous in K-*ras* gene alterations. Hiyama et al. reported interesting data in which K-*ras* mutations were detected in 3.0% in the background mucosa without cancer and in 10.9% in those with cancer, thus indicating a significant difference. In addition, most (70%) of the patterns of K-*ras* mutations detected in chronic gastritis patients were G to C transitions (GCT, Ala) (Hiyama et al., 2002). However, their data do not show K-*ras* gene alterations in only GIM, and thus their findings are different from those of our investigation. In the current study, we used a laser capture microdissection system to extract DNA from GIM. This method allows the procurement of relatively pure metaplastic cell populations from the complex heterogeneous cell mixtures (Bonner et al., 1997). Therefore, it is considered that the specificity of genetic alterations in DNA extracted selectively from GIM (Dillon et al., 2001). Our results may suggest that the mutations with AGT (Ser) is important in gastric tumorigenesis, but not in others. We investigated here on K-*ras* oncogene alterations in GIM using only one biopsy sample obtained from the antrum. It will be necessary to study whether the patients with mutations have the same mutation in multiple GIM foci in each patient in order to confirm more clearly the role of K-*ras* mutation in GIM.

H. pylori eradication dramatically improved the inflammation scores, i.e. neutrophils and mononuclear cells, but not the degree of GIM, thus confirming the findings of previous studies in which the effect of *H. pylori* eradication therapy led to an improvement in the severity of inflammation (Witteman et al., 1995; van der Hulst et al., 1997). However, no significant improvement in the inflammation scores was found in patients with gastric cancer (Group DYS). Although the reason cannot be clearly explained, one possibility for this finding may be the small number patients investigated in comparison to those of Group IM. Interestingly, the score of mononuclear cells in Group IM showed a significantly higher level than that in Group DYS at the pretreatment assessment although no significant differences in the neutrophil scores were observed between Groups IM and DYS. Recently, Brembeck et al have reported a fascinating data that they generated a novel mouse model in which the cytokeratin 19 promotor, specifically active in pancreatic ductal cells, is fused to mutant K-*ras* (Brembeck et al., 2003). These results showed dramatic evidence of lymphocytic infiltration around the periductal area, in both the interlobular and intralobular pancreas of transgenic mice, which may thus act as an adaptive immune response to activated ras-mediated signaling. Taking both our findings and previous results into consideration, a frequent K-*ras* mutation in GIM may therefore be associated with evidence of lymphocyte infiltration but not with gastric carcinogenesis, even though the K-*ras* gene is considered to be an oncogene.

In the present study, we first found the cellular proliferation of GIM to significantly be up-regulated in patients with gastric cancer more than in those without gastric cancer. As for apoptosis, there was a similar tendency even though no significant difference was seen. This finding supports the report of Shiotani et al that GIM results in proliferation-dominant cell kinetics may be one of the components of gastric carcinogenesis (Shiotani et al., 2005). Commonly, an imbalance of cell proliferation and apoptosis is known to play a role in cancer development, and tumor progression should be thus be considered in the context of both proliferative activity and cell loss (Wyllie, 1996). One of the pathways by which *H. pylori* is linked to gastric carcinogenesis may be related to the disruption of the cell kinetics. Uemura et al. reported that *H. pylori* eradication inhibited the development of new cancers in patients who underwent EMR for 2 years after EMR, while 9% of the patients who were not treated with this treatment developed new early stage gastric cancers after 3 years of follow-up (Uemura et al., 1997). From the standpoint of this clinical report by Uemura et al and our results, the increase of apoptosis in GIM by the clearance of *H. pylori* may be associated with the prevention of cancer development. To our knowledge, there has only been one study that has assessed the cell kinetics in *H. pylori*-associated GIM in patients with gastritis both before and after *H. pylori* eradication, although the sample size investigated in that study was small (14 cases) (Leung et al., 2001). They demonstrated a remarkable reduction in proliferation whereas the degree of apoptosis remained unaltered in GIM by treatment, by which the clearance of *H. pylori* may retard gastric carcinogenesis. However, we failed to detect such an association in the current study. This discrepancy seems to be derived from a few factors: namely, the difference in the sample number and the sampling error. As mentioned in the results, the severity of GIM was significantly higher in patients with cancer (Group DYS-1) than in those with chronic gastritis (Group IM) prior to treatment. Hence, an evaluation of the cell kinetics in GIM from the Group IM cases was therefore particularly difficult.

We recently found microsatellite instability (MSI) as a genetic alteration in *H. pylori*-related GIM to play a role in the early events leading to gastric carcinogenesis. *H. pylori* eradication reduced MSI during the one-year post-treatment period (Tanaka et al., 2006). In this prospective study, however, our current results suggest that K-*ras* codon 12 mutations in GIM may not be associated with gastric carcinogenesis. There are early events in K-*ras* mutations, which are influenced by inflammation-related *H. pylori* infection, and some mutations such as AGT (Ser) may thus be selected by eradication. Furthermore, these unstable K-*ras* mutations in GIM may be related to the lymphocyte infiltration caused by *H. pylori* infection. If *H. pylori* is eradicated before the development of stable mutations, then the risk of gastric cancer will likely be prevented. Furthermore, apoptosis in GIM showed the increase based on the treatment. Our 1-year prospective study may explain that the prevention of gastric cancer by *H. pylori* therapy is not associated with an improvement of K-*ras* mutations and the degree of GIM, but up-regulation in apoptosis control in GIM contributes to retard gastric carcinogenesis.

5. Conclusions

H. pylori eradication does not reduce the histologic GIM score, but changes the cellular phenotype of GIM. This change of phenotype may be an important factor in the reduction of cancer incidence after eradication of *H. pylori*. Furthermore, K-*ras* mutations in GIM do not always play a role in gastric carcinogenesis but cell kinetics, especially apoptosis, in GIM may contribute it.

6. Acknowledgements

This work was supported in part by a research grant (National Institute of Diabetes and Digestive and Kidney Disease, RO1DK63618 to K.M.D.) from the National Institutes of Health (Bethesda, MD). The authors would like to thank Ms. Harumi Suzuki for valuable help in preparing the slide sections.

7. References

Arber, N.; Shapira, I. & Ratan, J., et al. (2000). Activation of c-K-ras mutations in human gastrointestinal tumors. *Gastroenterology*, Vol. 118, No. 6, pp. 1045-1050

Asaka, M.; Sugiyama, T. & Nobuta, A., et al. (2001). Atrophic gastritis and intestinal metaplasia in Japan: results of a large multicenter study. *Helicobacter*, Vol. 6, No. 4, pp. 294-299.

Biancone, L.; Mandal, A. & Yang, H., et al. (1995). Production of immunoglobulin G and G1 antibodies to cytoskeletal protein by lamina propria cells in ulcerative colitis. *Gastroenterology*, Vol. 109, No. 1, pp. 3-12

Bonner, RF.; Emmert-Buck, M. & Cole, K., et al. (1997). Laser capture microdissection: molecular analysis of tissue. *Science*, Vol. 278, No. 5342, pp. 1481-1483.

Brembeck, FH.; Schreiber, FS. & Deramaudt, TB., et al. (2003). The mutant K-ras oncogene causes pancreatic periductal lymphocytic infiltration and gastric mucous neck cell hyperplasia in transgenic mice. *Cancer Res*, Vol. 63, No. 9, pp. 2005-2009

Chaubert, P.; Benhattar, J. & Saraga, E., et al. (1994). K-ras mutations and p53 alterations in neoplastic and nonneoplastic lesions associated with longstanding ulcerative colitis. *Am J Pathol*, Vol. 144, No. 4, pp. 767-775

Cooper, GM. (1995). Guanine nucleotide binding proteins. In: Oncogenes. Ed. 2, Sudbury, MA: Jones and Bartlett Publishers, pp. 222-242

Correa, P. (1988). A human model of gastric carcinogenesis. *Cancer Res*, Vol. 48, No. 13, pp. 3554-3560

Correa, P.; Fox, J. & Fontham, E., et al. (1990). Helicobacter pylori and gastric carcinoma. Serum antibody prevalence in populations with contrasting cancer risks. *Cancer*, Vol. 66, No. 12, pp. 2569-2574

Correa, P.; Haenszel, W. & Cuello, C., et al. (1990). Gastric precancerous process in a high risk population: cohort follow-up. *Cancer Res*, Vol. 50, No. 15, pp. 4737-4740

Correa, P. & Shiao, YH. (1994). Phenotypic and genotypic events in gastric carcinogenesis. *Cancer Res*, Vol. 54 (7 suppl), pp. 1941s-1943s

Correa, P. (1995). Helicobacter pylori and gastric carcinogenesis. *Am J Surg Pathol*, Vol. 19 (Suppl 1), pp. S37-S43

Correa, P.; Fontham, ET. & Bravo, JC., et al. (2000). Chemoprevention of gastric dysplasia: randomized trial of antioxidant supplements and anti-Helicobacter pylori therapy. *J Natl Cancer Inst*, Vol. 92, No. 23, pp. 1881-1888

Das-Bhattacharya, S.; Walton, K. & Watari, J., et al. (2001). Expression of a novel human tropomyosin isoform, TC22, in gastric intestinal metaplasia associated with gastric carcinoma. *Gastroenterology*, Vol. 122, A129

Das, KM.; Sakamaki, S. & Vecchi, M., et al. (1987). The production and characterization of monoclonal antibodies to a human colonic antigen associated with ulcerative colitis: cellular localization of the antigen by using the monoclonal antibody. *J Immunol*, Vol. 139, No. 1, pp. 77-84

Das, KM.; Dasgupta, A. & Mandal, A., et al. (1993). Autoimmunity to cytoskeletal protein tropomyosin: a clue to the pathogenetic mechanism for ulcerative colitis. *J Immunol*, Vol. 150, No. 3, pp. 2487-2493

Das, KM.; Prasad, I. & Garla, S., et al. (1994). Detection of a shared colon epithelial epitope on Barrett epithelium by a novel monoclonal antibody. *Ann Intern Med*, Vol. 120, No. 9, pp. 753-756

Dillon D, Zheng K, Costa J. (2001). Rapid, efficient genotyping of clinical tumor samples by laser-capture microdissection/PCR/SSCP. *Exp Mol Pathol*, Vol. 70, No. 3, pp. 195-200

Dixon, MF.; Genta, RM. & Yardley, JH., et al. (1996). Classification and grading of gastritis. The updated Sydney System. International Workshop on the Histopathology of Gastritis, Houston 1994. *Am J Surg Pathol*, Vol. 20, No. 10, pp. 1161-1181

El-Omar, EM.; Oien, K. & Murray, LS., et al. (2000). Increased prevalence of precancerous changes in relatives of gastric cancer patients: critical role of H. pylori. *Gastroenterology*, Vol. 118, No. 1, pp. 22-30

El-Zimaity, HM.; Ramchatesingh, J. & Saeed, MA., et al. (2001). Gastric intestinal metaplasia: subtypes and natural history. *J Clin Pathol*, Vol. 54, No. 9, pp. 679-683

Farinati, F.; Foschia, F. & Di Mario, F., et al. (1998). H. pylori eradication and gastric precancerous lesions. *Gastroenterology*, Vol. 115, No. 2, pp. 512-514

Filipe, MI. & Jass, JR. (1986). Intestinal metaplasia subtypes and cancer risk. In: Filipe MI, Jass JR, eds. Gastric carcinoma. Edinburgh: Churchill Livingstone, pp. 212-236.

Filipe, MI.; Munoz, N. & Matko, I., et al. (1994). Intestinal metaplasia types and the risk of gastric cancer: a cohort study in Slovenia. *Int J Cancer*, 1994;Vol. 57, No. 3, pp. 324-329

Forbes, GM.; Warren, JR. & Glaser, ME., et al. (1996). Long-term follow-up of gastric histology after Helicobacter pylori eradication. *J Gastroenterol Hepatol*, Vol. 11, No. 7, pp. 670-673

Gavrieli, Y.; Sherman, Y. & Ben-Sasson, SA. (1992). Identification of programmed cell death in situ via specific labeling of nuclear DNA fragmentation. *J Cell Biol*, Vol. 119, No. 3, pp. 493-501

Geng, X.; Biancone, L. & Dai, HH., et al. (1998). Tropomyosin isoforms in intestinal mucosa: production of autoantibodies to tropomyosin isoforms in ulcerative colitis. *Gastroenterology*, Vol. 114, No. 5, pp. 912-922

Genta, RM.; Lew, GM. & Graham, DY. (1993). Changes in the gastric mucosa following eradication of Helicobacter pylori. *Mod Pathol*, Vol. 6, No. 3, pp. 281-289

Gong, C.; Mera, R. & Bravo, JC., et al. (1999). KRAS mutations predict progression og preneoplastic gastric lesions. *Cancer Epidemiol Biomark Prev*, Vol. 8, No. 2, pp. 167-171

Graham, DY. (2000). Helicobacter pylori infection is the primary cause of gastric cancer. *J Gastroenterol*, Vol. 35 (suppl 12), pp. 90-97

Griffel, LH.; Amenta, PS. & Das, KM. (2000). Use of a novel monoclonal antibody in diagnosis of Barrett's esophagus. *Dig Dis Sci*, Vol. 45, No. 1, pp. 40-48

Halstensen, TS.; Das, KM. & Brandtzaeg, P. (1993). Epithelial deposits of immunoglobulin G1 and activated complement colocalise with the M(r) 40 kD putative autoantigen in ulcerative colitis. *Gut*, Vol. 34, No. 5, pp. 650-657

Hamamoto, T.; Yokozaki, H. & Semba, S., et al. (1997). Altered microsatellites in incomplete-type intestinal metaplasia adjacent to primary gastric cancers. *J Clin Pathol*, Vol. 50, No. 10, pp. 841-846

Hibi, K.; Mitomi, H. & Koizumi, W., et al. (1997). Enhanced cellular proliferation and p53 accumulation in gastric mucosa chronically infected with Helicobacter pylori. *Am J Clin Pathol*, Vol. 108, No. 1, pp. 26-34

Hiyama, T.; Haruma, K. & Kitadai, Y., et al. (2002). K-ras mutation in Helicobacter pylori-associated chronic gastritis in patients with and without gastric cancer. *Int J Cancer*, Vol. 97, No. 5, pp. 562-566

Hoshi, T.; Sasano, H. & Kato, K., et al. (1999). Cell damage and proliferation in human gastric mucosa infected by Helicobacter pylori-A comparison before and after H pylori eradication in eradication in non-atrophic gastritis. *Hum Pathol*, Vol. 30, No. 12, pp. 1412-1417

Imatani, A.; Sasano, H. & Yabuki, N., et al. (1996). In situ analysis of tissue dynamics and p53 expression in human gastric mucosa. *J Pathol*, Vol. 179, No. 1, pp. 39-42

International Agency for Research on Cancer. (1994). IARC monographs on the evaluation of carcinogenic risks to humans. Schistosomes, liver flukes and Helicobacter pylori. Lyon: IARC, vol. 61, pp. 177-240

Jones, NL.; Shannon, PT. & Cutz, E., et al. (1997). Increase in proliferation and apoptosis of gastric epithelial cells early in the natural history of Helicobacter pylori infection. *Am J Pathol*, Vol. 151, No. 6, pp. 1695-1703

Kim, N.; Lim, SH. & Lee, KH., et al. (2000). Long-term effects of Helicobacter pylori eradication on intestinal metaplasia in patients with duodenal and benign gastric ulcers. *Dig Dis Sci*, Vol. 45, No. 9, pp. 1754-1762

Kokkola, A.; Sipponen, P. & Rautelin, H., et al. (2002). The effect of Helicobacter pylori eradication on the natural course of atrophic gastritis with dysplasia. *Aliment Pharmacol Ther*, Vol. 16, No. 3, pp. 515-520

Kuipers, EJ.; Nelis, GF. & Klinkenberg-Knol, EC., et al. (2004). Cure of Helicobacter pylori infection in patients with reflux oesophagitis treated with long term omeprazole reverses gastritis without exacerbation of reflux disease: results of a randomised controlled trial. *Gut*, Vol. 53, No. 1, pp. 12-20

Lee, KH,: Lee, JS. & Suh, C., et al. (1995). Clinicopathologic significance of the K-ras gene codon 12 point mutation in stomach cancer. An analysis of 140 cases. *Cancer*, Vol. 75, No. 12, pp. 2794-2801

Lees-Miller, JP. & Helfman, DM. (1991). The molecular basis for tropomyosin isoform diversity. *Bioessays*, Vol. 13, No. 9, pp. 429-437

Leung, WK.; Yu, J. & To, KF., et al. (2001). Apoptosis and proliferation in Helicobacter pylori-associated gastric intestinal metaplasia. *Aliment Pharmacol Ther*, Vol. 15, No. 9, pp. 1467-1472

Levi, S.; Urbano-Ispizua, A. & Gill, R., et al. (1991). Multiple K-ras codon 12 mutations in cholangiocarcinomas demonstrated with a sensitive polymerase chain reaction technique. *Cancer Res*, Vol. 51, No. 13, pp. 3497-3502

Ley, C.; Mohar, A. & Guarner, J., et al. (2004). Helicobacter pylori eradication and gastric preneoplastic conditions: a randomized, double-blind, placebo-controlled trial. *Cancer Epidemiol Biomarkers Prev*, Vol. 13, No. 1, pp. 4-10

Lin, JJ.; Warren, KS. & Wamboldt, DD., et al. (1997). Tropomyosin isoforms in nonmuscle cells. *Int Rev Cytol*, Vol. 170, pp. 1-38

Lin, JL.; Geng, X. & Bhattacharya, SD., et al. (2002). Isolation and sequencing of a novel tropomyosin isoform prefentially associated with colon cancer. *Gastroenterology*, Vol. 123, No. 1, pp. 152-162

Mera, R.; Fontham, ET. & Bravo, LE., et al. (2005). Long term follow up of patients treated for Helicobacter pylori infection. *Gut*, Vol. 54, No. 11, pp.1536-1540

Miehlke, S.; Hackelsberger, A. & Meining, A., et al. (1998). Severe expression of corpus gastritis is characteristic in gastric cancer patients infected with Helicobacter pylori. *Br J Cancer*, Vol. 78, No. 2, pp. 263-266

Mirza, ZK.; Das, KK. & Slate, J., et al. (2003). Gastric intestinal metaplasia as detected by a novel biomarker is highly associated with gastric adenocarcinoma. *Gut*, Vol. 52, No.6, pp. 807-812

Moss, SF.; Calam, J. & Agarwal, B., et al. (1996). Induction of gastric epithelial apoptosis by Helicobacter pylori. *Gut*, Vol. 38, No. 4, pp. 498-501

Nardone, G.; Staibano, S. & Rocco, A., et al. (1999). Effect of Helicobacter pylori infection and its eradication on cell proliferation, DNA status, and oncogene expression in patients with chronic gastritis. *Gut*, Vol. 44, No. 6, pp. 789-799

Novy, RE.; Lin, JL. & Lin CS, et al. (1993). Human fibroblast tropomyosin isoforms: characterization of cDNA clones and analysis of tropomyosin isoform expression in human tissues and in normal and transformed cells. *Cell Motil Cytoskeleton*, Vol. 25, No. 3, pp. 267-281

Ohkusa, T.; Fujiki, K. & Takashimizu, I., et al. (2001). Improvement in atrophic gastritis and intestinal metaplasia in patients in whom Helicobacter pylori was eradicated. *Ann Int Med*, Vol. 134 No. 5, pp. 380-386

Onuma, EK.; Amenta, PS. & Ramaswamy, K., et al. (2000). Autoimmunity in ulcerative colitis (UC): a predominant colonic mucosal B cell response against human tropomyosin isoform 5. *Clin Exp Immunol*, Vol. 121, No. 3, pp. 466-471

Onuma, EK.; Amenta, PS. & Jukkola, AF., et al. (2001). A phenotypic change of small intestinal epithelium to that of colonocytes in small intestinal adenomas and adenocarcinomas. *Am J Gastroenterol*, Vol. 96, No. 8, pp. 2480-2485

Parkin, DM.; Whelan, SL. & Ferlay, J., et al. (1997). eds. Cancer incidence in five countries. Vol. VII, ARC Scientific Publication No. 143. Lyon: International Agency for Research on Cancer, World Health Organization and International Association of Cancer Registries

Pittenger, MF. & Helfman, DM. (1992). In vitro and in vivo characterization of four fibroblast tropomyosins produced in bacteria: TM-2, TM-3, TM-5a, and TM-5b are co-localized in interphase fibroblasts. *J Cell Biol*, Vol. 118, No. 4, pp. 841-858

Rugge, M.; Correa, P. & Dixon, MF., et al. (2000). Gastric dysplasia: The Padova international classification. *Am J Surg Pathol*, Vol. 24, No. 2, pp. 167-176

Sakaki, N.; Kozawa, H. & Egawa, N., et al. (2002). Ten-year prospective follow-up study on the relationship between Helicobacter pylori infection and progression of atrophic gastritis, particularly assessed by endoscopic findings. *Aliment Pharmacol Ther*, Vol. 16 (Suppl 2), pp. 198-203

Sakamaki, S.; Takayanagi, N. & Yoshizaki, N., et al. (2000). Autoantibodies against the specific epitope of human tropomyosin(s) detected by a peptide based enzyme immunoassay in sera of patients with ulcerative colitis show antibody dependent cell mediated cytotoxicity against HLA-DPw9 transfected L cells. *Gut*, Vol. 47, No. 2, pp. 236-241

Sanger, F.; Nicklen, S. & Coulson, AR. (1997). DNA sequencing with chain-terminating inhibitors. *Proc Natl Acad Sci USA*, Vol. 74, No. 12, pp. 5463-5467

Satoh, K.; Kihira, K. & Kawata, H., et al. (2001). p53 expression in the gastric mucosa before and after eradication of Helicobacter pylori. *Helicobacter*, Vol. 6, No. 1, pp. 31-36

Satoh, K.; Kimura, K. & Takimoto, T., et al. (1998). A follow-up study of atrophic gastritis and intestinal metaplasia after eradication of Helicobacter pylori. *Helicobacter*, Vol. 3, No. 4, pp. 236-240

Shiao, YH.; Rugge, M. & Correa, P., et al. (1994). p53 alteration in gastric precancerous lesions. *Am J Pathol*, Vol. 144, No. 3, pp. 511-517

Shiotani, A.; Iishi, H. & Ishiguro, S., et al. (2005). Epithelial cell turnover in relation to ongoing damage of the gastric mucosa in patients with early gastric cancer: increase of cell proliferation in paramalignant lesions. *J Gastroenterol* 2005;40, No. 4, pp.337-344

Sipponen, P. & Hyvarinen, H. (1993). Role of Helicobacter pylori in the pathogenesis of gastritis, peptic ulcer and gastric cancer. *Scand J Gastroenterol*, Vol. 196 (suppl), pp. 3-6

Soh, K.; Yanagisawa, A. & Hiratsuka, H., et al. (1993). Variation in K-ras codon 12 point mutation rate with histological atypia within individual colorecral tumors. *Jpn J Cancer Res*, Vol. 84, No. 4, pp. 388-393

Sung, JJ.; Lin, SR. & Ching, JY., et al. (2000). Atrophy and intestinal metaplasia one year after cure of H. pylori Infection: a prospective, randomized study. *Gastroenterology*, Vol. 119, No. 1, pp. 7-14

Tahara E. (1993). Molecular mechanism of stomach carcinogenesis. *Cancer Res Clin Oncol*, Vol. 119, No. 5, pp. 265-272

Take, S.; Mizuno, M. & Ishiki, K., et al. (2005). The effect of eradicating Helicobacter pylori on the development of gastric cancer in patients with peptic ulcer disease. *Am J Gastroenterol*, Vol. 100, No. 5, pp. 1037-1042

Tanaka, A.; Watari, J. & Tanabe, H., et al. (2006). Effect of eradication of Helicobacter pylori on genetic instabilities in gastric intestinal metaplasia. *Aliment Pharmacol Ther*, Vol. 24 (Suppl 4), pp. 194-202

Taniguchi, M.; Geng, X. & Glazier, KD., et al. (2001). Cellular immune response against tropomyosin isoform 5 in ulcerative colitis. *Clin Immunol*, Vol. 101, No. 3, pp. 289-295

Tepes, B.; Kavcic, B. & Zaletel, LK., et al. (1999). Two- to four-year histological follow-up of gastric mucosa after Helicobacter pylori eradication. *J Pathol*, Vol. 188, No. 1, pp. 24-29

Tucci, A.; Poli, L. & Tosetti, C., et al. (1998). Reversal of fundic atrophy after eradication of Helicobacter pylori. *Am J Gastroenterol*, Vol. 93, No. 9, pp. 1425-1431

Uemura, N.; Mukai, T. & Okamoto, S., et al. (1997). Effect of Helicobacter pylori eradication on subsequent development of cancer after endoscopic resection of early gastric cancer. *Cancer Epidemiol Biomarkers Prev*, Vol. 6, No. 8, pp. 639-642

Uemura, N.; Okamoto, S., & Yamamoto, S., et al. (2001). Helicobacter pylori infection and the development of gastric cancer. *N Engl J Med*, Vol. 345, No. 11, pp. 784-789

van der Hulst, RW.; van der Ende, A. & Dekker, FW., et al. (1997). Effect of Helicobacter pylori eradication on gastritis in relation to cagA: a prospective 1-year follow-up study. *Gastroenterology*, Vol. 113, No. 1, pp. 25-30

Vogelstein, B.; Fearon, ER. & Hamilton, SR., et al. (1988). Genetic alterations during colorectal-tumor development. *N Engl J Med*,1988;319, No. 9, pp. 525-532

Wagner, S.; Beil, W. & Westermann, J., et al. (1997). Regulation of gastric epithelial cell growth by Helicobacter pylori: evidence for a major role of apoptosis. *Gastroenterology*, Vol. 113, No. 6, pp. 1836-1847

Watari, J.; Saitoh, Y. & Obara T., et al. (2002), Natural history of colorectal nonpolypoid adenomas: a prospective colonoscopic study and relation with cell kinetics and K-ras mutations. *Am J Gastroenterol*, Vol. 97, No. 8, pp. 2109-2115

Watari, J.; Tanaka, A. & Tanabe, H., et al. (2007). K-ras mutations and cell kinetics in Helicobacter pylori associated gastric intestinal metaplasia: a comparison before and after eradication in patients with chronic gastritis and gastric cancer. *J Clin Pathol*, Vol. 60, No. 8, pp. 921-926

Watari, J.; Das, KK. & Amenta, PS., et al. (2008). Effect of eradication of Helicobacter pylori on the histology and cellular phenotype of gastric intestinal metaplasia. *Clin Gastroenterol Hepatol*, Vol. 6, No. 4, pp. 409-417

Witteman, EM.; Mravunac, M. & Becx, MJ., et al. (1995). Improvement of gastric inflammation and resolution of epithelial damage one year after eradication of Helicobacter pylori. *J Clin Pathol*, Vol. 48, No. 3, pp. 250-256

Wong, BC.; Lam, SK. & Wong, WM., et al. (2004). Helicobacter pylori eradication to prevent gastric cancer in a high-risk region of China: a randomized controlled trial. *JAMA*, Vol. 291, No. 2, pp. 187-194

Wright, NA. (1998). Gastric carcinogenesis: when is the point of no return? In: Hunt RH, Tytgat GNJ, eds. Helicobacter pylori: Basic Mechanisms to Clinical Cure. Boston, Mass: Kluwer Academic Publishers, pp. 325-335

Wyllie, AH. (1996). The biology of cell death in tumors. *Anticancer Res*, Vol. 5, No. 1, pp. 131-136

Yanagisawa, A.; Ohtake, K. & Ohashi, K., et al. (1993). Frequent c-Ki-ras oncogene activation in mucous cell hyperplasias of pancreas suffering from chronic inflammation. *Cancer Res*, Vol. 53, No. 5, pp. 953-956

You, WC.; Brown, LM. & Zhang, L., et al. (2006). Randomized double-blind factorial of three treatments to reduce the precancerous gastric lesion. *J Natl Cancer Inst*, Vol. 98, No. 14, pp. 974-983

13

Helicobacter pylori Lipopolysaccharide as a Possible Pathogenic Factor for Gastric Carcinogenesis

Shin-ichi Yokota[1], Ken-ichi Amano[2] and Nobuhiro Fujii[1]
[1]*Department of Microbiology, Sapporo Medical University School of Medicine, Sapporo*
[2]*Bioscience Education and Research Center, Akita University, Akita*
Japan

1. Introduction

Helicobacter pylori is now recognized as being a causative factor of gastroduodenal diseases such as chronic gastritis, gastric ulcer, duodenal ulcer, gastric cancer and gastric low-grade mucosa-associated lymphoma tissue (MALT). Long-term persistent inflammation, injury and reconstitution of gastric mucosa, and immunological reactions against the infected *H. pylori* are thought to be the causes of lesion formation. Various causative factors of *H. pylori* for inflammation and injury of gastric mucosa have been proposed. The most studied bacterial pathogenic factors are vacuolating toxin (VacA) produced by *H. pylori*, ammonium ion generated by *H. pylori* urease, and monochloramines formed from hypochlorite produced by phagocytic cells and the ammonium ion (Hofman et al., 2004; Xia & Talley, 2001). These agents cause directly injury to the host gastric mucosa. Proinflammatory cytokines, such as interleukin (IL)-1, tumor necrosis factor-α (TNF-α), IL-6 and IL-8, are also induced by *H. pylori*. *H. pylori* activates the transcription factor NF-κB, which has a key role on inducing various inflammatory reaction including cytokine production, through type IV secretion system (Glocker et al., 1998). The type IV secretion system consisits of proteins encoded by genes located on *cag* pathogenicity island.

In addition, lipopolysaccharide (LPS) is believed to contribute to the pathogenicity of this bacterium. LPS is a major component of Gram-negative bacterial outer membrane. It is known as an endotoxin and is a strong inducer of inflammatory reaction. *H. pylori* LPS, however, has much lower endotoxic activity than that of other typical Gram-negative bacteria, such as member of the *Enterobacteriaceae* family (Matsuyama et al., 2001; Muotiala et al., 1992; Nielsen et al., 1994; Perez-Perez et al., 1995; Semeraro et al., 1996). Strong endotoxin at infection sites, such as the systemic circulation system and digestive tract, should lead to sepsis, namely systemic inflammatory response syndrome (SIRS), and severe local inflammation, respectively. The weak endotoxic activity is considered to be important for chronic infection. Weakly endotoxic LPSs are also reported for *Chlamydia/Chlamydophila* (Heine et al., 2003) and *Porphyromonas gingivalis* (Ogawa et al., 2000). These bacteria commonly infected humans chronically.

Typical LPS acts as a pathogen-associated molecular pattern (PAMP). PAMPs are recognized by pattern recognition receptors (PRRs) of which the most studies are the Toll-like receptors (TLRs). Typical highly endotoxic LPS are recognized by the TLR4/MD2/CD14 complex, whereas the TLR that recognizes the weakly exdotoxic *H. pylori* LPS is controversial as discussed below. Bacterial flagella also act as a PAMP, and they are recognized by TLR5. Like the LPS, *H. pylori* flagella also show less activity as a TLR5 agonist (Andersen-Nissen et al., 2005). The PAMPs of *H. pylori*, therefore, share low potency as TLR agonists, namely they are weak inducers of inflammation.

In addition to low endotoxic activity, *H. pylori* LPS has several unique features, for example structures that mimic host Lewis blood group antigens (Moran, 2008). In this review, the chemical characteristics, biological activities, and role in gastric carcinogenesis of *H. pylori* LPS will be described. In particular we will focus on our recent research into LPS as a pathogenic factor for carcinogenesis.

2. General architecture of *H. pylori* LPS

Like other typical bacterial LPS, *H. pylori* LPS consists of three region, namely lipid A, core oligosaccharide and O-polysaccharide (Fig. 1). The weakly endotoxic activity is due to the chemical structure of lipid A portion. In *H. pylori* LPS, the carbohydrate portion of lipid A consists of a glucosaminyl-β-1-6-glucosamine disaccharide backbone, as well as the typical lipid A. Whereas the lipid A of typical LPS derived from *E. coli* contains six fatty acid residues with relatively short carbon chain, such as C14 and C12, *H. pylori* lipid A contains three to five fatty acids with long carbon chain of C18 and C16 (Moran et al., 1997; Suda et al., 1997). Netea et al. (2002) describe that the molecular shapes, such as conical, cylindrical and intermediate, of lipid A are different between the highly endotoxic typical LPS and the weakly endotoxic LPS. The diversity of molecular shapes may cause the difference of endotoxic activity and usage of TLRs. Remodeling of lipid A structures occur in *H. pylori* by the action of phosphatase, ethanolamine phosphate transferase, 3-deoxy-D-*manno*-octulosonic acid (KDO) hydrolase and deacylase (Tran et al., 2005). Hildebrandt & McGee (2009) report structural modifications of lipid A occur in an exogenous cholesterol-dependent manner. Thus lipid A structures may vary among strains or change depending on culture conditions.

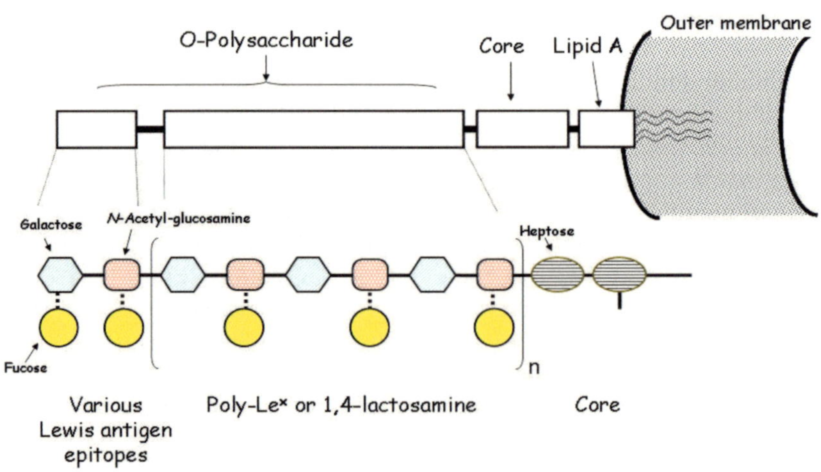

Fig. 1. General architecture of *H. pylori* LPS

The core oligosaccharide region of *H. pylori* LPS has a characteristic structure among *H. pylori* strains, however, the detailed structure is distinct from the typical LPS (Aspinall et al., 1997; Monteiro, 2001). It contains KDO and heptose residues similar to typical gram-negative bacterial LPS. There is some heterogeneity among *H. pylori* strains. For example, heptose oligomer (heptan) or glucose oligomer (glucan) is found in some strains.

One of the important features of *H. pylori* LPS is the O-polysaccharide region that bears the mimicking structures of the host carbohydrate antigens, Lewis antigens (Moran, 2008). It is interesting that *Campylobacter* species, which also belongs to spirillum, also shares host carbohydrate structures in gangliosides, such as GM1 and GQ1b (Yuki, 1999). Host Lewis antigens are recognized as a tumor antigen. Le^x is also known as CD15, which is a marker for neutrophils. The existence of Lewis antigens, such as Le^x, Le^y, Le^a and Le^b, varies among *H. pylori* strains. Lewis antigns are considered to contribute to escape from a host immune response and to induction of an autoimmune response. The O-polysaccharide of most *H. pylori* strains consists of a lactosamine (galacotosyl-β1-4-*N*-acetyl-glucosamine) unit as the backbone chain. L-Fucose residues are partially substituted in the backbone chain and form a polymeric Le^x structure. In addition, a high level of variability occurs in the non-reducing terminal end of the O-polysaccharide chain. For example, β1-3- or β1-4-linked galactose and α1-3- or α1-4-linked fucose can substitute on the *N*-acetyl-glucosamine residue, and α1-2-linked fucose can occur on the galactose residue. The variable substitutions form various Lewis antigen structures (Fig. 2).

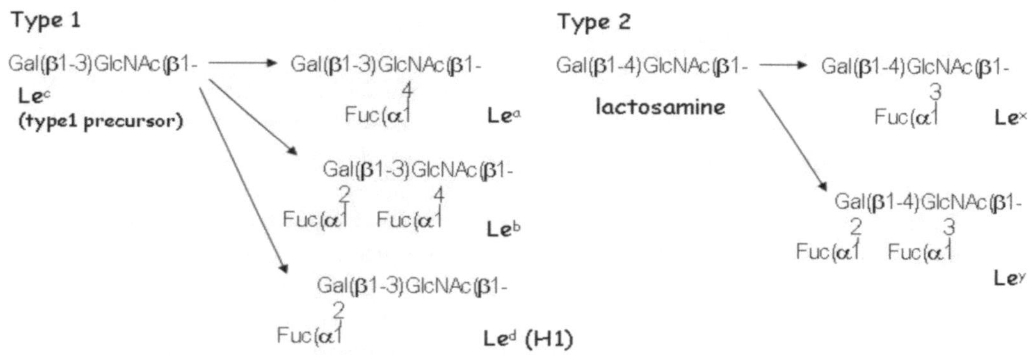

Fig. 2. Structures of Lewis antigens
Abbreviations. Fuc: L-fucose, Gal: D-galactose, GlcNAc: *N*-acetyl-D-glucosamine.

3. Biological roles of Lewis antigens *H. pylori* LPS

As described above, *H. pylori* Lewis antigens mimic host antigens and can thus modulate various host physiological responses, especially immunological reactions.

The O-polysaccharide, in particular the polymeric Le^x structure, has been shown to contribute to adhesion of *H. pylori* to human antral gastric mucosa. Galectin-3 is a gastric receptor for *H. pylori* Le^x antigen (Fowler et al., 2006). Lewis antigens can interact with other host lectins. Interaction with two particular C-type lectins is important for the modulation of immunological responses. One is Dendritic Cell Specific ICAM-3 Grabbing Non-integrin (DC-SIGN; CD209). Whereas Lewis antigen-negative *H. pylori* cells predominantly promotes a strong Th1 cell response, Lewis antigen-bearing cells interact with DC-SIGN on dendritic cells and induce IL-10, which promotes a Th2 response in a mouse infection model (Bergman et al., 2004). The other C-type lectin that interact with *H. pylori* LPS is surfactant protein D (SP-D) (Khamri et al., 2005; Murray et al., 2002). SP-D is involved in antibody-independent clearance of bacteria. Levels of SP-D are increased in gastric mucosa with *H. pylori*-associated antral gastritis compared to normal gastric mucosa. The fucose residues of the O-polysaccharide chain are shown to be important for the recognition of SP-D. On the other hand, our recent study showed that D-galactose residue of *H. pylori* LPS is involved in interaction with SP-D as described below.

Another important issue is formation of anti-Lewis antigen autoantibodies. Anti-Le^y autoantibodies have been implicated in the pathogenesis of atrophic gastritis. The anti-Le^y autoantiboides are found both in patients with atrophic gastritis and gastric cancer (Heneghan et al., 2001; Negrini et al., 1996). A candidate for the target of the autoantibodies is the β-chain of the H^+,K^+-ATPase, which is a proton pump (Appelmelk et al., 1996). Anti-Le^x autoantibodies are also found in *H. pylori*-infected patients (Heneghan et al., 2001; Negrini et al., 1996). Anti-Le^x antibodies have been shown to activate neutrophils and enhance their adhesion to endothelium (Stockl et al., 1993) which could lead to inflammation and tissue damage. However, these antibodies induced by *H. pylori* do not react with synthetic Lewis antigens (Amano et al., 1997; Heneghan et al., 2001). The actual specificity of the anti-Lewis antigen antibodies has not been clear yet.

4. Antigenic epitopes of *H. pylori* LPS

Whereas anti-Lewis antigen autoantibodies have been shown to be raised in response to *H. pylori* infection and to contribute to generation of diseases, we did not found significantly increased levels of any anti-Lewis antigen antibodies in *H. pylori*-infected gastroduodenal disease patients, *H. pylori*-positive individuals, and *H. pylori*-negative individuals (Amano et al., 1997). The reactivity of human antisera to *H. pylori* LPS derived from various strains was examined and a classification of *H. pylori* LPS has been proposed based on the antigenicity of O-polysaccharides to humans, namely highly-antigenic-epitope-carrying LPS and weakly-antigenic-epitope-carrying LPS (Yokota et al., 1998; Yokota et al., 2000b). The two epitopes were clearly characterized by examining serum absorption by LPS (Fig. 3). All *H. pylori* strains carrying the O-polysaccharide chain (namely, smooth strains) isolated in Japan have either one or the other epitope, but not both. The existence of these epitopes does not relate to that of the Lewis antigen structures. Most (over 95%) of *H. pylori*-infected individuals, including gastroduodenal patients and asymptomatic individuals, have a high titer of antibodies against the anti-highly-antigenic epitope in their sera. It is therefore proposed that the highly-antigenic epitope-carrying LPS are applicable to diagnosis of *H. pylori* infection (Amano et al., 1998) (Table 1). As an advantage, the LPS antigen is more stable against heat, drying and humidity than protein antigens. On the other hand, about half of *H. pylori*-infected individuals have antibodies against the weakly-antigenic epitope at a lower titer than those against the highly-antigenic epitope. The antibody titer against the weakly-antigenic epitope is significantly higher in gastroduodenal patients than in asymptomatic individuals with *H. pylori* infection (Yokota et al., 2000a). The antibodies against the weakly-antigenic epitope could relate to chronic and active infection of *H. pylori*.

Human serum containing:	No. of sera
anti-highly antigenic epitope antibody only	31 (52.5%)
anti-weakly antigenic epitope antibody only	4 (6.8%)
both antibodies	24 (40.7%)

Table 1. Frequency of anti-*H. pylori* LPS epitope antibodies in 59 sera derived from *H. pylori*-infected individuals.

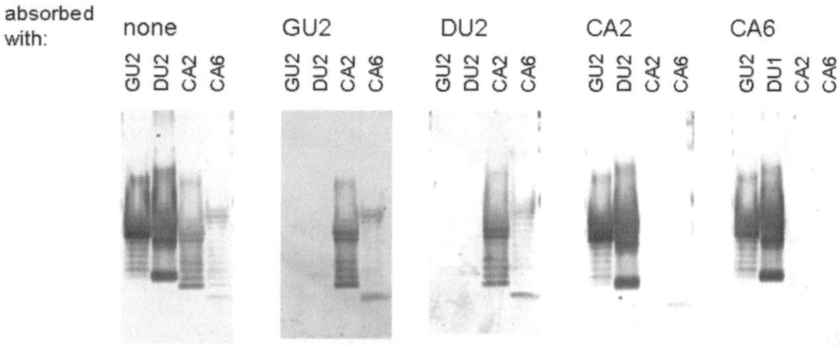

Fig. 3. Reactivity of human serum containing antibodies against both highly-antigenic epitope and weakly-antigenic epitope in *H. pylori* LPS determined by Western blotting and absorption with LPS.
Serum from one individual containing antibodies against both epitopes was absorbed with the indicated LPS at 37 C for 1 h, and used in Western blotting. LPS derived from strains GU2 and DU2 are highly-antigenic epitope-containing. LPS derived from strains CA2 and CA6 are weakly-antigenic epitope-containing.

5. Usage of TLRs by *H. pylori* LPS

TLR usage by *H. pylori* LPS remains controversial. An important issue to consider in these kinds of studies is the presence of contaminants with endotoxin-like activities, for example lipopeptides of *H. pylori* and other bacterial LPS, in the *H. pylori* LPS preparations. The extremely low level activity of *H. pylori* LPS means that very low level contamination cannot be ignored. Alternatively, as described above, structural heterogeneity exists in *H. pylori* lipid A and therefore different TLR usage could depend on lipid A structural variation.

Whereas the weakly endotoxic activity of *H. pylori* LPS is widely accepted, TLR usage has been controversial with some researchers reporting that *H. pylori* LPS transduces signaling via the TLR4/MD2/CD14 complex like a typical LPS and others reporting signaling transduction via TLR2 as summarized in Table 2. Another report describes antagonistic activity of *H. pylori* LPS derived from some strains to TLR4-mediated typical LPS signaling (Lepper et al., 2005).

Strains having the highly-antigenic epitope-carrying LPS are frequently found in those derived from patients with chronic gastritis. Strains having the weakly-antigenic epitope-carrying LPS are predominantly found in those derived from patients with gastric cancer (Yokota et al., 2000b; Yokota et al., 1997) (Fig. 4).

Report	Usage of TLR	*H. pylori* strain	Purification method of LPS	Experimental evidences
Kawahara et al,(2001)	TLR4	Various strains	Hot phenol water/ ultracentrifugation	Using primary gastric mucosa cells derived from guinea pig. The cells are negative for TLR2.
Ogawa et al. (2000), (2003)	TLR4	206-1	Synthetic lipid A	Using human peripheral blood mononuclear cells. The activities are neutralized by anti-TLR4 antibodies.
Ishihara et al. (2004)	TLR2	26695	Reextraction method described by (Hirschfeld et al., 2000)	Luciferase reporter gene assay using HEK293 cells transfected with TLRs.
Lepper et al. (2005)	TLR2	Various strains	Reextraction method described by (Hirschfeld et al., 2000)	Luciferase reporter gene assay using HEK293 and COS cells transfected with TLRs. LPS derived from some strains shares activity that antagonized TLR4.
Yokota et al. (2007)	TLR2	Various clinical isolates	Reextraction (treatment with proteinase K and lipoprotein lipases / HIC[a])	Luciferase reporter gene assay using HEK293 cells transfected with TLRs. Effect of the expression of dominant negative mutants of TLRs.
Chochi et al. (2008)	TLR4	A clinical isolate	Not described (donated from Ohtsuka Co.)	Using 4 gastric cancer cell lines. The activities are neutralized by anti-TLR4 antibodies.
Smith et al. (2011)	TLR2	3 reference strains and 4 clinical strains	Hot phenol water/proteinase K and nuclease treatment / ultracentrifugation	Using HEK293 cells transfected with TLR2. Using TLR2-negative gastric cell line AGS.

Table 2. Interaction between *H. pylori* LPS and TLRs.
[a]HIC: hydrophobic interaction chromatography.

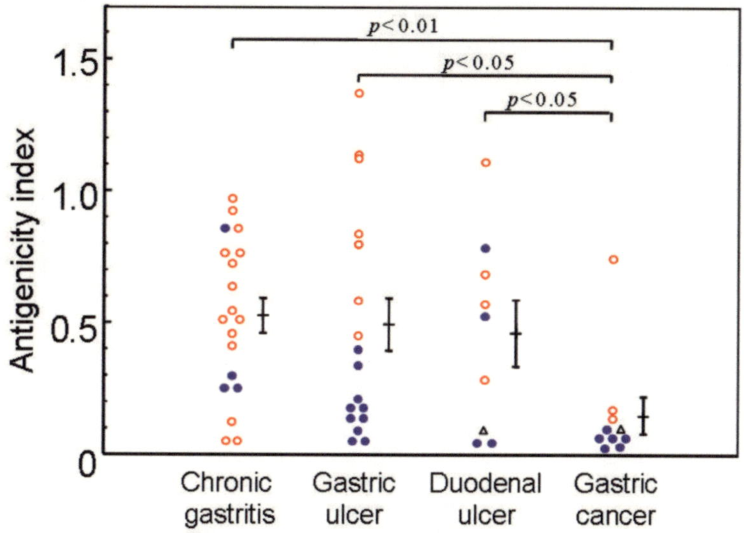

Fig. 4. Antigenicity and antigenic type of *H. pylori* isolated from various clinical sources. Antigenicity index is expressed as the mean values of ELISA reading for 15 randomly selected serum samples from *H. pylori*-infected individuals. Red open circle: Strains with LPS carrying the highly-antigenic epitope. Blue close circle: Strains with LPS carrying the weakly-antigenic epitope. Triangle: Rough strains.

6. Novel biological activities of *H. pylori* LPS

While a consensus has gotten on that *H. pylori* LPS share low toxicity as an endotoxin, some important biological activities have been observed. Chochi et al. (2008) reported that both *H. pylori* and *E. coli* LPS enhance the proliferation rate of gastric cancer cell lines. However, they also showed that *H. pylori* LPS, but not *E. coli* LPS, attenuates the cytotoxicity of mononuclear cells against gastric cancer cells, and downregulates perforin production in $CD56^+$ natural killer cells cocultured with gastric cancer cells. Both the mitogenic activity, in common with *E. coli*, and the *H. pylori*-specific decrease in cytotoxicity of natural killer cells are likely to promote tumorigenesis. Grebowska et al. report that *H. pylori* LPS suppress phagocytic activity of human peripheral blood granulocytes (Grebowska et al., 2008) and *H. pylori* LPS-chased macrophages have low activity of lymphocyte proliferation (Grebowska et al., 2010). They speculate that these activities contribute to chronic infection of *H pylori*.

Slomiany et al. reported that *H. pylori* LPS disrupts gastric mucin synthesis, increases caspase-3 activity, causes apoptosis, and upregulates endothelin-1 and TNF-α via p38 and ERK MAP kinase cascade activation (Slomiany et al., 1999; Slomiany & Slomiany, 2002). Furthermore, it inhibits glycation and sulfation in gastric mucin biosynthesis (Slomiany et al., 1992). Kawahara et al. (2001) reported that the LPS of *H. pylori*, as well as that of *E. coli*, upregulates mitogen oxidase 1 (Mox1), which leads to the generation of superoxide anions. Young et al. (1992) report that it stimulates gastric mucosal pepsinogen secretion. These are likely to lead to injury of gastric mucosa.

We found that pretreatment of gastric epithelial cell lines with *H. pylori* LPS enhanced the expression of TLR4 and also the responsiveness to *E. coli* LPS (Fig. 5-C) (Yokota et al., 2010). These gastric epithelial cell lines express markedly low levels of TLR4. *H. pylori* LPS

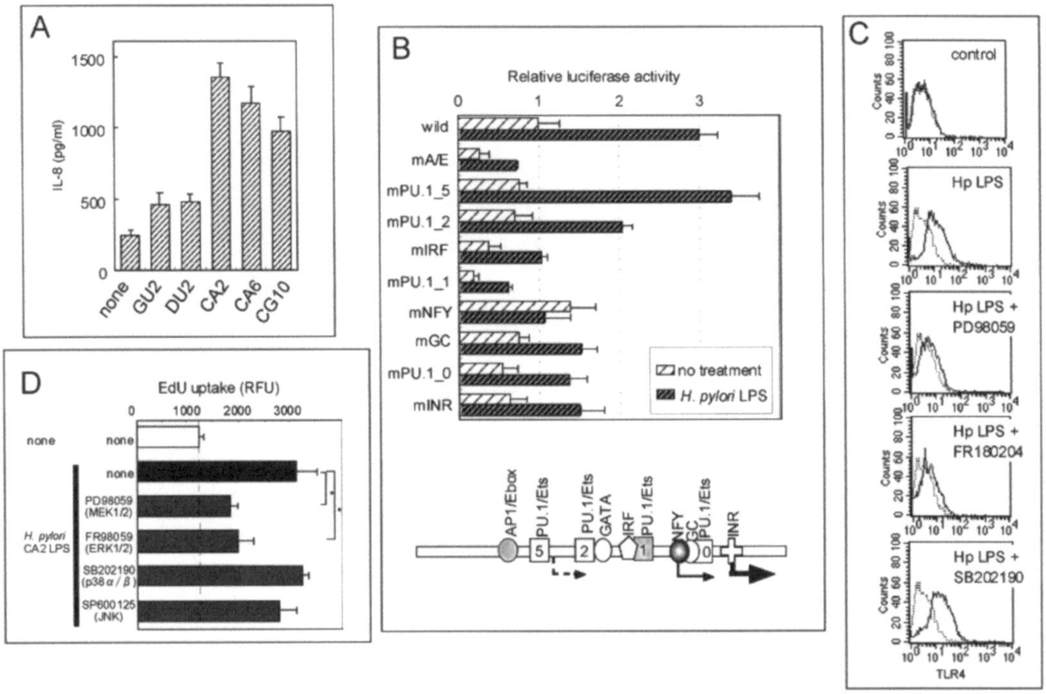

Fig. 5. A. Pretreatment with *H. pylori* LPS enhanced *E. coli* LPS-induced IL-8 production. Gastric cancer cell line MKN28 was treated with *H. pylori* LPS (100 ng/ml) for 24 h, then treated with *E. coli* LPS (1000 ng/ml) for 24 h, and IL-8 in the culture supernatants was measured by ELISA. LPS derived from GU2 and DU2 *H. pylori* strains is highly-antigenic epitope-carrying. LPS derived from CA2 and CA6 strains is weakly-antigenic LPS-carrying. LPS derived from CG10 strain is rough-type.

B. TLR4 promoter activity with *H. pylori* CA2 LPS treatment determined by the luciferase reporter assay. Luciferase gene-conjugated promoters with a series of mutations introduced in the transcription factor binding motifs indicated were used. NF-Y binding motif is indicated to be important for transcriptional induction of TLR4 by *H. pylori* LPS.

C. Enhancement of TLR4 expression by *H. pylori* LPS and effect of inhibitors for MAP kinases. MKN28 cells were treated with *H. pylori* CA2 LPS (100 ng/ml) for 24 h, and then TLR4 on the cell surface was analyzed by flow cytometry.

D. Enhancement of gastric epithelial cell growth by *H. pylori* LPS and effect of MAP kinase inhibitors. MKN28 cells were treated with *H. pylori* CA2 LPS (100 ng/ml) for 18 h, and then cell proliferation rate was measured by the uptake of 5-ethinyl-2′-deoxyuridine into DNA. MAP kinase inhibitors used were PD98059 (MEK1/2 inhibitor; 50 μM), FR180204 (ERK1/2 inhibitor; 5 μM), SB202190 (p38 inhibitor; 5 μM), and SP600125 (JNK inhibitor; 10 μM).

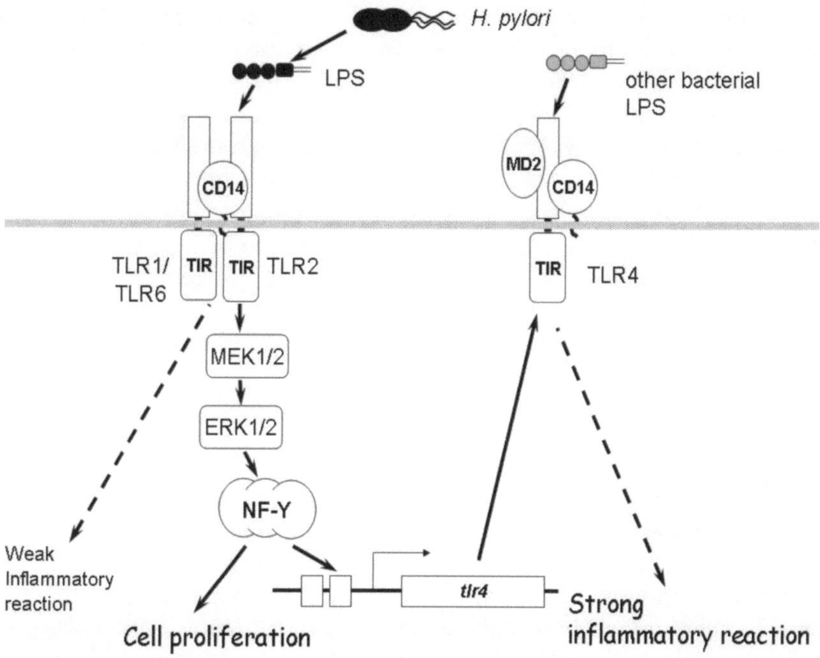

Fig. 6. Proposed action of *H. pylori* LPS on gastric epithelial cells.
H. pylori LPS upregulates TLR4 and augments cell proliferation via TLR2 and the MEK1/2-ERK1/2 MAP kinase pathway in gastric epithelial cells. These activities are likely to enhance the inflammatory response, by increasing the activity of highly endotoxic typical LPS derived from other bacteria, and tumorigenesis.

recognized by TLR2, preferentially as a TLR2/TLR1 complex, activated MEK-ERK MAP kinase cascade and the transcription factor NF-Y, and upregulated transcription of the TLR4 gene (Fig. 5-B). In consistent with the in vitro observation, Asahi et al. (2007) indicate that higher expression of TLR4 is observed in biopsy specimens in the antral and corpus mucosa from *H. pylori*-infected patients than *H. pylori*-negative individuals. Backhed et al. (2003) report that primary gastric antral cells do not express TLR4, in contrast, several epithelial cell lines derived form gastric cancer do. The upregulated TLR4 in the gastric epithelial cells causes more efficient transduction of inflammatory signals by typical LPS, such as LPS derived from *Enterobacteriaceae* (Fig. 5-A).

In concordance with the report of Chochi et al. (2008), *H. pylori* LPS was shown to upregulate the cell growth rate of gastric epithelial cell lines (Yokota et al., 2010) (Fig. 5-D). Activation of the MEK-ERK MAP kinase pathway via TLR2 activates NF-Y, and the NF-Y transcriptionally activates various cell cycle regulation genes, such as cyclin A1, cyclin B2, and E2F1. However, there are some contradictions between our report (Yokota et al., 2010) and the report of Chochi et al. (2008). We found that the mitogenic activity was *H. pylori*-specific. With respect to TLR usage, Chochi et al. (2008) showed that anti-TLR4 antibody can neutralize the activity; however, we found that downregulation of TLR2 expression by siRNA diminished the activity (Yokota et al., 2010).

The novel activities of *H. pylori* LPS reported by us (Yokota et al., 2010) (Fig. 6) are more potent in weakly-antigenic epitope-carrying LPS frequently isolated from gastric cancer, than in highly-antigenic LPS-carrying strains. The weakly-antigenic LPS-carrying *H. pylori* strains are suggested to be more potent inducers of gastric cancer. The potent activities of the weakly-antigenic LPS may be due to interaction of *H. pylori* LPS with host SP-D. A recent study indicates that SP-D enhances *E. coli* LPS-induced proinflammatory cytokine production upregulated by *H. pylori* LPS pretreatment (Yokota et al. unpublished results). SP-D interacts more strongly with weakly-antigenic epitope-carrying LPS than highly-antigenic epitope-carrying LPS. The β-linked *N*-acetyl-glucosamine residue is suggested to be important for the highly-antigenic epitope, and digestion of the residue by a β-*N*-acetyl-glucosamindase abolished the reactivity with anti-highly antigenic epitope antibody and appeared reactivity with anti-weakly antigenic epiotpe antibodies (Yokota et al., unpublished results). The β-galacotose residue is implicated in the weakly antigenic epitope and interaction with SP-D.

7. Concluding remarks

We propose the existence of two antigenic epitopes in *H. pylori* LPS. One of these, the weakly-antigenic epiotpe-carrying LPS, appears to occur frequently in strains derived from gastric cancer patients, as compared with chronic gastritis patients. The anti-weakly-antigenic epitope antibody titers are higher in gastroduodenal patients than in asymptomatic *H. pylori*-infected individuals. The weakly-antigenic epitope-carrying LPS has stronger biological activity than the highly-antigenic epitope-carrying LPS. From these lines of evidence, strains carrying highly-antigenic epitope may change to strains carrying weakly-antigenic epitope during infection periods and disease progression status (Fig. 7). This phenotypic change leads to an escape strategy for *H. pylori* from host immune response

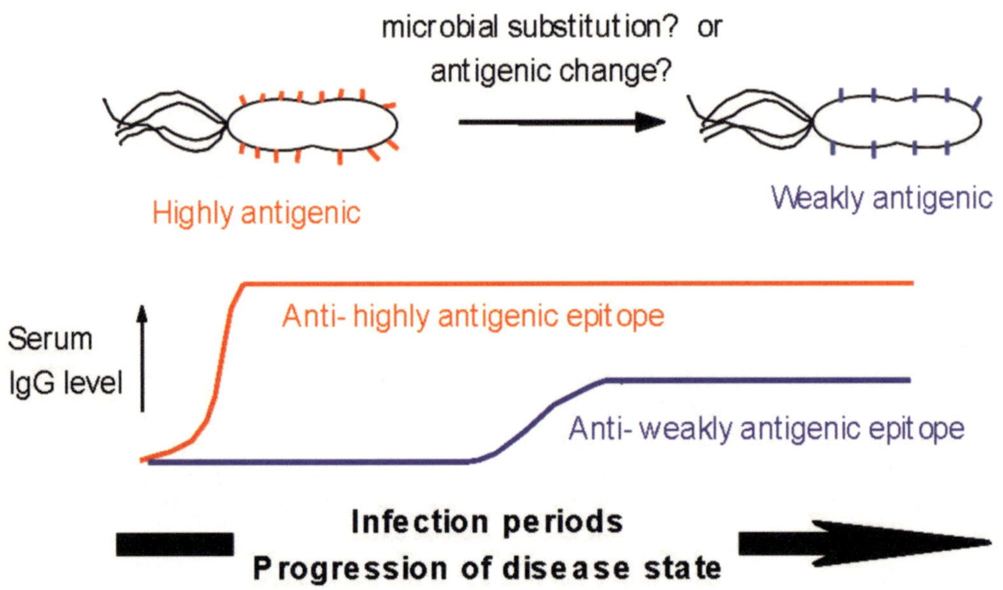

Fig. 7. Relationship between changes of antigenic epitopes of *H. pylori* LPS, serum antibody titers to *H. pylori* LPS epitopes, and infection periods.

and to an increase in virulence. It is not clear whether the phenotypic change occurs by antigenic change of one strain or by microbial substitution. But the presence or not of a β-*N*-acetyl-glucosamine residue of the polysaccharide chain of LPS appears to determine the antigenic conversion. Molecular studies of biosynthesis of LPS, for example glycosyltransferase expressions, are now required to elucidate these changes.

We propose that *H. pylori* LPS enhances the inflammatory reaction induced by other bacterial LPS and upregulates the growth rate of epithelial cells via activation of the MEK1/2-ERK1/2 MAP kinase cascade. A putative role for *H. pylori* LPS as a pathogenic factor is shown in Fig. 8. In an *H. pylori*-uninfected gastric mucosa, Gram-negative bacteria invading orally do not cause a strong inflammatory response in gastric mucosa because the expression levels of TLR4 are low in gastric epithelial cells. On infection with *H. pylori, H. pylori* LPS upregulates TLR4 via TLR2 signaling in gastric epithelial cells. The upregulation of TLR4 leads to increased susceptibility of epithelial cells to typical LPS derived from other bacteria. Although the acids of gastric juice kill orally invading bacteria, LPS should be still stable. *H. pylori* LPS itself showed extremely weak endotoxic activity and therefore does not cause acute and systemic inflammatory reaction, such as sepsis. This strategy enables *H. pylori* to escape the host immune system and establish chronic infection. On the other hand, *H. pylori* LPS sets the stage for inflammatory response and tumorigenesis in the gastric mucosa during chronic infection, in other words, colonization.

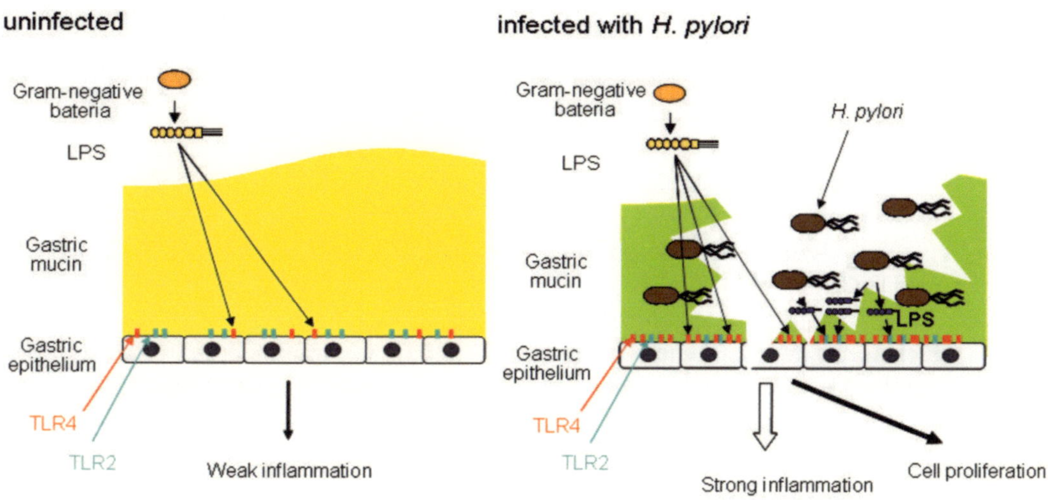

Fig. 8. Hypothesis for a pathogenic role of weakly-endotoxic *H. pylori* LPS in gastric mucosa. Uninfected state: Expression of TLR4 on the epithelial cells in gastric mucosa is low. So LPS derived from orally invaded bacteria does not induce a strong inflammatory response.
H. pylori-infected state: *H. pylori* LPS itself causes low-level direct inflammation and tissue injury. At the same time, *H. pylori* LPS induces TLR4 expression on the epithelial cells in gastric mucosa, and therefore LPS with high endotoxic activity derived from orally invading bacteria causes higher level inflammation than in the *H. pylori*-uninfected state.

8. References

Amano, K., Hayashi, S., Kubota, T., Fujii, N. & Yokota, S. (1997). Reactivities of Lewis antigen monoclonal antibodies with the lipopolysaccharides of *Helicobacter pylori* strains isolated from patients with gastroduodenal diseases in Japan. *Clinical and Diagnostic Laboratory Immunology* Vol. 4, No. 5, pp. 540-544, ISSN 1556-679X.

Amano, K., Yokota, S., Ishioka, T., Hayashi, S., Kubota, T. & Fujii, N. (1998). Utilization of proteinase K-treated cells as lipopolysaccharide antigens for the serodiagnosis of *Helicobacter pylori* infections. *Microbiology and Immunology* Vol. 42, No. 7, pp. 509-514, ISSN 1348-0421.

Andersen-Nissen, E., Smith, K. D., Strobe, K. L., Barrett, S. L., Cookson, B. T., Logan, S. M. & Aderem, A. (2005). Evasion of Toll-like receptor 5 by flagellated bacteria. *Proceedings of the National Academy of Sciences of the United States of America* Vol. 102, No. 26, pp. 9247-9252., ISSN 1091-6490.

Appelmelk, B. J., Simoons-Smit, I., Negrini, R., Moran, A. P., Aspinall, G. O., Forte, J. G., de Vries, T., Quan, H., Verboom, T., Maaskant, J. J., Ghiara, P., Kuipers, E. J., Bloemena, E., Tadema, T. M., Townsend, R. R., Tyagarajan, K., Crothers, J. M., Jr., Monterio, M. A., Savio, A. & de Graaff, J. (1996). Potential role of molecular mimicry between *Helicobacter pylori* lipopolysaccharide and host Lewis blood group antigens in autoimmunity. *Infection and Immunity* Vol. 64, No. 6, pp. 2031-2040, ISSN 1098-5522.

Asahi, K., Fu, H. Y., Hayashi, Y., Eguchi, H., Murata, H., Tsujii, M., Tsuji, S., Tanimura, H. & Kawano, S. (2007). *Helicobacter pylori* infection affects Toll-like receptor 4 expression in human gastric mucosa. *Hepato-gastroenterology* Vol. 54, No. 79, pp. 1941-1944, ISSN 0172-6390.

Aspinall, G. O., Monteiro, M. A., Shaver, R. T., Kurjanczyk, L. A. & Penner, J. L. (1997). Lipopolysaccharides of *Helicobacter pylori* serogroups O:3 and O:6. Structures of a class of lipopolysaccharides with reference to the location of oligomeric units of D-*glycero*-α-D-*manno*-heptose residues. *European Journal of Biochemistry* Vol. 248, No. 2, pp. 592-601, ISSN 1432-1033.

Backhed, F., Rokbi, B., Torstensson, E., Zhao, Y., Nilsson, C., Seguin, D., Normark, S., Buchan, A. M. & Richter-Dahlfors, A. (2003). Gastric mucosal recognition of *Helicobacter pylori* is independent of Toll-like receptor 4. *Journal of Infectious Diseases* Vol. 187, No. 5, pp. 829-836, ISSN 0022-1899.

Bergman, M. P., Engering, A., Smits, H. H., van Vliet, S. J., van Bodegraven, A. A., Wirth, H. P., Kapsenberg, M. L., Vandenbroucke-Grauls, C. M., van Kooyk, Y. & Appelmelk, B. J. (2004). *Helicobacter pylori* modulates the T helper cell 1/T helper cell 2 balance through phase-variable interaction between lipopolysaccharide and DC-SIGN. *Journal of Experimental Medicine* Vol. 200, No. 8, pp. 979-990, ISSN 1540-9538.

Chochi, K., Ichikura, T., Kinoshita, M., Majima, T., Shinomiya, N., Tsujimoto, H., Kawabata, T., Sugasawa, H., Ono, S., Seki, S. & Mochizuki, H. (2008). *Helicobacter pylori* augments growth of gastric cancers via the lipopolysaccharide-toll-like receptor 4 pathway whereas its lipopolysaccharide attenuates antitumor activities of human mononuclear cells. *Clinical Cancer Research* Vol. 14, No. 10, pp. 2909-2917, ISSN 1557-3265.

Fowler, M., Thomas, R. J., Atherton, J., Roberts, I. S. & High, N. J. (2006). Galectin-3 binds to *Helicobacter pylori* O-antigen: it is upregulated and rapidly secreted by gastric epithelial cells in response to *H. pylori* adhesion. *Cellular Microbiology* Vol. 8, No. 1, pp. 44-54, ISSN 1462-5822.

Glocker, E., Lange, C., Covacci, A., Bereswill, S., Kist, M. & Pahl, H. L. (1998). Proteins encoded by the cag pathogenicity island of *Helicobacter pylori* are required for NF-κB activation. *Infection and Immunity* Vol. 66, No. 5, pp. 2346-2348., ISSN 1098-5522.

Grebowska, A., Moran, A.P., Matusiak, A., Bak-Romaniszyn, L., Czkwianianc, E., Rechcinski, T., Walencka, M., Płaneta-Małecka, I., Rudnicka, W. & Chmiela, M. (2008). Anti-phagocytic activity of *Helicobacter pylori* lipopolysaccharide (LPS)-possible modulation of the innate immune response to these bacteria. *Polish Journal of Microbiology* Vol. 57, No. 3, pp. 185-192, ISSN 1733-1331.

Grebowska, A., Moran, A.P., Bielanski, W., Matusiak, A., Rechcinski, T., Rudnicka, K., Baranowska, A., Rudnicka, W. & Chmiela, M. (2010). *Helicobacter pylori* lipopolysaccharide activity in human peripheral blood mononuclear leukocyte cultures. *Journal of Physiology and Pharmacology* Vol. 61, No. 4, pp. 437-442, ISSN 0867-5910.

Heine, H., Muller-Loennies, S., Brade, L., Lindner, B. & Brade, H. (2003). Endotoxic activity and chemical structure of lipopolysaccharides from *Chlamydia trachomatis* serotypes E and L2 and *Chlamydophila psittaci* 6BC. *European Journal of Biochemistry* Vol. 270, No. 3, pp. 440-450., ISSN 1432-1033.

Heneghan, M. A., McCarthy, C. F., Janulaityte, D. & Moran, A. P. (2001). Relationship of anti-Lewis x and anti-Lewis y antibodies in serum samples from gastric cancer and chronic gastritis patients to *Helicobacter pylori*-mediated autoimmunity. *Infection and Immunity* Vol. 69, No. 8, pp. 4774-4781, ISSN 1098-5522.

Hildebrandt, E. & McGee, D.J. (2009). *Helicobacter pylori* lipopolysaccharide modification, Lewis antigen expression, and gastric colonization are cholesterol-dependent. *BMC Microbiology* Vol. 9, (December 14), Article ID 258, ISSN 1471-2180.

Hirschfeld, M., Ma, Y., Weis, J. H., Vogel, S. N. & Weis, J. J. (2000). Cutting edge: repurification of lipopolysaccharide eliminates signaling through both human and murine toll-like receptor 2. *Journal of Immunology* Vol. 165, No. 2, pp. 618-622, ISSN 1550-6606.

Hofman, P., Waidner, B., Hofman, V., Bereswill, S., Brest, P. & Kist, M. (2004). Pathogenesis of *Helicobacter pylori* infection. *Helicobacter* Vol. 9, Suppl. 1, pp. 15-22, ISSN 1523-5378.

Ishihara, S., Rumi, M. A., Kadowaki, Y., Ortega-Cava, C. F., Yuki, T., Yoshino, N., Miyaoka, Y., Kazumori, H., Ishimura, N., Amano, Y. & Kinoshita, Y. (2004). Essential role of MD-2 in TLR4-dependent signaling during *Helicobacter pylori*-associated gastritis. *Journal of Immunology* Vol. 173, No. 2, pp. 1406-1416., ISSN 1550-6606.

Kawahara, T., Teshima, S., Oka, A., Sugiyama, T., Kishi, K. & Rokutan, K. (2001). Type I *Helicobacter pylori* lipopolysaccharide stimulates toll-like receptor 4 and activates mitogen oxidase 1 in gastric pit cells. *Infection and Immunity* Vol. 69, No. 7, pp. 4382-4389., ISSN 1098-5522.

Khamri, W., Moran, A. P., Worku, M. L., Karim, Q. N., Walker, M. M., Annuk, H., Ferris, J. A., Appelmelk, B. J., Eggleton, P., Reid, K. B. & Thursz, M. R. (2005). Variations in *Helicobacter pylori* lipopolysaccharide to evade the innate immune component surfactant protein D. *Infection and Immunity* Vol. 73, No. 11, pp. 7677-7686, ISSN 1098-5522.

Lepper, P. M., Triantafilou, M., Schumann, C., Schneider, E. M. & Triantafilou, K. (2005). Lipopolysaccharides from *Helicobacter pylori* can act as antagonists for Toll-like receptor 4. *Cellular Microbiology* Vol. 7, No. 4, pp. 519-528., ISSN 1462-5822.

Matsuyama, N., Kirikae, T., Kirikae, F., Hashimoto, M., Amanot, K., Hayashi, S., Hirai, Y., Kubota, T. & Nakano, M. (2001). Non-standard biological activities of lipopolysaccharide from *Helicobacter pylori*. *Journal of Medical Microbiology* Vol. 50, No. 10, pp. 865-869., ISSN 1473-5644.

Monteiro, M. A. (2001). *Helicobacter pylori*: a wolf in sheep's clothing: the glycotype families of *Helicobacter pylori* lipopolysaccharides expressing histo-blood groups: structure, biosynthesis, and role in pathogenesis. *Advances in Carbohydrate Chemistry and Biochemistry* Vol. 57, No. 99-158, ISBN 978-0-12-380854-7.

Moran, A. P. (1999). *Helicobacter pylori* lipopolysaccharide-mediated gastric and extragastric pathology. *Journal of Physiology and Pharmacology* Vol. 50, No. 5, pp. 787-805., ISSN 0867-5910.

Moran, A. P. (2008). Relevance of fucosylation and Lewis antigen expression in the bacterial gastroduodenal pathogen *Helicobacter pylori*. *Carbohydrate Research* Vol. 343, No. 12, pp. 1952-1965, ISSN 0008-6215.

Moran, A. P., Lindner, B. & Walsh, E. J. (1997). Structural characterization of the lipid A component of *Helicobacter pylori* rough- and smooth-form lipopolysaccharides. *Journal of Bacteriology* Vol. 179, No. 20, pp. 6453-6463, ISSN 1098-5530.

Muotiala, A., Helander, I. M., Pyhala, L., Kosunen, T. U. & Moran, A. P. (1992). Low biological activity of *Helicobacter pylori* lipopolysaccharide. *Infection and Immunity* Vol. 60, No. 4, pp. 1714-1716, ISSN 1098-5522.

Murray, E., Khamri, W., Walker, M. M., Eggleton, P., Moran, A. P., Ferris, J. A., Knapp, S., Karim, Q. N., Worku, M., Strong, P., Reid, K. B. & Thursz, M. R. (2002). Expression of surfactant protein D in the human gastric mucosa and during *Helicobacter pylori* infection. *Infection and Immunity* Vol. 70, No. 3, pp. 1481-1487, ISSN 1098-5522.

Negrini, R., Savio, A., Poiesi, C., Appelmelk, B. J., Buffoli, F., Paterlini, A., Cesari, P., Graffeo, M., Vaira, D. & Franzin, G. (1996). Antigenic mimicry between *Helicobacter pylori* and gastric mucosa in the pathogenesis of body atrophic gastritis. *Gastroenterology* Vol. 111, No. 3, pp. 655-665, ISSN 0016-5805.

Netea, M. G., van Deuren, M., Kullberg, B. J., Cavaillon, J. M. & Van der Meer, J. W. (2002). Does the shape of lipid A determine the interaction of LPS with Toll-like receptors? *Trends in Immunology* Vol. 23, No. 3, pp. 135-139., ISSN 1471-4906.

Nielsen, H., Birkholz, S., Andersen, L. P. & Moran, A. P. (1994). Neutrophil activation by *Helicobacter pylori* lipopolysaccharides. *Journal of Infectious Diseases* Vol. 170, No. 1, pp. 135-139, ISSN 1537-6613.

Ogawa, T., Asai, Y., Sakai, Y., Oikawa, M., Fukase, K., Suda, Y., Kusumoto, S. & Tamura, T. (2003). Endotoxic and immunobiological activities of a chemically synthesized lipid A of *Helicobacter pylori* strain 206-1. *FEMS Immunology and Medical Microbiology* Vol. 36, No. 1-2, pp. 1-7., ISSN 1574-695X.

Ogawa, T., Asai, Y., Yamamoto, H., Taiji, Y., Jinno, T., Kodama, T., Niwata, S., Shimauchi, H. & Ochiai, K. (2000). Immunobiological activities of a chemically synthesized lipid A of *Porphyromonas gingivalis*. *FEMS Immunology and Medical Microbiology* Vol. 28, No. 4, pp. 273-281., ISSN 1574-695X.

Smith, S.M., Moran, A.P., Duggan, S.P., Ahmed, S.E., Mohamed, A.S., Windle, H.J., O'Neill, L.A. & Kelleher, D.P. (2011). Tribbles 3: a novel regulator of TLR2-mediated signaling in response to *Helicobacter pylori* lipopolysaccharide. *Journal of Immunology* Vol. 186, No. 4, pp. 2462-2471, ISSN 1550-6606.

Perez-Perez, G. I., Shepherd, V. L., Morrow, J. D. & Blaser, M. J. (1995). Activation of human THP-1 cells and rat bone marrow-derived macrophages by *Helicobacter pylori* lipopolysaccharide. *Infection and Immunity* Vol. 63, No. 4, pp. 1183-1187, ISSN 1098-5522.

Semeraro, N., Montemurro, P., Piccoli, C., Muolo, V., Colucci, M., Giuliani, G., Fumarola, D., Pece, S. & Moran, A. P. (1996). Effect of *Helicobacter pylori* lipopolysaccharide (LPS) and LPS derivatives on the production of tissue factor and plasminogen activator inhibitor type 2 by human blood mononuclear cells. *Journal of Infectious Diseases* Vol. 174, No. 6, pp. 1255-1260., ISSN 1537-6613.

Slomiany, B. L., Liau, Y. H., Lopez, R. A., Piotrowski, J., Czajkowski, A. & Slomiany, A. (1992). Effect of *Helicobacter pylori* lipopolysaccharide on the synthesis of sulfated gastric mucin. *Biochemistry International* Vol. 27, No. 4, pp. 687-697., ISSN 0518-5231.

Slomiany, B. L., Piotrowski, J. & Slomiany, A. (1999). Gastric mucosal inflammatory responses to *Helicobacter pylori* lipopolysaccharide: down-regulation of nitric oxide synthase-2 and caspase-3 by sulglycotide. *Biochemical Biophysical Research Communications* Vol. 261, No. 1, pp. 15-20., ISSN 0006-291X.

Slomiany, B. L. & Slomiany, A. (2002). Disruption in gastric mucin synthesis by *Helicobacter pylori* lipopolysaccharide involves ERK and p38 mitogen-activated protein kinase participation. *Biochemical Biophysical Research Communications* Vol. 294, No. 2, pp. 220-224., ISSN 0006-291X.

Stockl, J., Majdic, O., Rosenkranz, A., Fiebiger, E., Kniep, B., Stockinger, H. & Knapp, W. (1993). Monoclonal antibodies to the carbohydrate structure Lewisx stimulate the adhesive activity of leukocyte integrin CD11b/CD18 (CR3, Mac-1, αmβ2) on human granulocytes. *Journal of Leukocyte Biology* Vol. 53, No. 5, pp. 541-549, ISSN 1938-3673.

Suda, Y., Ogawa, T., Kashihara, W., Oikawa, M., Shimoyama, T., Hayashi, T., Tamura, T. & Kusumoto, S. (1997). Chemical structure of lipid A from *Helicobacter pylori* strain

206-1 lipopolysaccharide. *Journal of Biochemistry* Vol. 121, No. 6, pp. 1129-1133, ISSN 1083-351X.

Tran, A. X., Stead, C. M. & Trent, M. S. (2005). Remodeling of *Helicobacter pylori* lipopolysaccharide. *Journal of Endotoxin Research* Vol. 11, No. 3, pp. 161-166, ISSN 1743-2839.

Xia, H. H. & Talley, N. J. (2001). Apoptosis in gastric epithelium induced by *Helicobacter pylori* infection: implications in gastric carcinogenesis. *American Journal of Gastroenterology* Vol. 96, No. 1, pp. 16-26, ISSN 1572-0241.

Yokota, S., Amano, K., Fujii, N. & Yokochi, T. (2000a). Comparison of serum antibody titers to *Helicobacter pylori* lipopolysaccharides, CagA, VacA and partially purified cellular extracts in a Japanese population. *FEMS Microbiology Letts* Vol. 185, No. 2, pp. 193-198., ISSN 1574-6968.

Yokota, S., Amano, K., Hayashi, S. & Fujii, N. (1997). Low antigenicity of the polysaccharide region of *Helicobacter pylori* lipopolysaccharides derived from tumors of patients with gastric cancer. *Infection and Immunity* Vol. 65, No. 9, pp. 3509-3512, ISSN 1098-5522.

Yokota, S., Amano, K., Hayashi, S., Kubota, T., Fujii, N. & Yokochi, T. (1998). Human antibody response to *Helicobacter pylori* lipopolysaccharide: presence of an immunodominant epitope in the polysaccharide chain of lipopolysaccharide. *Infection and Immunity* Vol. 66, No. 6, pp. 3006-3011, ISSN 1098-5522.

Yokota, S., Amano, K., Shibata, Y., Nakajima, M., Suzuki, M., Hayashi, S., Fujii, N. & Yokochi, T. (2000b). Two distinct antigenic types of the polysaccharide chains of *Helicobacter pylori* lipopolysaccharides characterized by reactivity with sera from humans with natural infection. *Infection and Immunity* Vol. 68, No. 1. pp. 151-159, ISSN 1098-5522.

Yokota, S., Ohnishi, T., Muroi, M., Tanamoto, K., Fujii, N. & Amano, K. (2007). Highly-purified *Helicobacter pylori* LPS preparations induce weak inflammatory reactions and utilize Toll-like receptor 2 complex but not Toll-like receptor 4 complex. *FEMS Immunology and Medical Microbiology* Vol. 51, No. 1, pp. 140-148, ISSN 1574-695X.

Yokota, S., Okabayashi, T., Rehli, M., Fujii, N. & Amano, K. (2010). *Helicobacter pylori* lipopolysaccharides upregulate toll-like receptor 4 expression and proliferation of gastric epithelial cells via the MEK1/2-ERK1/2 mitogen-activated protein kinase pathway. *Infection and Immunity* Vol. 78, No. 1, pp. 468-476, ISSN 1098-5522.

Young, G. O., Stemmet, N., Lastovica, A., van der Merwe, E. L., Louw, J. A., Modlin, I. M. & Marks, I. N. (1992). *Helicobacter pylori* lipopolysaccharide stimulates gastric mucosal pepsinogen secretion. *Alimentary Pharmacology and Therapeutics* Vol. 6, No. 2, pp. 169-177., ISSN 1365-2036.

Yuki, N. (1999). Pathogenesis of Guillain-Barre and Miller Fisher syndromes subsequent to *Campylobacter jejuni* enteritis. *Japanese Journal of Infectious Diseases* Vol. 52, No. 3, pp. 99-105., ISSN 1884-2836.

14

Virulence Factors of *Helicobacter pylori* and Their Relationship with the Development of Early and Advanced Distal Intestinal Type Gastric Adenocarcinoma

Bruna Maria Roesler, Sandra Cecília Botelho Costa
and José Murilo Robilotta Zeitune
State University of Campinas
Brazil

1. Introduction

The first isolation of *Helicobacter pylori* (*H. pylori*) in 1980s by Marshall and Warren (Marshall & Warren, 1984) ushered in a new era in gastric microbiology, and, in conjunction with increased interest in the pathogenesis of gastroduodenal diseases, has led to important breakthroughs in medical care (Dunn et al., 1997).

H. pylori is a spiral-shaped gram-negative flagellate bacterium that demonstrates bluntly rounded ends in gastric biopsy specimens (Goodwin et al., 1987). *H. pylori* organisms are 2.5 to 5.0 μm long and 0.5 to 1.0 μm wide, with four to six polar sheathed flagellas, which are essential for bacterial motility (Goodwin & Armstrong, 1990).

H. pylori was the first pathogenic microorganism that had its genome sequenced in two different strains. In 1997, *H. pylori* strain 26695 was firstly isolated from an English patient with chronic gastritis and then sequenced. It had a circular chromosome composed of 1.667.867 base pairs (Tomb et al., 1997). In 1999, strain J99 was isolated from an American patient with duodenal ulcer and then sequenced. This presented a similar, overall genomic organization, gene order and prediction of proteomes when compared to strain 26695 (Alm et al., 1999). In 2006, a chronic atrophic gastritis strain, HPAG1, was isolated and sequenced from a Swedish old patient (Oh et al., 2006). More recently, strain G27 was isolated from an Italian patient and had a similar size to the other three strains (Baltrus et al., 2009). Finally, other strains were sequenced, such as Shi470, B128 and 98-10 (McClain et al., 2009; Thiberge et al., 2010).

The finding of strain-specific genes from the comparison of the sequenced strains is in agreement with the earlier studies which demonstrated the high diversity of the *H. pylori* genome (Akopyanz et al., 1992; Han et al., 2003). Consequently, this high level of genetic diversity can be an important factor in its adaptation to the host stomach and also for the clinical outcome of the infection, an aspect that remains unclear. However, it is thought to involve an interplay between the virulence of the infecting strain, host genetics and environmental factors (Kabir, 2009) and experience with other bacterial pathogens suggests that *H. pylori*-specific factors may exist that influence the microorganism pathogenicity.

According to Yamaoka (2008), many putative virulence genes of *H. pylori* have been reported to determine clinical outcomes, and these are generally classified into three categories. The first one contains strain-specific genes, which are present in only some *H. pylori* strains. Among them, the best studied is the cag pathogenicity island (PAI), which encodes a bacterial type IV secretory apparatus (Censini et al., 1996). The second group is the phase-variable genes which the gene status can be changed during growth or in different conditions. Based on the comparison of the three first sequenced genomes of *H. pylori,* six genes encoding outer-membrane proteins (oipA, sabA, sabB, babB, babC and hopZ) are thought to undergo phase variation (Tomb et al., 1997; Alm et al., 1999; Oh et al., 2006). The last group of genes is with variable structures and genotypes depending on the strain, as example the vacA gene. Besides, the structure of many genes differs between Western strains and East Asian strains, and the structural differences in some genes are reported to influence virulence (Lu et al., 2007; Yamaoka, 2008). So, in this chapter, among virulence factors are described and analysed urease, vacA, cagA, cagT and dupA genes.

H. pylori urease is a potent stimulus of mononuclear phagocyte activation and inflammatory cytokine production (Harris et al., 1996). It appears to function as both a colonization factor and a virulence factor (Dun et al., 1997). The urease C gene, or glmM gene (Foxall et al., 1992), a particular region of the urease gene, is specific to *H. pylori* and can be used for primary identification of the microorganism (Moore et al., 1993). The urease gene can also be used to prove the heterogeneity of *H. pylori* strains. For instance, its heterogeneity can be seen by the diversity of patterns obtained by a restriction fragment length polymorphism (RFLP) of urease C and urease B genes, which is able to differentiate many strains presented in diverse pathologies, such as chronic gastritis and peptic ulcer, caused by this bacterium (Roesler et al., 2009).

Other of the major determinants of *H. pylori* virulence is VacA (vacuolating cytotoxin), a toxin that induces cytoplasmic vacuolation in gastric cells (Figura et al., 1989), membrane channel formation, apoptosis and immunomodulation (Atherton et al., 1995; Cover & Blanke, 2005). The vacA gene is present in all strains and comprises of two variable parts. The s-region encodes the signal peptide and is located at the 5´end of the gene which exists as an s1 or s2 allele, while the m-region (middle) occurs as an m1 or m2 allele (van Door et al. 1998). The production of vacuolating cytotoxin is related to the mosaic combination of s and m allelic types and has been associated to specific genotypes with different outcomes (Telford et al., 1994; van Door et al., 1998).

The cytotoxin-associated gene (cag) pathogenicity island (PAI) is approximately a 40-kb cluster of genes in the *H. pylori* chromosome and can be divided into two regions, cag I and cag II (Censini et al., 1996), according to a novel insertion sequence. This gene encodes a type IV secretion system, which delivers CagA into the cytosol of gastric epithelial cells through a rigid needle structure covered by CagY, a VirB10-homologous protein and CagT, a VirB7-homologous protein, at the base (Covacci & Rappuoli, 2000; Rohde et al., 2003). *H. pylori* cagA positive strains are associated with higher grades of inflammation and a significantly increased risk of developing gastric cancer (Parsonnet et al., 1997). cagT gene is found at the base of the outgrowing pilus of the type IV secretion system and is supposed to be responsible for binding to a cellular receptor to induce interleukine-8 secretion and eject CagA (Rohde et al., 2003).

Finally, the duodenal ulcer promoting gene (dupA) was the first putative disease specific marker whose association was described using *H. pylori* strains obtained in both Asian

(Japan and Korea) and Western (Colombia) regions (Lu et al., 2005). dupA gene is suggested to be a vir homologue and encompasses the sequences jhp0917 and jhp0918, as described in strain J99. This gene is associated with interleukin-8 induction (Schmidt et al., 2009) and is possibly part of a yet unidentified type IV secretion system (Lu et al., 2005). The original description of dupA reported that its presence was inversely related to mucosal atrophy and gastric cancer (Zhang et al., 2008, Yamaoka, 2008).

H. pylori is an universal distribution bacterium which affects more than half of the world population, and is considered an important public health problem. Even though its transmission pathways are not completely clarified (Rothenbacher et al., 1998), infection by *H. pylori* is usually acquired during childhood and is characterized as being chronic, with greater prevalence in developing countries in all ages (Kodaira et al., 2002).

Colonization with *H. pylori* is not actually a disease but a condition that affects the relative risk of developing various clinical disorders of the upper gastrointestinal tract (Kusters et al., 2006) and, possibly, extradigestive disorders (Gasbarrini et al., 1999; Figura et al., 2010). In the first case, *H. pylori* infection is responsible for the development of chronic gastritis, peptic ulcers, mucosa associated lymphoid tissue (MALT lymphoma) and gastric adenocarcinoma (Ahmed & Sechi, 2005). Regarding to extradigestive diseases, *H. pylori* infection has been associated with iron-deficiency anemia (Capurso et al., 2001), idiopathic thrombocytopenic purpura (Pellicano et al., 2009; Arnold et al., 2009), cardiovascular diseases (Franceschi et al., 2009), hepatobiliary diseases (Isaeva et al., 2009; Pirouz et al., 2009) and amongst others.

Especially with regards to gastric cancer, the interest in *H. pylori* as a cause of this illness began after the pioneering discoveries of Marshall and Warren. Prior to the discovery of the organism, it was known that gastric adenocarcinomas typically arose in areas of gastritis. When the relationship between *H. pylori* and chronic gastritis was established, investigators began to take interest in the causal role of the bacterium in gastric cancer (Herrera & Parsonnet, 2009). Therefore, on the basis of numerous epidemiological studies, *H. pylori* infection has been shown to be associated with an increased risk of gastric adenocarcinoma development (Parsonnet et al., 1997; Sugiyama & Asaka, 2004). Evidence that the presence of *H. pylori* increases the risk of developing gastric cancer through atrophy and intestinal metaplasia has also been reported (Asaka et al., 1994; Kuipers, 1995), suggesting that *H. pylori* positive patients developed these conditions in a greater proportion than control subjects. Besides, research conducted in animal models (Zhou et al., 2004) demonstrated that the eradication of the bacteria could reduce the incidence of gastric cancer in mice that developed the disease by inoculation of strains of *H. pylori* and administration of low doses of carcinogenic agents. These findings suggest that eradication of these bacteria during precancerous lesions of the disease significantly can reduce the incidence of gastric cancer also in humans (Sugiyama & Asaka, 2004). Consequently, in 1994 the International Agency for Research on Cancer, World Health Organization, concluded that *H. pylori* has a causal link with gastric carcinogenesis and was defined as type I carcinogen, a definite cause of cancer in humans (IARC, 1994).

Gastric cancer continues to be a major global health problem (Malfertheiner et al., 2010) and, despite the decreasing incidence and mortality rates observed worldwide over the last 50 years, it still ranks as a leading cause of cancer-related deaths in many parts of the world (Nardone et al., 2004). As symptoms are often absent or nonspecific in patients with the early stages of the disease, gastric cancer is usually diagnosed in an advanced stage, when curative options are limited. With exceptions in countries that have developed screening programs for early diagnoses, most patients reach treatment with cancers already in advanced stages (Hohenberger & Gretschel, 2003). Consequently, gastric cancer carries a poor prognosis, with an overall five-year survival rate of less than 20% (Bowles & Benjamin, 2001).

The vast majority of gastric cancers are adenocarcinomas, which can be prevalently divided into two types, the intestinal and the diffuse (Lauren, 1965), which corresponds, respectively, to the well-differentiated type and to the poorly-differentiated type, in the Japanese classification (Sugiyama & Asaka, 2004). In contrast to the diffuse type (**Figure 1**), often associated with familial distribution and developed in the stomach following chronic inflammation, especially in the cardia (Nardone et al., 2004), intestinal type adenocarcinomas (**Figure 2**) are generally thought to be preceded by a sequence of precursor lesions (Correa, 1975). The basic components of this process are chronic inflammation of the gastric mucosa, which slowly progresses through the premalignant stages of atrophic gastritis, intestinal metaplasia and dysplasia to gastric cancer (**Figure 3**) (Correa & Houghton, 2007). In respect to localization in the stomach, premalignant lesions are most frequently localized in the antrum in the transitional zone between the antrum and corpus (de Vries et al., 2007).

Unlike patients with advanced gastric cancer, patients diagnosed in an early stage of the disease present an excellent prognostic, in which a five-year survival rate is more than 90%. This disorder is defined as the adenocarcinoma that is confined to the mucosa or submucosa, irrespective of lymph-node invasion (Everett & Axon, 1998). Many early gastric cancers are believed to go through a life cycle consisting of ulcerations, followed by healing, then reulceration, and some tumours remain at this early stage for years even without treatment (Everett & Axon, 1998). Nevertheless, some early tumours rapidly became advanced and it is one of the principal questions concerning gastric carcinogenesis **(Figure 4).**

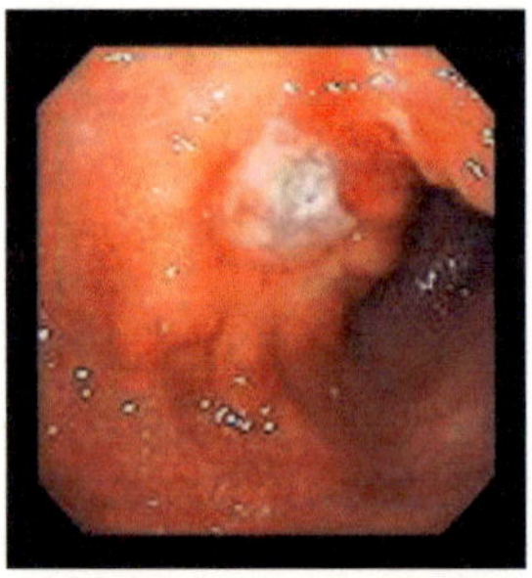

Fig. 1. Diffuse type adenocarcinoma

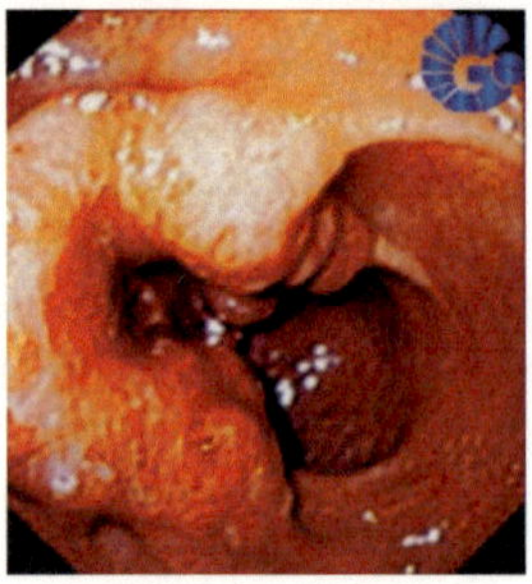

Fig. 2. Intestinal type adenocarcinoma

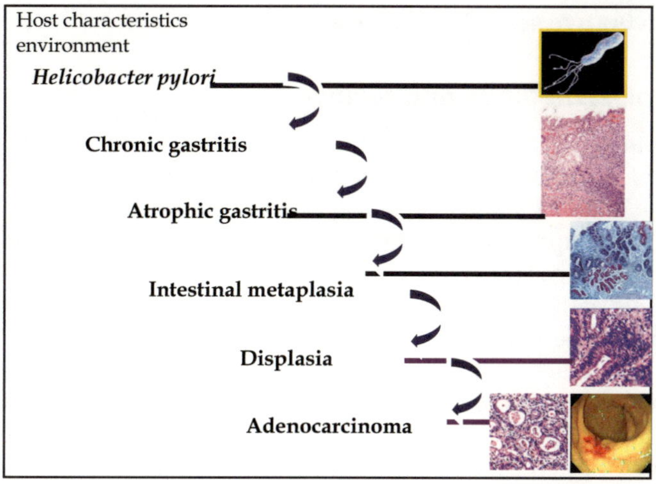

Fig. 3. Sequence of precursor lesions of the intestinal type adenocarcinoma development

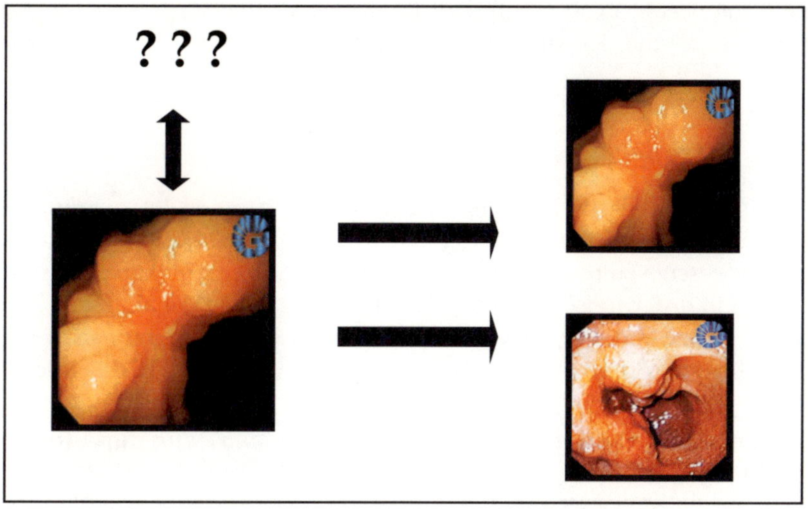

Fig. 4. Early gastric cancer: healing, maintenance or progression.

Have *H. pylori* virulence factors influenced this alteration? Why any tumour remains at an early stage for years even without treatment, or why they are able to heal by themselves, we do not know. Obviously, gastric carcinogenesis involves the interaction of the etiologic agent (*H. pylori*), the host characteristics and the external environment (Kabir, 2009), and, in this relationship, it should be considered the different strains of *H. pylori* and their virulence factors, important keys in the role of gastric carcinogenesis. Consequently, with the aim to try and understand better the mechanism of gastric carcinogenesis, especially concerning about the act of *H. pylori* , in which present studies have identified and analysed possible and essential differences among *H. pylori* strains derived from patients with early and advanced distal intestinal type gastric adenocarcinoma. Molecular biology techniques were used in order to amplify genes of this bacterium that act as virulence factors, comparing the results obtained in the two severities of illness.

2. Clinical samples, methods and results

2.1 Clinical samples

Clinical isolates of *H. pylori* used in this study were obtained from the Laboratory of Pathology of the Centre of Diagnosis of Digestive Diseases, Faculty of Medical Sciences, State University of Campinas (UNICAMP), São Paulo, Brazil. Eighty nine paraffin wax-embedded specimens of gastric tissue were analysed from a total of 89 patients: 31 of these were diagnosed with early distal type intestinal gastric adenocarcinoma (group one) and 58 with advanced distal type intestinal gastric adenocarcinoma (group two). The mean ages of group one were 61.0 years, with 20 male cases (64.5%) and 11 female cases (35.5%). For group two the mean ages was 64.5 years, with 40 male cases (69.0%) and 18 female cases (31.0%). All the gastric tissue samples were obtained from endoscopic biopsy and had positive results for *H. pylori* by histological analysis. Samples from gastric tissues obtained by endoscopic biopsy of patients with chronic gastritis and peptic ulcers were used as a control for all the reactions performed in this study. Primer pairs were chosen in order to amplify final products with similar length (base pairs) and, with this aim, only for the cagA gene, we used the nested PCR. Finally, all the stages of this study were approved by the Ethics Committee of the Faculty of Medical Sciences, State University of Campinas (UNICAMP).

2.2 Methods

2.2.1 DNA extraction

Paraffin wax-embedded tissue DNA extraction was performed by carrying out the pre-extraction treatment of fixed tissues, using xylene and ethanol washes for paraffin removal. Subsequently, successive steps using proteinase K, phenol, chloroform and isoamyl alcohol were carried out, in order to isolate and purify the DNA (Goelz et al., 1985). Quantification of the extracted DNA and polymerase chain reaction (PCR) for human betaglobin gene (Saiki et al., 1988) were carried out in order to guarantee the quality of this research.

2.2.2 PCR for urease C, vacA (regions s and m), cagA, cagT and dupA (regions jhp0917 and jhp0918) genes

Primer pairs for all the genes are described in **Table 1**, as well as the length of the fragments amplified for each reaction: urease C (Lage et al., 1995), vacA s1/s2 (Atherton et al., 1997), vacA m1/m2 (Atherton et al., 1999; Thomazini et al., 2006), cagA (Faundez et al., 2002), cagT (Mattar et al., 2007) and dupA jhp0917 and jhp0918 (Lu et al., 2005). PCR for urease C gene was performed with the aim to identify the bacterium DNA in samples.

After amplification, each PCR product was submitted to eletrophoresis on a 2% agarose gel stained by ethidium bromide with a 0.5 X tris-acetate-EDTA buffer. A 100-bp ladder was used as standard.

Then, for each specific reaction, after being tested positive for urease C gene, products obtained were classified in vacA s1m1, s2m1, s1m2 or s2m2, cagA positive or negative, cagT positive or negative, dupA jhp0917 positive or negative and dupA jhp0918 positive or negative; dupA gene was considered positive when its two regions were positive simultaneously.

Gene	Strand	Primer sequence (5´ - 3´)	Length (bp)
Betaglobin	+	ACACAACTGTGTTCACTAGC	110
	-	CAACTTCATCCACGTTTCACC	
Urease C	+	AAGCTTTTAGGGGTGTTAGGGGTTT	294
	-	AAGCTTACTTTCTAACACTAACGC	
vacA s (s1/s2)	+	ATGGAAATACAACAAACACAC	S1,259; s2: 286
	-	CTGCTTGAATGCGCCAAAC	
vacA m1	+	GGTCAAAATGCGGTCATGG	290
	-	CCATTGGTACCTGTAGAAAC	
vacA m2	+	ATGCTTTAATATCGTTGAGA	198
	-	GAA CAT GTT TTA GTG AAA GC	
cagA (1st PCR)	+	GATAACAGGCAAGCTTTTGAGAGGG A	393
	-	CCATGAATTTTTGATCCGTTCGG	
cagA (nested)	+	GATAACAGGCAAGCTTTTGAGG	349
	-	CTGCAAAAGATTGTTTGGCAGA	
cagT	+	CCATGTTTATACGCCTGTGT	301
	-	CATCACCACACCCTTTTGAT	
dupA (jhp0917)	+	TGGTTTCTACTGACAGAGCGC	307
	-	AACACGCTGACAGGACAATCTCCC	
dupA (jhp0918)	+	CCTATATCGCTAACGCGCGCTC	276
	-	AAGCTGAAGCGTTTGTAACG	

Table 1. Sequence of synthetic oligonucleotide primers used to characterization of *H. pylori* strains

2.2.3 Statistical analysis

After all amplification reactions, the results were analysed by a chi-square test at the Statistical Service of the Faculty of Medical Sciences at UNICAMP. Results were then related to the diseases in study, observing possible differences among *H. pylori* strains encountered in early and in advanced distal type intestinal gastric adenocarcinoma. Values of $p<0.05$ were considered to be statistically significant. The results as a whole, after comparison between the two groups, were depicted. Odd ratios with a confidence interval of 95% were also observed. Tables with absolute frequencies (n) and percentages (%) were made in order to determine genotypes combinations. Then, Exact Fischer´s Test was used in order to compare the genotypes combinations between early and advanced gastric cancer. Values of $p<0.05$ were considered to be statistically significant.

2.3 Results

PCR for the urease C gene of *H. pylori* was positive in all 89 samples, identifying the bacterium DNA (**Table 2; Figure 5**). For the vacA gene, with regard to region s, of 31 samples from patients with early gastric cancer, 71.0% (22 cases) were s1 and 29.0% (9 cases) s2. Fifty eight samples from patients with advanced gastric cancer, 70.7% (41 cases) were s1 and 29.3% (17 cases) s2 ($p = 0.978$) (**Table 2; Figure 6**). In conclusion, 63 (70.8%) samples were diagnosed with vacA subtype s1 and 26 (29.2%) samples were with subtype vacA s2. Related to the vacA gene subunit m, no positive results were observed for the vacA gene subunit m2. From all 89 samples, 31 patients with early gastric cancer and 58 patients with

advanced gastric cancer were m1 positive (**Table 2; Figure 7**). Following this analysis, samples were classified into s1m1 or s2m1. For patients with early gastric cancer, 71.0% (22 cases) were s1m1 and 29.0% (9 cases) were s2m1. From 58 samples of patients with advanced gastric cancer, 70.7% (41 cases) were s1m1 and 29.3% (17 cases) s2m1 (table 3). Results were not statistically significant (p = 0.978). In conclusion, 63 (70.8%) samples were vacA s1m1 and 26 (29.2%) were vacA s2m1 (**Table 2**).
Analyzing the cagA gene, from patients with early gastric cancer, 61.3% (19 cases) were positive and from patients with advanced gastric cancer, 82.8% (48 cases) were positive (p = 0.025), with an odds ratio of 3.032, 95% confidence interval (1.123-8.185) **(Table 2; Figure 8)**. In the group as a whole, there were 67 positive cases (75.3%) for the cagA gene. On the other hand, analyzing the cagT gene of *H. pylori*, from patients with early gastric adenocarcinoma 54.8% (17 cases) were positive and in patients with advanced gastric adenocarcinoma, 65.5% (38 cases) were positive (p = 0.323) (**Table 2; Figure 9**). In the group there were 55 positive cases (61.8%) for the cagT gene.
Results of dupA jhp0917 in patients with early gastric cancer, 35.5% (11 cases) presented positive results and in patients with advanced gastric cancer, 39.7% (23 cases) presented positive (p = 0.700) (**Table 2; Figure 10**). In the group as a whole, there were 34 positive cases (38.2%) and 55 negative cases (61.8%) for jhp0917. Tests of dupA jhp0918 in patients with early gastric cancer, 51.6% (16 cases) had positive results and In patients with advanced gastric cancer, 55.2% (32 cases) were positive (p = 0.748) (**Table 2; Figure 11**). The p value obtained was 0.748, which was not statistically significant. In the group there were 48 cases (53.9%) that were positive for dupA jhp0918 gene and 41 cases (46.1%) that were negative.

Classification	Early gastric cancer	Advanced gastric cancer	Total	p value
urease C	31 (100.0%)	58 (100.0%)	89 (100.0%)	
s1	22 (71.0%)	41 (70.7%)	63 (70.8%)	
s2	9 (29.0%)	17 (29.3%)	26 (29.2%)	p = 0.978
m1	31 (100.0%)	58 (100.0%)	89 (100.0%)	
m2	0 (0.0%)	0 (0.0%)	0 (0.0%)	
s1m1	22 (71.0%)	41 (70.7%)	63 (70.8%)	
s2m1	9 (29.0%)	17 (29.3%)	26 (29.2%)	p = 0.978
cagA positive	19 (61.3%)	48 (82.8%)	67 (75.3%)	
cagA negative	12 (38.7%)	10 (17.2%)	22 (24.7%)	p = 0.025*
cagT positive	17 (54.8%)	38 (65.5%)	55 (61.8%)	
cagT negative	14 (45.2%)	20 (34.5%)	34 (38.2%)	p = 0.323
dupA jhp0917 positive	11 (35.5%)	23 (39.7%)	34 (38.2%)	
dupA jhp0917 negative	20 (64.5%)	35 (60.3%)	55 (61.8%)	P = 0.700
dupA jhp0918 positive	16 (51.6%)	32 (55.2%)	48 (53.9%)	
dupA jhp0918 negative	15 (48.4%)	26 (44.8%)	41 (46.1%)	P = 0.748
Total	31 (100.0%)	58 (100.0%)	89 (100.0%)	

* cagA gene (p = 0.025), OR = 3.032 (95% CI, 1.123-8.185)

Table 2. General results obtained after reactions for urease C, vacA (s/m), cagA, cagT and dupA jhp0917 and jhp0918 genes of *Helicobacter pylori*

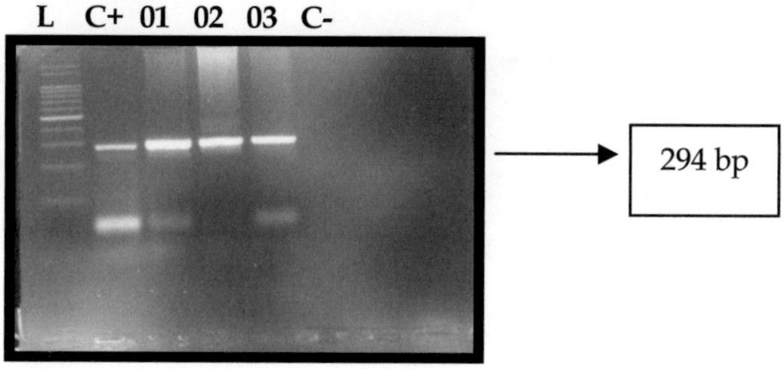

Fig. 5. Amplification of the urease C gene of *H. pylori* (294 bp); L, ladder 100 bp; C+, positive control; 01 to 03, positive samples; C-, negative control.

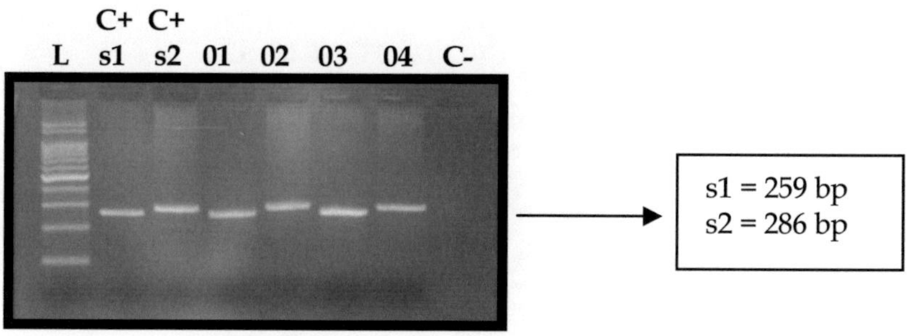

Fig. 6. Amplification of the vacA region s gene of *H. pylori* (s1, 259 bp; s2, 286 bp); L, ladder 100 bp; C+s1, positive control for vacA s1; C+s2, positive control for vacA s2; 01 and 03, positive samples for s1; 02 and 04, positive samples for s2; C-, negative control.

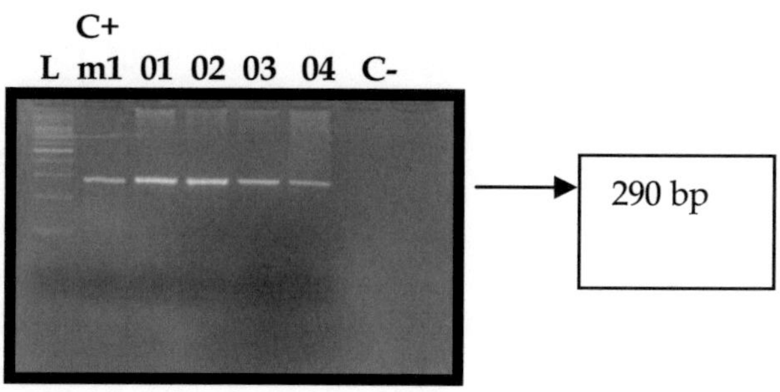

Fig. 7. Amplification of the vacA m1 region of *H. pylori* (290 bp). L, ladder 100 bp; C+ m1, positive control for vacA m1; 01 to 04, positive samples; C-, negative control.

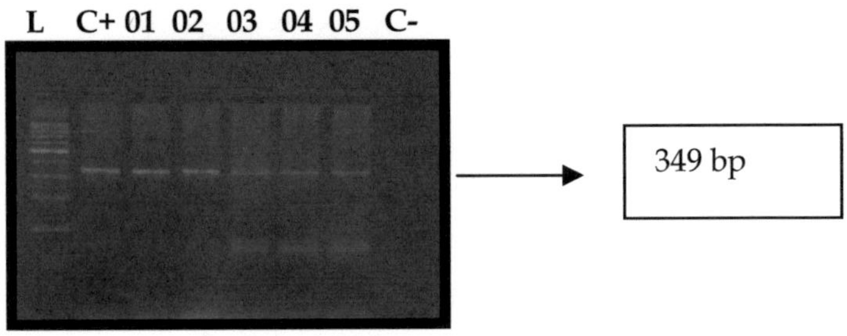

Fig. 8. Amplification of cagA gene of *H. pylori* (349 bp). L, ladder 100 bp; C+, positive control; 01 to 05, positive samples; C-, negative control.

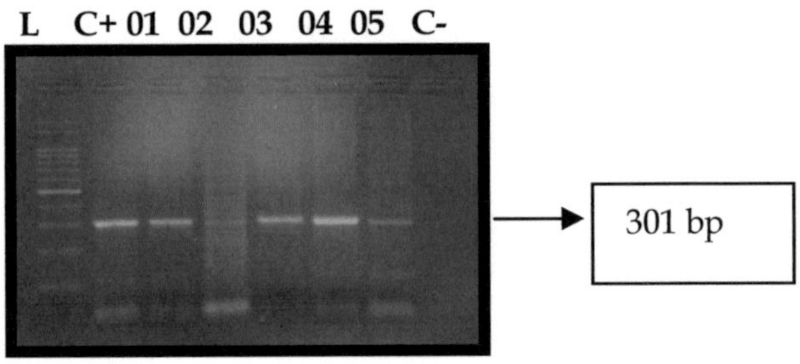

Fig. 9. Amplification of cagT gene of *H. pylori* (301 bp). L, ladder 100 bp; C+, positive control; 01 to 05, positive samples; C-, negative control.

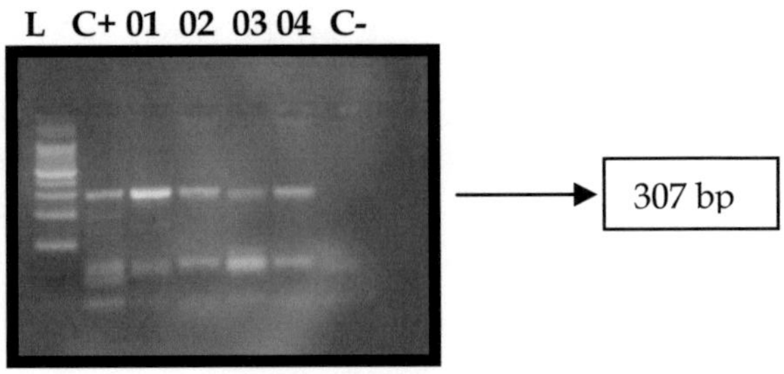

Fig. 10. Amplification of dupA jhp0917 gene of *H. pylori* (307 bp). L, ladder 100 bp; C+, positive control; 01 to 04, positive samples; C-, negative control.

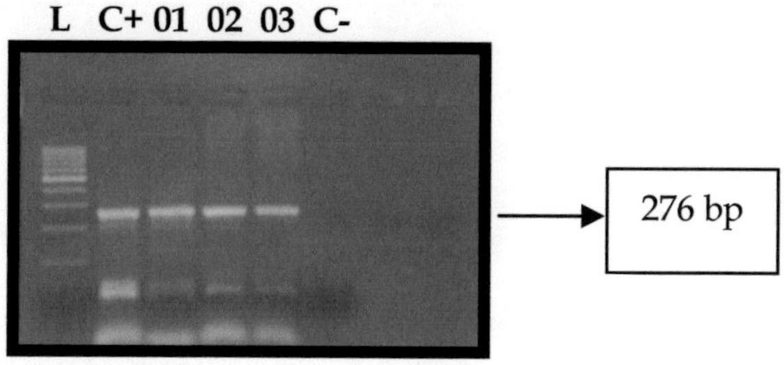

Fig. 11. Amplification of dupA jhp0918 gene of *H. pylori* (276 bp). L, ladder 100 bp; C+, positive control; 01 to 03, positive samples; C-, negative control.

After this analysis, tables with absolute frequencies (n) and percentages (%) were made in order to compare the genotypes combinations. vacA s1m1, cagA positive, cagT positive and dupA negative were, individually, the most frequent genotypes (**Table 3**). In order to specify better the results obtained, the dupA gene was considered positive when its two continuous regions (jhp0917 and jhp0918) were positive simultaneously. So, the combinations of genotypes were made and then compared between the two groups of patients, with early and advanced gastric cancer (**Tables 4 and 5, respectively**). The most prevalent genotype for all the samples, in both groups of patients, was vacA s1m1, cagA positive, cagT positive and dupA negative. The percentage was 29.21%. About the comparison of genotypes combinations between the two groups of samples, there was not a significant difference ($p = 0.116$).

Genomic region		Frequence (n)	Percentage (%)
vacA s/m gene	s1m1	63	70.79
	s2m1	26	29.21
cagA gene	positive	67	75.28
	negative	22	24.72
cagT gene	positive	55	61.80
	negative	34	38.20
dupA jhp0917 gene	positive	34	38.20
	negative	55	61.80
dupA jhp0918 gene	positive	48	53.93
	negative	41	46.07
dupA jhp0917/0918 gene	positive	28	31.46
	negative	61	68.54

Table 3. Descriptive analysis of genomic regions of *H. pylori*

Genotypes combinations: vacA s/m, cagA, cagT, dupA (jhp0917/0918)	Frequency (n)	Percentage (%)
s1m1 neg neg neg	8	8.99
s1m1 neg neg pos	1	1.12
s2m1 neg neg neg	3	3.37
s2m1 neg neg pos	2	2.25
s1m1 neg pos neg	3	3.37
s1m1 neg pos pos	1	1.12
s2m1 neg pos neg	2	2.25
s2m1 neg pos pos	2	2.25
s1m1 pos neg neg	9	10.11
s1m1 pos neg pos	6	6.74
s2m1 pos neg neg	4	4.49
s2m1 pos neg pos	1	1.12
s1m1 pos pos neg	26	29.21
s1m1 pos pos pos	9	10.11
s2m1 pos pos neg	6	6.74
s2m1 pos pos pos	6	6.74

Table 4. Genotype combinations, according to the results obtained for vacA s/m, cagA, cagT and dupA (jhp0917/0918) genes of *H. pylori*

Genotype combinations: vacA s/m, cagA, cagT, dupA (jhp0917/0918)	Early gastric câncer	Advanced gastric cancer	Total
s1m1 neg neg neg	4 12.90	4 6.90	8
s1m1 neg neg pos	1 3.23	0 0.00	1
s2m1 neg neg neg	1 3.23	2 3.45	3
s2m1 neg neg pos	0 0.00	2 3.45	2
s1m1 neg pos neg	2 6.45	1 1.72	3
s1m1 neg pos pos	1 3.23	0 0.00	1
s2m1 neg pos neg	2 6.45	0 0.00	2
s2m1 neg pos pos	1 3.23	1 1.72	2
s1m1 pos neg neg	3 9.68	6 10.34	9
s1m1 pos neg pos	2 6.45	4 6.90	6
s2m1 pos neg neg	2 6.45	2 3.45	4

Genotype combinations: vacA s/m, cagA, cagT, dupA (jhp0917/0918)	Early gastric câncer	Advanced gastric cancer	Total
s2m1 pos neg pos	1 3.23	0 0.00	1
s1m1 pos pos neg	5 16.13	21 36.21	26
s1m1 pos pos pos	4 12.90	5 8.62	9
s2m1 pos pos neg	2 6.45	4 6.90	6
s2m1 pos pos pos	0 0.00	6 10.34	6
Total	31	58	89

$p = 0.116$

Table 5. Comparison of genotypes combinations between early and advanced gastric cancer.

3. Conclusions

The understanding of gastric carcinogenesis has advanced considerably in recent decades, especially as regards to the role of *Helicobacter pylori* in the progression of chronic gastritis in precancerous lesions and cancer (de Vries et al., 2007). The risk of development of gastric cancer is also related to genetic characteristics of the host and environmental factors, which, associated with specific bacterial strain characteristics, influence the severity of the chronic inflammatory response (Peek et al., 1999). Thus, although infection with *H. pylori* almost always results in chronic active gastritis, many infected patients do not develop any complication, even those not showing clinical symptoms of infection (Blaser & Atherton, 2004). This leads to the conclusion that some strains are more virulent than others (Kusters et al., 2006), expressing, in different manners, specific bacterial products.

In the present study, we compared the *H. pylori* strains obtained from patients with early and advanced distal type intestinal gastric adenocarcinoma with the aim to identify possible differences among strains present in one or other case, using the polymerase chain reaction (PCR) for several bacterial genome regions. The primary detection of *H. pylori* in the samples was performed using the urease C region, present in all strains. After this, PCR was used for amplifying two genes from the cagPAI (cagA and cagT), the vacA gene (regions s and m) and the dupA gene (jhp0917/0918).

Strains with an s1-type signalling-sequence allele produce functional VacA toxin, whereas those with an s2-type signalling sequence have little cytotoxic activity (Peek & Blaser, 2002). Moreover, mosaic s1m1 strains are more toxic than s1m2 strains and are associated with more severe forms of gastritis, atrophy and intestinal metaplasia (Björkholm et al., 2003). The presence of s1 m1 vacA alleles is also strongly correlated with the expression of the cag-PAI (Covacci et al., 1993; Tummuru et al., 1993). Although located on a different loci of the *H. pylori* chromosome, cagA is strongly linked with VacA cytotoxic activity (Hocker & Hohenberger, 2003) and strains expressing the combination of these alleles and cag-PAI show enhanced epithelial cell injury (Ghiara et al., 1995). In our study, for patients with advanced gastric cancer, we found prevalent cagA positive (82.8%) and vacA s1m1 (70.7%) strains, corroborating the results of other studies (Miehlke et al., 2000; Leanza et al., 2004), and demonstrating that this combination can result in more virulent strains. These results are also similar to those obtained in China (Qiao et al., 2003), where *H. pylori* strains were cagA positive in 95% of samples in the gastric cancer group and the expression of type s1 vacA was more than type s2. Nevertheless, with respect to type m, the expression of type m1 was equal to type m2, even in the gastric cancer group. In our study we did not find a positive result for m2.

With regards to early gastric cancer patients, unless we found strains with the same characteristics to those of advanced gastric cancer, some samples (cagA positive for 61.3% of samples and vacA s1m1 for 71.0% of samples), were positive for cagA and vacA s2m1 (29.0%), which may contribute for the maintenance of the early stage of disease. In addition, one possible explanation would be that the strains found in early lesions, in relation to the cagA gene, could be different which respects to their EPYIA motifs (polymorfisms of the cagA gene) (Nguyen et al., 2009; Truong et al., 2009), leading to the maintenance of early stage disease, without its progression to advanced lesions.

As regards to the cagA gene, in an isolate analysis, our results were similar to those of in which strains cagA positive were related to the development of gastric cancer. cagA positive strains tend to be more virulent and induce higher levels of expression of cytokines such as interleukin 1b and 8 (El-Omar et al., 2000). Some studies have shown that patients with strains that express CagA are three times more likely to develop gastric cancer [Parsonnet et al., 1997; Huang et al., 2003) than those infected with cagA negative strains (Husson et al., 1995; Yamaoka et al., 1999). In the present study the same characteristics were observed and patients infected with cagA positive strains demonstrated a high risk of advanced gastric cancer development (OR = 3.032, 95%CI). Besides, studies conducted in Western countries (Crabtree et al., 1994; Blaser et al., 1995) and in Asian countries (Mizushima et al., 2001) reported that most patients with gastric cancer are infected with *H. pylori* cagA positive strains.

Like the cagA gene, the cagT also belongs to the cag pathogenicity island and it is assumed that it is related to the type IV secretion system, responsible for binding to cell receptors and inducing the release of interleukin-8 and also by ejecting the CagA protein (Rohde et al., 2003). The cagT gene has been linked to the development of peptic ulcer, and strains with the absence of this gene were generally related to chronic gastritis (Mattar et al., 2007). In this study, values were not found to be statistically significant between the two studied groups (p = 0.323). However, the cagT gene was found, in the group as a whole, in 61.8% of the samples, which reflects a significant result, showing that this gene, like cagA, or acting together with cagA, may be related to gastric cancer development.

Finally, for the dupA gene, which was originally considered a marker for duodenal ulcer disease and a protective factor against gastric cancer in strains isolated from Japan, Korea and Colombia (Lu et al., 2005), we did not find any statistically significant difference between the two studied groups. Thus, although the dupA gene can not be considered as a marker for duodenal ulcer disease, the presence of this gene was found in few samples of patients with gastric cancer, suggesting that it is not an important gene for the development of this disease, by itself. Conversely, dupA genotyping of samples obtained from four populations (Argent et al., 2008), from Belgium, South Africa, China and the United States of America, showed no association of this gene with duodenal ulcer, but suggested an association with gastric cancer. Another study carried out in Brazilian patients (Gomes et al., 2008) also did not find any association between dupA and either of the two diseases. Finally, in India, a study demonstrated a significant association of dupA gene with duodenal ulcer disease in the population (Arachchi et al., 2007). These different results demonstrate that further studies are required to elucidate the roles of dupA gene in the development of gastric diseases.

There are a number of studies that have investigated the virulence factors of *H. pylori* strains, but a gene marker for gastric cancer disease has not yet been found. Our study has demonstrated an interaction between some virulence factors found in gastric tissue samples obtained by early and advanced distal type intestinal gastric adenocarcinoma and a significant statistically value for cagA gene, which is more present in patients with advanced cancer. In the group gastric cancer as a whole, we found a prevalence of cagA positive, cagT positive, vacA s1m1 strains genotypes and a low number of dupA positive samples. Between the two groups, there were no statistically differences about the most prevalent combination of genotypes. In conclusion, the identification of a disease specific *H. pylori* virulence factor could be useful in clinical practice, helping to identify patients infected with strains that are able to develop a serious disease, such as gastric cancer.

4. Acknowledgment

The authors thank the "Coordenação de Aperfeiçoamento de Pessoal de Nível Superior" (CAPES) and the "Fundação de Amparo à Pesquisa do Estado de São Paulo" (FAPESP) for their financial support; and Centre of Diagnosis of Digestive Diseases, State University of Campinas, for the concession of the use of figures utilized here.

5. References

Ahmed, N. & Sechi, L.A. (2005). *Helicobacter pylori* and gastroduodenal pathology: New threats of the old friend. *Annals of Clinical Microbiology and Antimicrobials*, Vol.4, (January 2005), pp. 1-10, ISSN 1476-0711.

Akopyanz, N.; Bukanov, N.O.; Westblom, T.U; Kresovich, S. & Berg, D.E. (1992). DNA diversity among clinical isolates of *Helicobacter pylori* detected by PCR-based RAPD fingerprinting. *Nucleic Acids Research*, Vol.20, No.19, (October 1992), pp. 5137-5142, ISSN 1362-4962.

Alm, R.A.; Ling, L.S.; Moir, D.T.; King, B.L.; Brown, E.D.; Doig, P.C.; Smith, D.R.; Noonan, B.; Guild, B.C.; deJonge, B.L.; Carmel, G.; Tummino, P.J.; Caruso, A.; Uria-Nickelsen, M.; Mills, D.M.; Ives, C.; Gibson, R.; Merberg, D.; Mills, S.D.; Jiang, Q.; Taylor, D.E.; Vovis, G.F. & Trust, T.J. (1999). Genomic-sequence comparison of two unrelated isolates of the human gastric pathogen *Helicobacter pylori*. *Nature*, Vol.397, No.6715, (January 1999), pp. 176-180, ISSN 0028-0836.

Arachich, H.S.; Kalra, V.; Lal, B.; Bhatia, V.; Baba, C.S.; Chakravarthy, S.; Rohatgi, S., Sarma, P.M.; Mishra, V.; Das, B. & Ahula, V. (2007). Prevalence of duodenal-ulcer promoting gene (dupA) of *Helicobacter pylori* in patients with duodenal ulcer in North Indian population. *Helicobacter*, Vol.12, No.6, (December 2007), pp. 591-597, ISSN 1523-5378.

Argent, R.H.; Thomas, R.J.; Letley, D.P.; Rittig, M.G.; Hardie, K.R. & Atherton, J.C. (2008). Functional association between the *Helicobacter pylori* virulence factors VacA and CagA. *Journal of Medical Microbiology*, Vol.57, No.2, (February 2008), pp. 145-150, ISSN 1473-5644.

Arnold, D.M.; Bernotas, A.; Nazi, I.; Stasi, R.; Kuwana, M.; Liu, Y.; Kelton, J.G. & Crowther, M.A. (2009). Platelet count response to *H. pylori* treatment in patients with immune thrombocytopenic purpura with and without *H. pylori* infection: a systematic review. *Haematologica*, Vol.94; No.6, (June 2009), pp. 850-856, ISSN 1592-8721.

Asaka, M.; Kimura, T.; Kato, M.; Kudo, M.; Miki, K.; Ogoshi, K.; Kato, T.; Tatsuta, M. & Graham, D.Y. (1994). Possible role of *Helicobacter pylori* infection in early gastric cancer development. *Cancer*, Vol.73, No.11, (June 1994), pp. 2691-2694, ISSN 1097-0142.

Atherton, J.C.; Cao, P.; Peek Jr, R.M.; Tummuru, M.K.; Blaser, M.J. & Cover, T.L. (1995). Mosaicism in vacuolating cytotoxin alleles of *Helicobacter pylori*. Association of specific vacA types with cytotoxin production and peptic ulceration. *The Journal of Biological Chemistry*, Vol.270, No.30, (July 1995), pp. 1771-1777, ISSN 1083-351X.

Atherton, J.C.; Peek, R.M.; Tham, K.T.; Cover, T.L.& Blaser, M.J. (1997). Clinical and pathological importance of heterogenicity in vacA, the vacuolating cytotoxin gene of *Helicobacter pylori*. *Gastroenterology*, Vol.112, No.1, (January 1997), pp. 92-97, ISSN 0016-5085.

Atherton, J.C.; Cover, T.L.; Twells, R.J.; Morales, M.R.; Hawkey, C.J. & Blaser, M.J. (1997). Simple and accurate PCR-based system for typing vacuolating cytotoxin alleles of *Helicobacter pylori*. *Journal of Clinical Microbiology*, Vol.37, No.9, (September 1999), pp. 2979-2982, ISSN 1098-660X.

Baltrus, D.A; Amieva, M.R.; Covacci, A; Lowe, T.M.; Merrell, D.S; Ottemann, K.M.; Stein, M.; Salama, N.R. & Guillemin, K. (2009). The complete genome sequence of *Helicobacter pylori* strain G27. *Journal of Bacteriology*, Vol.191, No.1, (January 2009), pp. 447-448, ISSN 0021-9193.

Björkholm, B.; Falk, P.; Engstrand, L; & Nyrén, O. (2003). *Helicobacter pylori:* resurrection of the cancer link. *Journal of Internal Medicine*, Vol. 253, No.2, (February 2003), pp. 102-119, ISSN 0954-6820.

Blaser, M.J.; Perez-Perez, G.I.; Kleanthous, H.; Cover, T.L.; Peek, R.M.; Chyou, P.H.; Stemmermann, G.N. & Nomura, A. (1995). Infection with *Helicobacter pylori* strains possessing cagA is associated with an increased risk of developing adenocarcinoma of the stomach. *Cancer Research*, Vol.55, No.10, (May 1995), pp. 2111-2115, ISSN 1538-7445.

Blaser, M.J. & Atherton, J.C. (2004). *Helicobacter pylori* persistence: biology and disease. The *Journal of Clinical Investigation*, Vol.113, No.3, (February 2004), pp. 321-333, ISSN 0021-9738.

Bowles, M.J. & Benjamin, I.C. (2001) ABC of the upper gastrointestinal tract. Cancer of the stomach and pancreas. BMJ, Vol.323, No.7326, (December 2001), pp. 1413-1416, ISSN 1982-9000.

Capurso, G.; Lahner, E.; Marcheggiano, A.; Caruana, P.; Carnuccio, A.; Bordi, C. Delle Fave, G. & Annibale, B. (2001). Involvement of the corporal mucosa and related changes in gastric acid secretion characterize patients with iron deficiency anemy associated with *Helicobacter pylori* infection. *Alimentary Pharmacology & Therapeutics*, Vol.15, No.11, (November 2001), pp. 1753-1761, ISSN 1365-2036.

Censini, S.; Lange, C.; Xiang, Z.; Crabtree, J.E.; Ghiara, P.; Borodovsky, M.; Rappuoli, R. & Covacci, A. (1996). Cag, a pathogenicity island of *Helicobacter pylori*, encodes type I-specific and disease-associated virulence factors. *Proceedings of the National Academy of Sciences of the United States of America*, Vol.93, No.25, (December 1996), pp. 14648-14653, ISSN 1091-6490.

Correa, P.; Haenszel, W.; Cuello, C.; Tannenbaum, S. & Archer, M. (1975). A model for gastric cancer epidemiology. *Lancet*, Vol.2, No.7924, (July 1975), pp. 58-60, ISSN 0140-6736.

Correa, P. & Hughton, J. (2007). Carcinogenesis of *Helicobacter pylori. Gastroenterology*, Vol.133, No.2, (August 2007), pp. 659-672, ISSN 0016-5085.

Covacci, A.; Censini, S.; Bugnoli, M.; Petracca, R.; Burroni, D.; Macchia, G.; Massone, A.; Papini, E.; Xiang, Z. & Figura, N. (1993). Molecular characterization of the 128-kDa immunodominant antigen of *Helicobacter pylori* associated with citotoxicity and duodenal ulcer. *Proceedings of the National Academy of Sciences of the United States of America*, Vol.90, No.12, (June 1993), pp. 5791-5795, ISSN 1091-6490.

Covacci, A. & Rappuoli, R. (2000). Tyrosine-phosphorylated bacterial proteins: Trojan horses for the host cell. *The Journal of Experimental Medicine*, Vol.191, No.4, (February 2000), pp. 587-592, ISSN 1540-9538.

Cover, T.L. & Blanke, S.R. (2005). *Helicobacter pylori* VacA, a paradigm for toxin multifunctionality. *Nature Reviews. Microbiology*, Vol.3, No.4, (April 2005), pp. 320-332, ISSN 1740-1526.

Crabtree, J.E; Farmery, S.M.; Lindley, I.J.; Figura, N.; Peichl, P. & Tompkins, D.S. (1994). CagA/cytotoxic strains of *Helicobacter pylori* and interleukin-8 in gastric epithelial cell lines. *Journal of Clinical Pathology*, Vol.47, No.10, (October 1994), pp. 945-950, ISSN 1472-4146.

de Vries, A.C.; Haringsma, J.; & Kuipers, E.J. (2007). The detection, surveillance and treatment of premalignant gastric lesions related to *Helicobacter pylori* infection. *Helicobacter*, Vol.12, No.1, (February 2007), pp. 1-15, ISSN 1523-5378.

Dunn, B.E.; Cohen, H. & Blaser, M.J. (1997). *Helicobacter pylori. Clinical Microbiology Reviews*, Vol.10, No.4, (October 1997), pp. 720-741, ISSN 1098-6618.

El-Omar, E.M.; Carrington, M.; Chow, W.H.; McColl, K.E.; Bream, J.H.; Young, H.A.; Herrera, J.; Lissowska, J.; Yuan, C.C.; Rothman, N.; Lanyon, G.; Martin, M.; Fraumeni, J.F. Jr.; & Rabkin, C.S. (2000). Interleukin-1 polymorphisms associated with increased risk of gastric cancer. *Nature*, Vol.404, No.6776, (March 2000), pp. 398-402, ISSN 0028-0836.

Everett, S.M. & Axon, A.T.R. (1998). Early gastric cancer: disease or pseudo-disease? *Lancet*, Vo.351, No.9112, (May 1998), pp. 1350-1352, ISSN 0140-6736.

Faundez, G.; Troncoso, M. & Figueroa, G. (2002). cagA and vacA in strains of *Helicobacter pylori* from ulcer and non-ulcerative dyspepsia patients. *BMC Gastroenterology*, Vol.2, (September 2002), pp. 20-24, ISSN 1471-230X.

Figura, N.; Guglielmetti, P.; Rossolini, A.; Barberi, A.; Cusi, G.; Musmanno, R.A.; Russi, M. & Quaranta, S. (1989). Cytotoxin production by *Campylobacter pylori* strains isolated from patients with peptic ulcers and from patients with chronic gastritis only. *Journal of Clinical Microbiology*, Vol.27, No.1, (January 1989), pp. 225-226, ISSN 1098-660X.

Figura, N.; Franceschi, F.; Santucci, A.; Bernardini, G.; Gasbarrini, G.; & Gasbarrini, A. (2010). Extragastric manifestations of *Helicobacter pylori* infection. *Helicobacter*, Vol.15, Suppl.1, (January 2010), ISSN 1523-5378.

Foxall, P.A.; Hu, L.T. & Mobley, H.L. (1992). Use of polymerase chain reaction-amplified *Helicobacter pylori* urease structural genes for differentiation of isolates. *Journal of Clinical Microbiology,* Vol.30, No.3, (March 1992), pp. 739-741, ISSN 1098-660X.

Franceschi, F.; Navarese, E.P.; Mollo, R.; Giupponi, B.; De Marco, G.; Merra, G. Gasbarrini, G. & Silveri, N.G. (2009). *Helicobacter pylori* and atherosclerosis. A review of the literature. *Recenti Progress in Medicine,* Vol.100; No.2, (February 2009), pp. 91-96, ISSN 0034-1193.

Gasbarrini, A.; Franceschi, F.; Armuzzi, A.; Ojetti, V.; Candelli, M.; Sanz Torre, E.S.; De Lorenzo, A.; Anti, M.; Pretolani, S. & Gasbarrini, G. (1999). Extradigestive manifestations of *Helicobacter pylori* gastric infection. *Gut,* Vol.45, Suppl.1, (July 1999), pp. 9-12, ISSN 1468-3288.

Ghiara, P., Marchetti, M.; Blaser, M.J.; Tummuru, M.K.; Cover, T.L.; Segal, E.D.; Tompkins, L.S. & Rapuolli, R. (1995). Role of the *Helicobacter pylori* virulence factors vacuolating cytotoxin, CagA, and urease in a mouse model of disease. *Infection and immunity,* Vol. 63, No.10, (October 1995), pp. 4154-4160, ISSN 1098-5522.

Goelz, S.E; Hamilton, S.R. & Vogelstein, B. (1985). Purification of DNA from formaldehyde fixed and paraffin embedded human tissue. *Biochemical and Biophysical Research Communications,* Vol. 130, No.1, (July 1985), pp. 118-126, ISSN 0006-291X.

Gomes, L.I.; Rocha, G.A.; Rocha, A.M.; Soares, T.F.; Oliveira, C.A.; Bittencourt, P.F. & Queiroz, D.M. (2008). Lack of association between *Helicobacter pylori* infection with dupA-positive strains and gastroduodenal diseases in Brazilian patients. *International Journal of Medical Microbiology,* Vol.298, No.3-4, (April 2008), pp. 223-230, ISSN 1438-4221.

Goodwin, C.S.R.; McCulloch, R.K.; Armstrong, J.A. & Wee, S.W. (1987). Unusual cellular fatty acids and distinctive ultrastructure in a new spiral bacterium (Campylobacter pyloridis) from the human gastric mucosa. *Journal of Medical Microbiology,* Vol.19, (April 1985), pp. 257-267. ISSN 1473-5644.

Goodwin, C.S.R. & Armstrong, J.A. (1990). Microbiological aspects of *Helicobacter pylori* (*Campylobacter pylori*). *European Journal of Clinical Microbiology,* Vol.9, No.1, (January 1990), pp. 1-13. ISSN 1435-4373.

Han, F.C.; Ng, H.C. & Ho, B. (2003). Stability of randomly amplified polymorphic DNA fingerprinting in genotyping clinical isolates of *Helicobacter pylori. World Journal of Gastroenterology,* Vol.9, No.9, (September 2009), pp. 2021-2024, ISSN 1007-9327.

Harris, P.R.; Mobley, H.L.; Perez-Perez, G.I.; Blaser, M.J. & Smith, P.D. (1996). *Helicobacter pylori* urease is a potent stimulus of mononuclear phagocyte activation and inflammatory cytokine production. *Gastroenterology,* Vol.111, No.2, (August 1996), pp. 419-425, ISSN 0016-5085.

Herrera, V. & Parsonnet, J. (2009). *Helicobacter pylori* and gastric adenocarcinoma. *Clinical Microbiology and Infection,* Vol. 15, No.11, (November 2009), pp. 971-976, ISSN 1469-0691.

Höcker, M. & Hohenberger, P. (2003). *Helicobacter pylori* virulence factors – one part of a big picture. *Lancet,* Vol.362, No. 9391, (October 2003), pp. 1231-1233, ISSN 0140-6736.

Hoehnberger, P. & Gretschel, S. (2003). Gastric cancer. *Lancet,* Vol.362, No.9380, (July 2003), pp. 305-315, ISSN 0140-6736.

Huang, J.Q.; Zheng, G.F.; Sumanac, K.; Irvine, E.J. & Hunt, R.H. (2003). Meta-analyisis of the relationship between cagA seropositivity and gastric cancer. *Gastroenterology*, Vol. 125, No.6, (December 2003), pp. 1636-1644, ISSN 0016-5085.

Husson, M.O.; Gottrand, F.; Vachee, A.; Dhaenens, L.; de la Salle, E.M.; Turck, D.; Houcke, M. &Leclerc, H. (1995). Importance in diagnosis of gastritis of detection by PCR of the cagA gene in *Helicobacter pylori* strains isolated from children. *Journal of Clinical Microbiology*, Vol.33, No.12, (December 1995), pp. 3300-3303, ISSN 1098-660X.

International Agency for Research on Cancer. Schistosomes, liver flukes and *Helicobacter pylori*. IARC Working Group on the Evaluation of Carcinogenic Risks to Humans. IARC monographs on the evaluation of carcinogenic risks to humans. *World Health Organization, International Agency for Research on Cancer*, Vol.61, pp. 1-241.

Isaeva, G.Sh.; Abuzarova, E.R.; Valeeva, Iu.V.; Pozdeev, O.K. & Murav´eva, E.V. (2009). *Helicobacter pylori* in patients with disorders of hepatobiliary system. *Zhurnal Mikrobiologii Epidemiologii i Immunobioogiil*, Vol.2, (March-April), pp. 96-101, ISSN 0378-9311.

Kabir, S. (2009). Effect of *Helicobacter pylori* eradication on incidence of gastric cancer in human and animal models: underlying biochemical and molecular events. *Helicobacter*, Vol.14, No.3, (June 2009), pp. 159-171, ISSN 1523-5378.

Kodaira, M.S.; Escobar, A.M.U. & Grisi, S. (2002). Aspectos epidemiológicos do *Helicobacter pylori* na infância e adolescência. *Revista de Saúde Pública*, Vol.36, pp. 356-369, ISSN 0034-8910.

Kuipers, E.J.; Perez-Perez, G.I.; Meuwissen, S.G. & Blaser, M.J. (1995). *Helicobacter pylori* and atrophic gastritis. Importance of the cagA status. *Journal of the National Cancer Institute*, Vol.87, No.23, (December 1995), pp. 1777-1780, ISSN 0027-8874.

Kusters, J.G.; van Vliet, A.H.M & Kuipers, E.J. (2006). Pathogenesis of *Helicobacter pylori* infection. *Clinical Microbiology Reviews*, Vol.19; No.3, (July 2006), pp. 449-490, ISSN 1098-6618.

Lage, A.P.;Godfroid, P.; Fauconnier, A., Burette, A.; Butzler, J.P.; Bollen, A. & Glupczynski, Y. (1995). Diagnosis of *Helicobacter pylori* infection by PCR: comparison with other invasive techniques and detection of cagA gene in gastric biopsy specimens. *Journal of Clinical Microbiology*, Vol.33, No.10, (October 1995), pp. 2752-2756, ISSN 1098-660X.

Lauren, P. (1975). The two histological main types of gastric carcinoma: Diffuse and so-called intestinal type carcinoma. *Acta Pathologica et Microbiologica Scandinavica*, Vol.64, (1975), pp. 31-49, ISSN 0365-5571.

Leanza, A.G.; Matteo, M.J.; Crespo, O.; Antello, P.; Olmos, J.; & Catalano, M. (2004). Genetic characterization of *Helicobacter pylori* isolates from na Argentinean adult population based on cag pathogenicity island right-end motifs, IspA-glmM polymorphism and iceA and vacA genotypes. *Clinical microbiology and infection*, Vol.10, No.9, (September 2004), pp. 811-819, ISSN 1469-0691.

Lu, H.; Hsu, P.; Graham, D.Y. & Yamaoka, Y. (2005). Duodenal ulcer promoting gene of *Helicobacter pylori*. *Gastroenterology*, Vol.128, No.4, (April 2005), pp. 844-848, ISSN 0016-5085.

Lu, H.; Wu, J.Y.; Beswick, E.J.; Ohno, T.; Odenbreit, S., Haas, R.; Reyes, V.E.; Kita, M.; Graham, D.Y. & Yamaoka, Y. (2007). Functional and intracellular signaling differences associated with the *Helicobacter pylori* AlpAB adhesin from Western and

East Asian strains. *The Journal of Biological Chemistry*, Vol.282, No.9, (March 2007), pp. 6242-6254, ISSN 1083-351X.

Malfertheiner, P.; Bornschein, J. & Selgrad, M. (2010). Role of *Helicobacter pylori* infection in gastric cancer pathogenesis: a chance for prevention. *Journal of Digestive Diseases*, Vol.11, No.1, (February 2010), pp. 2-11, ISSN 1751-2972.

Marshall, B.J., & Warren, J.R. (1984). Unidentified curved bacilli in the stomach of patients with gastritis and peptic ulceration. *Lancet*, Vol.1, No.8390, (June 1984), pp. 1311-1315, ISSN 0140-6736.

Mattar, R.; Marques, S.B.; Monteiro, M.S.; Santos, A.F.; Iriya, K. & Carrilho, F.J. (2007) *Helicobacter pylori* cag pathogenicity island genes: clinical relevance for peptic ulcer disease development in Brazil. *Journal of Medical Microbiology*, Vol.56, No.1, (January 2007), pp. 9-14, ISSN 1473-5644.

McClain, M.S.; Shaffer, C.L.; Israel, D.A.; Peek Jr, R.M. & Cover, T.L. (2009). Genome sequence analysis of *Helicobacter pylori* strains associated with gastric ulceration and gastric cancer. *BMC Genomics*, Vol.10, (January 2009), pp. 3-16, ISSN 1471-2164.

Miehlke, S.; Kirsch, C.; Agha-Amiri, K.; Günther, T.; Lehn, N.; Malfertheiner, P.; Stolte, M.; Ehninger, G. & Bayerdörffer, E. (2000). The *Helicobacter pylori* vacA s1, m1 genotype and cagA is associated with gastric carcinoma in Germany. *International Journal of Cancer*, Vol.87, No.3, (August 2000), pp. 322-327, ISSN 1097-0215.

Mizushima, T.; Sugiyama, T; Komatsu, Y.; Ishituza, J.; Kato, M. & Asaka, M. (2001). Clinical relevance of the babA2 genotype of *Helicobacter pylori* in Japanese clnical isolates. *Journal of Clinical Microbiology*, Vol.39, No.7, (July 2001), pp.2463-2465, ISSN 1098-660X.

Moore, R.A.; Kureishi, A.; Wong, S. & Bryan, L.E. (1993). Categorization of clinical isolates of *Helicobacter pylori* on the basis of restriction digest analyses of polymerase chain reaction-amplified ureC genes. *Journal of Clinical Microbiology*, Vol.31, No.5, (May 1993), pp. 1334-1335, ISSN 1098-660X.

Nardone, G. Rocco, A. & Malfertheiner, P. (2004). Review article: *Helicobacter pylori* and molecular events in precancerous gastric lesions. *Alimentary pharmacology& therapeutics*, Vol.20, No.3, (August 2004), pp. 261-270, ISSN 0269-2813.

Nguyen, L.T.; Uchida, T.; Kuroda, A.; Tsukamoto, Y.; Trinh, T.D.; Ta, L.; Mai, H.B.; Ho, D.Q.; Hoang, H.H.; Vilaichone, R.K.; Mahachai, V.; Matsuhisa, T.; Kudo, Y.; Okimoto, T.; Kodama, M.; Murakami, K.; Fujioka, T.; Yamaoka, Y. & Moriyama, M. (2009). Evaluation of the anti-East Asian CagA-specific antibody for CagA phenotyping. *Clinical and vaccine immunology*, Vol.16, No.11, (November 2009), pp. 1687-1692, ISSN 1556-679X.

Oh, J.D.; Kling-Backhed, H.; Giannakis, M.; Xu, J.; Fulton, R.S; Fulton, L.A.; Cordum, H.S.; Wang, C.; Elliott, G.; Edwards, J.; Mardis, E.R.; Engstrand, L.G. & Gordon, J.L. (2006). The complete genome sequence of a chronic atrophic gastritis *Helicobacter pylori* strain: evolution during disease progression. *Proceedings of the National Academy of Sciences of the United States of America*, Vol.103, No.26, (June 2006), pp. 9999-1004, ISSN 1091-6490.

Parsonnet, J.; Friedman, G.D.; Orentreich, N. & Vogelman, H. (1997). Risk for gastric cancer in people with CagA positive or CagA negative *Helicobacter pylori* infection. *Gut*, Vol.40, No.3, (March 1997), pp. 297-301, ISSN 1468-3288.

Peek, R.M.; Blaser, M.J.; Mays, D.J.; Forsyth, M.H.; Cover, T.L; Song, S.Y.; Krishna, U. & Pietenpol, J.A. (1999). *Helicobacter pylori* strain-specific genotypes and modulation of the gastric epithelial cell cycle. *Cancer Research*, Vol.59, No.24, (December 1999), pp. 6124-6131, ISSN 1538-7445.

Peek Jr, R.M. & Blaser, M.J. (2002). *Helicobacter pylori* and gastrointestinal tract adenocarcinomas. *Nature Reviews. Cancer*, Vol.2, No.1, (January 2002), pp. 28-37, ISSN 1474-175X.

Pellicano, R.; Franceschi, F.; Saracco, G.; Fagoonee, S.; Roccarina, D. & Gasbarrini, A. (2009). Helicobacters and extragastric diseases. *Helicobacter*, Vol.14, Suppl.1, (September 2009), pp. 58-68, ISSN 1523-5378.

Pirouz, T.; Zounubi, L.; Keivani, H.; Rakhshani, N. & Hormazdi, M. (2009). Detection of *Helicobacter pylori* in paraffin-embedded specimens from patients with chronic liver diseases, using the amplification method. *Digestive Diseases and Sciences*, Vol.54, No.7 (July 2009), pp. 1456-1459, ISSN 1573-2568.

Qiao, W.; Hu, J.; Xiao, B.; Wu, K.C.; Peng, D.R.; Atherton, J.C. &Xue, H. (2003). CagA and vacA genotype of *Helicobacter pylori* associated with gastric diseases in Xi´an area. World *Journal of Gastroenterology*, Vol.9, No.8, (August 2003), pp. 1762-1766, ISSN 1007-9327.

Roesler, B.M.; Oliveira, T.B.; Bonon, S.H.A.; Monici, L.T.; Zeitune, J.M.R. & Costa, S.C.B. (2009). Restriction fragment length polymorphism of urease C and urease B gene of *Helicobacter pylori* strains isolated from Brazilian patients with peptic ulcer and chronic gastritis. *Digestive Diseases and Sciences*, Vol.54, No.7, (July 2009), pp. 1487-1493, ISSN 1573-2568.

Rohde, M.; Püls, J.; Buhrdorf, R.; Fischer, W. & Haas, R. (2003). A novel sheated surface organelle of the *Helicobacter pylori* cag type IV secretion system. *Molecular Microbiology*, Vol.49, No.1, (July 2003), pp. 219-234, ISSN 1365-2958.

Rothenbacher, D.; Bode, G.; Berg, G.; Gommel, R.; Gonser, T.; Adler, G. & Brenner, H. (1998). Prevalence and determinants of *Helicobacter pylori* infection in preschool children: a population-based study from Germany. *International Journal of Epidemiology*, Vol.27, No.1, (February 1998), pp. 135-141, ISSN 1464-3685.

Saiki, R.K.; Gelfand, D.H.; Stoffel, S.; Scharf, S.J.; Higuchi, R.; Horn, G.T.; Mullis, K.B. & Erlich, H.A. (1981). Primer-directed enzymatic amplification of DNA with a termostable DNA polymerase. *Science*, Vol.239, No.4839, (January 1981), pp. 487-491, ISSN 1095-9203.

Schmidt, H.M.A.; Andres, S.; Kaakoush, N.O.; Engstrand, L.; Eriksson, L.; Goh, K.L.; Fock, K.M.; Hilmi, I.; Dhamodaran, S.; Forman, D. & Mitchell, H. (2009). The prevalence of duodenal ulcer promoting gene (dupA) in *Helicobacter pylori* isolates varies by ethnic group and is not universally associated with disease development: a case-control study. *Gut Pathogens*, Vol.1, No.1, (March 2009), pp. 5-13, ISSN 1757-4749.

Sugiyama, T. & Asaka, M. (2004). *Helicobacter pylori* infection and gastric cancer. *Medical Electron Microscopy*, Vol.37, No.3, (September 2004), pp. 149-157, ISSN 1437-773X.

Telford, J.L.; Ghiara, P.; Dell´Orco, M.; Comanducci, M.; Burroni, D.; Bugnoli, M.; Tecce, M.F.; Censini, S.; Covacci, A. & Xiang, Z. (1994). Gene structure of the *Helicobacter pylori* cytotoxin and evidence of its key role in gastric disease. *The Journal of Experimental Medicine*, Vol.179, No.5, (May 1994), pp. 1653-1658, ISSN 1540-9538.

Thiberge, J.M.; Boursaux-Eude, C.; Lehours, P.; Dillies, M.A.; Creno, S.; Coppée, Y.; Rouy, Z.; Lajus, A.; Ma, L.; Burucoa, C.; Ruskoné-Foumestraux, A.; Courillon-Mallet, A.; De Reuse, H.; Boneca, I.G.; Lamarque, D.; Mégraud, F.; Delchier, J.C.; Médigue, C.; Bouchier, C.; Labigne, A. & Raymond, J. (2010). From array-based hybridization of *Helicobacter pylori* isolates to the complete genome sequence of an isolate associated with MALT lymphoma. *BMC Genomics*, Vol.11, (June 2010), pp. 368-379, ISSN 1471-2164.

Thomazini, C.M.; Pinheiro, N.A.; Pardini, M.I.; Naresse, L.E. & Rodrigues, M.A.M. (2006). Infecção por *Helicobacter pylori* e câncer gástrico: frequência de cepas patogênicas cagA e vacA em pacientes com câncer gástrico. *Jornal Brasileiro de Patologia e Medicina Laboratorial,* Vol.42, No.1, pp. 25-30, ISSN 1676-2444.

Tomb, J.F.; White, O.; Kerlavage, A.R.; Clayton, R.A.; Sutton, G.G.; Fleischmann, R.D.; Ketchum, K.A.; Klenk, H.P.; Gill, S.; Dougherty, B.A.; Nelson, K.; Quackenbush, J.; Zhou, L.; Kirkness, E.F.; Peterson, S.; Loftus, B.; Richardson, D.; Dodson, R.; Khalak, H.G.; Glodek, A.; McKenney, K.; Fitzegerald, L.M.; Lee, N.; Adams, M.D.; Hickey, E.K.; Berg, D.E.; Gocayne, J.D.; Utterback, T.R.; Peterson, J.D.; Kelley, J.M.; Cotton, M.D.; Weidman, J.M.; Fujii, C.; Bowman, C.; Watthey, L.; Wallin, E.; Hayes, W.S.; Borodovsky, M.; Karp, P.D.; Smith, H.O.; Fraser, C.M. & Venter, J.C. (1997). The complete genome sequence of the gastric pathogen *Helicobacter pylori. Nature,* Vol.388, No.6642, (August 1997), pp. 539-547, ISSN 0028-0836.

Truong, B.X.; Mai, V.T.; Tanaka, H.; Ly le, T.; Thong, T.M.; Hai, H.H.; Van Long, D.; Furumatsu, K.; Yoshida, M.; Kutsumi, H. & Azuma T. (2009). Diverse characteristics of the cagA gene of *Helicobacter pylori* strains collected from patients from southern Vietnam with gastric cancer and peptic ulcer. *Journal of Clinical Microbiology*, Vo.47, No.12, (December 2009), pp. 4021-4028, ISSN 1098-660X.

Tummuru, M.K.;Cover, T.L. & Blaser, M.J. (1993). Cloning and expression of a high-molecular-mass major antigen of *Helicobacter pylori*: evidence of linkage to cytotoxin production. *Infection and immunity*, Vol. 61, No.5, (May 1993), pp. 1799-1809, ISSN 1098-5522.

vanDoor, L.J.; Figueiredo, C.; Sanna, R.; Plaisier, A., Schneeberger, P. de Boer, W. & Quint, W. (1998). Clinical relevance of the cagA, vacA and iceA status of *Helicobacter pylori. Gastroenterology*, Vol.115, No.1, (July 1998), pp. 58-66, ISSN 0016-5085.

Yamaoka, Y.; Kodama, T.; Gutierrez, O.; Kim, J.G.; Kashima, K. & Graham, D. (1999). Relationship between *Helicobacter pylori* iceA, cagA and vacA status and clinical outcome: studies in four different countries. *Journal of Clinical Microbiology*, Vol.37, No.7, (July 1999), pp. 2274-2279, ISSN 1098-660X.

Yamaoka, Y. (2008). Roles of the plasticity regions of *Helicobacter pylori* in gastroduodenal pathogenesis. *Journal of Medical Microbiology*, Vol.57, No.5, (May 2008), pp. 545-553, ISSN 1473-5644.

Zhang, Z.; Zheng, Q.; Chen, X.; Xiao, S.; Liu, W. & Lu, H. (2008). The *Helicobacter pylori* duodenal ulcer promoting gene, dupA in China. *BMC Gastroenterology*, Vol.8, (October 2008), pp. 49-54, ISSN 1471-230X.

Zhou, J.; Zhang, J.; Xu, C. & He, L. cagA genotype and variants in Chinese *Helicobacter pylori* strains and relationship to gastroduodenal diseases. (2004). *Journal of Medical Microbiology*, Vol.53, No.3, (March 2004), pp. 231-235, ISSN 0022-2615.

15

Role of Gastrokine 1 in Gastric Cancer

Emilia Rippa[1], Paolo Mallardo[1] and Paolo Arcari[1,2]
[1]*Department of Biochemistry and Medical Biotechnologies, University of Naples Federico II,*
[2]*CEINGE, Advanced Biotechnologies scarl, Naples*
Italy

1. Introduction

Gastric cancer (GC) has high incidence (> 1.000.000 new cases/year) and mortality rate in several countries and is still one of the most frequent and lethal (> 600.000 dead/year) neoplasia with an average survival of five years (less than 20%) (Pisani et al., 1990; Lands et al., 1998). It is already well known that infection of gastric antrum mucosal with the bacterium *Helicobacter pylori* is the cause of the chronic inflammation that leads to intestinal-type gastric cancer in the majority of the cases. The *H. pylori* infection is widespread but only a small number of the total population of infected individuals might eventually develop adenocarcinoma (around 3/10,000 individuals per year or 2.1% for lifetime infection) (Correa & Piazuelo, 2008). Risk factors influencing the outcome of *H. pylori*–associated pathology include bacterial cytotoxic heterogeneity, diet, and geographic differences. The phenomenon of decreased gastric cancer incidence in Africa compared with other regions where *H. pylori* is endemic (Holcombe, 1992) is probably due to the different diet of these populations compared to the western countries. This discrepancy has been partially attributed to helminth co-infection that likely modifies the characteristic proinflammatory type 1 T-helper 1 cell response, to a T-helper 2–predominant response (Whary et al., 2005), typified by the release of non-inflammatory cytokines and reduced incidence of *H. pylori*–associated glandular atrophy, an early marker of cancer development. The identification of novel genes regulated by *H. pylori* in vivo, particularly those contributing to these early stages of gastric cancer, would facilitate improved understanding of the differential susceptibility to this pathogen. The different susceptibility among individuals to *H. pylori* infection is still not yet defined. Some works, however, suggested that the polymorphisms in host genetic factors like the proinflammatory cytokines interleukin-1, interleukin-8, and tumor necrosis factor may play a relevant role (El-Omar et al., 2003).
The evolution of intestinal tumours is characterized by a progression of several sequential steps that starts with gastritis and then progresses to mucosal atrophy (atrophic gastritis), intestinal metaplasia, dysplasia and carcinoma with subsequent metastatic dissemination (Correa, 1992, 1995). The diffuse-type has instead a poorer prognosis and develops through unknown genetic and morphological events from normal gastric epithelium. No preceding steps have been identified in the pathogenesis of diffuse carcinoma other than the chronic gastritis. The pathogenesis of gastric cancer remains poorly understood although it is

evident that several environmental factors, such as *H. pylori* infection can be one of the causes leading to this disease. In fact, the risk to develop gastric cancer is increased in patients with *H. pylori* infections probably as the result of a combination of genetic and environmental factors in which the infection by *H. pylori* is of particular relevance, especially when the inflammation involves the gastric body region with respect to the antrum (Correa, 1995; Goldstone et al., 1996; Nabewera & Logan, 1999). Generally, this condition is associated to different degrees of atrophy and alterations of the secretor function that, in the long term, became associated to gastric carcinoma (Forman et al., 1991; Parsonnet et al., 1997; Watanabe et al., 1998).

Diffuse adenocarcinoma shows an increased propensity for intra and transmural spread and is therefore associated with a poorer prognosis. Unfortunately, the histological classification of an individual gastric adenocarcinoma is not clear-cut with a tumour often comprising a mixture of intestinal and diffuse tissue types. Under these considerations, we think that there is an urgent necessity to dispose of an efficient tool for the detection of early stage gastric cancer like the identification of highly sensitive and specific biomarkers that will aid disease diagnosis and ensure early clinical intervention, thereby preventing mortality and reducing morbidity (Boussioutas & Taupin, 2001). Since most of GC (around 73%) is developed at antrum/pylorus, proteins secreted by antrum/pylorus mucosa might play a critical role in maintaining normal gastric mucosa structure and function.

2. Expression of gastrokine 1 in normal and malignant tissues

From a comparative proteomic analysis of human specimens of gastric mucosa from patients with and without *H. pylori* infection, we have shown the differential expression of several up- and down-regulated proteins (Rippa et al., 2007). One of these proteins, gastrokine 1 (GKN1), a novel stomach-specific protein also known as 18 kDa antrum mucosa protein (AMP-18 or foveolin) (Oien et al., 2004), was highly expressed in normal tissues and markedly down-regulated in samples derived from *H. pylori* infected patients (Nardone et al, 2007). To elucidate the biological function of GKN1, we have characterized its expression in normal and malignant gastric tissues also by immunohistochemical technique. The etiology of most gastric cancers is multifactorial and the pathogenesis is believed to involve a multi-step process in which the normal gastric epithelium evolves through intermediate pre-malignant lesions (intestinal metaplasia and dysplasia) leading to adenocarcinoma. These investigations were based on the hypothesis that GKN1 expression in pre-malignant gastric tissues and in gastric carcinomas is altered in terms of quantity (reduced amount or complete absence of the protein), quality (altered protein size), and distribution (abnormal cell-type and/or subcellular localization) compared to normal gastric tissues.

2.1 The gastrokine family

GKN1 belongs to a family of genes encoding stomach-specific secreted proteins consisting of 3 known members: gastrokine 1 (GKN1) (Martin et al., 2003), gastrokine 2 (GKN2) (Du et al., 2003), and gastrokine 3 (GKN3) (Menheniott et al., 2010). Although their mode of action remains unclear, the recent demonstration of a GKN2/trefoil factor (TFF1) heterodimer in gastric mucus suggests that gastrokines may regulate the extracellular function of TFFs (Westley *et al.*, 2005).

2.2 Gastrokine 1

GKN1 (also named as AMP18), a member of BRICHOS superfamily, is secreted by antrum mucosa (Oien et al., 2004). *GKN1* gene of about 6 kb was reported to be located at 2p13 and contains 6 exons (Martin et al., 2003). Bioinformatics analysis suggested the secretory signal peptide with 20-amino acids presented at the N-terminal and the processed protein consisted of 165-amino acids after cleavage. Despite several asparagine residues in the N-terminal domain, none seems to be the consensus site of traditional glycosylation (Martin et al., 2003). The *GKN1* gene encodes a small protein of 185 amino acids containing a N-terminal signal peptide (Yoshikawa et al., 2000). The BRICHOS domain consists of about 100 amino acids and it has been found in several unrelated proteins associated with major human diseases (Sanchez-Pulido et al., 2002) like BRI2, related to familial British and Danish dementia; chondromodulin-I (ChM-I), linked to chondrosarcoma; surfactant protein C (SP-C), associated with respiratory distress syndrome; and gastrokine 1 (also known as CA11, AMP18 & foveolin) (Shiozaki et al., 2001; Martin et al., 2003), linked to gastric cancer (Sanchez-Pulido et al., 2002; Shiozaki et al., 2001). Evaluation of GKN1 expression at mRNA and protein level, by RT-PCR and immunhistochemistry (IHC), was found only in stomach, gastric antrum, but not in esophagus, duodenum, or intestine (Oien et al., 2004).

2.3 Evaluation of GKN1 expression levels

The evaluation of GKN1 expression in normal and malignant cells was performed according the following strategy.

2.3.1 Patients enrolment and clinical characterization

In this study a population of 28 patients with gastric cancer (20 intestinal and 8 diffuse types) was enrolled. Interview focusing on diet and lifestyle habits, family history and other toxic environmental factors was performed. A family history positive for gastric cancer was also carefully verified. The biopsy specimens were taken during an upper video-endoscopy in the gastric body or collected immediately after surgical resection and soon delivered for diagnosis and tissue sampling. Specimens were used for culture test, histological and immunohistochemical tests and for molecular approach.

Gastric biopsy specimens were collected from normal subjects and patients with erosive gastritis, peptic ulcer or gastric cancer, either infected or not infected with *H. pylori*. None of the subjects had taken antibiotics, proton pump inhibitors or nonsteroidal antinflammatory drugs during the preceding 3 months. At least 65 gastric biopsy specimens were taken during upper endoscopy: one pinch was used to measure the urease activity (rapid urease test), and one pinch was used for a histological examination of *H. pylori* infection using hematoxylin-eosin stain. Three pinches and four pinches were used respectively for protein and RNA extraction. 36 patients (55%) showed to be negative for *H. pylori* infection and among these, 31 had normal mucosa while the remaining 5 had minimal infiltration of lymphomonocytes in the lamina propria. *H. pylori* infection was detected in 29/65 patients suffering from active gastritis (25 mild-moderate and 4 severe); 10 patients showed mild or moderate atrophy that was associated in 4 cases with focal antral complete IM. Anti-*H. pylori* and anti CagA IgG antibodies were not detected in any of the *H. pylori*-negative subjects but were found in 29 (100%) and 21 (72%) *H. pylori*-positive patients, respectively.

2.3.2 Proteomic analysis

In order to identify proteins differently expressed in human gastric mucosa without and with *H. pylori* infection, proteins extracted from biological specimens were analyzed by 2D electrophoresis in the pH range 3-10. Protein samples (100 μg) were focused on IPG strips and then separated by 12% SDS-PAGE. Proteins were stained with Comassie Brilliant Blue G-250. Comassie-stained protein spots were excised from 2-D gels and treated with 10 ng/μl of trypsin and digested overnight at 37°C according to Schevechencko et al., 1996. The peptide mixture obtained was then analyzed using a MALDI-TOF mass spectrometer Voyager DE™ PRO (Applied Biosystems), operating in positive-ion reflectron mode. Protein identification was achieved using MALDI mass spectral data for a data-base search against the NCBInr database using the Mascot search algorithm, a parameter representing the reliability of protein identification (see also http://www.matrixscience.com/) (Nardone et al., 2007).

Figure 1, shows the protein profiles observed in human gastric mucosa specimens. GKN1 was identified by MALDI-TOF analysis of tryptic fragments (Rippa et al., 2007). On 2D gels, the GKN1 protein spot was found in all samples from *H. pylori* non-infected patients and it was generally drastically reduced in several samples of *H. pylori* infected tissues. The amino acid sequence of GKN1 isolated from gel covered about 38% of the entire protein sequence. Mature GKN1 did not contain the first 20 amino acid leader peptide as confirmed by the amino acid sequence of the N-terminal performed by Edman's degradation. As expected from the isoelectric point of the mature protein (pI = 5.32), the migrating position of GKN1 on the 2D gel was toward acidic pH.

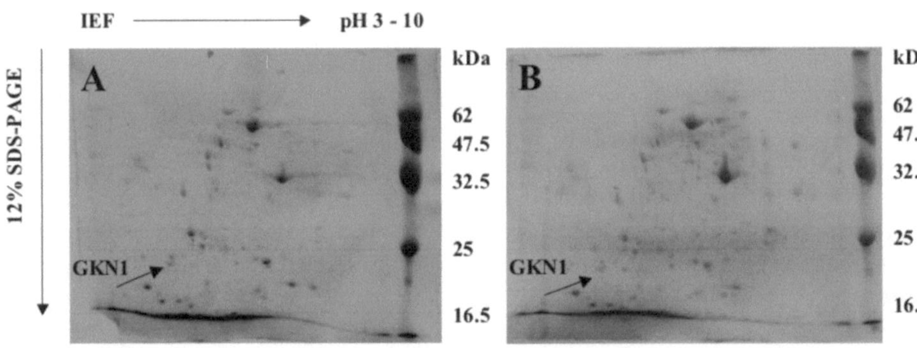

Fig. 1. Bidimensional gel electrophoresis of proteins extracted from gastric endoscopic mucosal samples. A) *H. pylori*-negative sample, B) *H. pylori*-positive sample. The first-dimension (isoelectric focusing, IEF) was performed using the Ettan IPGphor (Amersham Biosciences) equipped with 7 cm strip holders.

To analyze more quickly the expression levels of GKN1 in our collection of samples from patients with and without *H. pylori* infection (45 cases), we first tried to use mono-dimensional SDS-PAGE followed by staining of the gel with comassie blue. Figure 2 shows the position of the GKN1 stained band after electrophoresis at around 18 kDa however this approach resulted only qualitative and not quantitative.

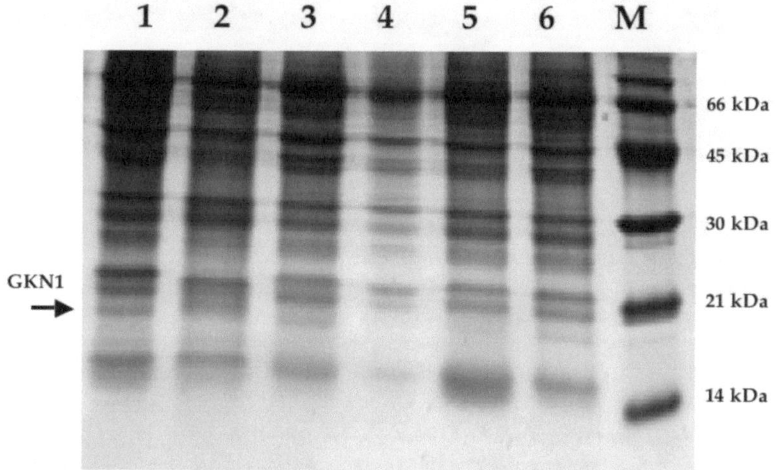

Fig. 2. Monodimensional gel electrophoresis of proteins extracted from gastric endoscopic mucosal samples. SDS-PAGE (14%) of proteins extracted from gastric endoscopic mucosal samples from *H. pylori*-negative patient (Lanes 1, 3, 5) and *H. pylori*-positive patient (Lanes 2, 4, 6). M, size markers.

2.3.3 Western blotting analysis of GKN1 expression

To detect more precisely the GKN1 expression levels, we adopted the Western blot procedure using a specific anti-GKN1 antibody (Abnova) raised against the intact protein. The analysis was carried out starting from three biopsies. Specimens were mixed with proteases inhibitor (Roche), homogenized and equivalent amounts of protein (10 μg) were separated by electrophoresis on sodium dodecyl sulfate-12% polyacrylamide gels. After electrophoresis, the proteins were electroblotted to a nitrocellulose membrane (Immobilon PQS). GKN1 protein was identified using a specific rabbit polyclonal antibody (Abnova, diluted 1/50000). Visualization was obtained with an ECL kit (Pirce).

As reported in Figure 3, the reduction in expression levels of GKN1 was not always observed in all patients with *H. pylori* associated gastritis but only in about 20% of samples. The evaluation has been based on the expression levels of β-tubulin. In all cases, the reduction of GKN1 levels was about two times that of non-infected samples. Densitometric evaluation of the bands showed a lower level in *H. pylori*-positive patients compared to the *H. pylori*-negative subjects (average: 0.19 ± 0.02 vs 0.44 ± 0.07, $p < 0.005$). This finding is in agreement to what observed also in another proteomic analysis regarding other proteins/enzymes differentially expressed by *H. pylori* infection (Baek et al., 2004).

We also analyzed the expression of GKN1 in human specimens derived from patients with gastric cancer. With respect to the non-tumoral area, it was observed that GKN1 expression was consistently down regulated or absent in tumoral area (Nardone et al., 2008). The 28 patients with Gastric Cancer (GC) (20 intestinal and 8 diffuse) showed the following characteristics: the intestinal type was well differentiated in 4, moderately differentiated in 8

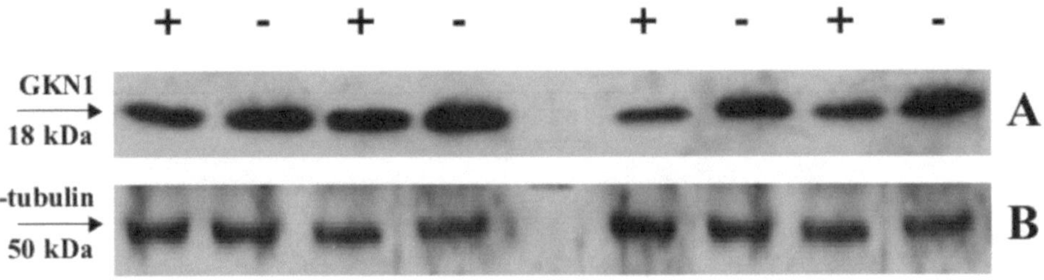

Fig. 3. Western blot analysis of human gastric mucosa samples. About 10 μg of protein extracts from samples of gastric mucosa from non-infected patient (-) and patients with *H. pylori* infection (+) were separated on SDS-PAGE and blotted against commercial antibody anti-GKN1 (A) and anti-β-tubulin (B) (control).

and poorly differentiated in the remaining 8 cases, while four were in the early stage and the remaining 16 in the advanced stage. Diffuse type GC was poorly differentiated and advanced in all cases. The non tumoural areas of intestinal type GC showed a variable degree of gastric atrophy with diffuse IM, instead, the peritumoural areas of diffuse type GC showed a variable degree of non-dysplastic inflammation. *H. pylori* infection was not revealed in all cases of tumoural areas. It is interesting to point out, however, that *H. pylori* infection was detected, in the peritumoral areas, in 6 cases (4 early and 2 advanced). Anti-*H. pylori* IgG antibodies were detected in 16/20 patients with intestinal histotype GC and in 6 out of 8 with diffuse type GC. Anti-CagA antibodies were detectable in 17/28 cases (14 intestinal and 3 diffuse histotype). Using Western blot (WB) analysis, GKN1 protein expression was not detected in any of the tumoural areas but was revealed instead in non-tumoural areas (Fig. 4).

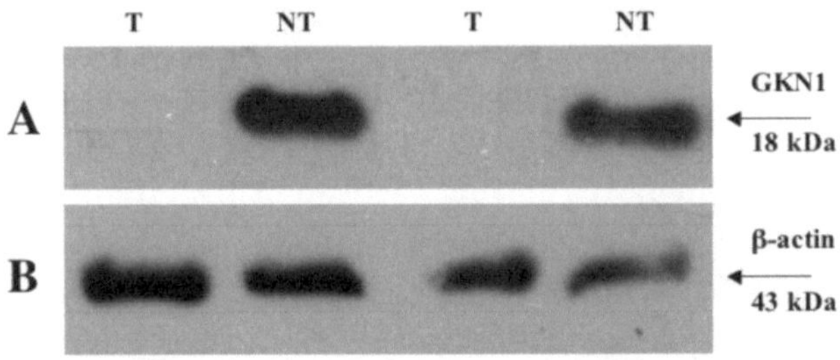

Fig. 4 Western blot analysis of GKN1 expression in human gastric specimens. About 20 μg of protein extracts from samples tumoral area (T) and non-tumoral area (NT) were separated on SDS-PAGE and blotted against commercial antibody anti-GKN1 (A) and anti--β-actin (B) (control).

2.3.4 Immunohistochemical analysis of GKN1 expression

The Immunohistochemical evaluation of GKN1 on surgical specimens was performed on 7-micron sections of frozen unfixed gastric tissues. The percentages of immunoreactive cells was scored as follows: 0-5% = negative; 5-25% = low staining; 25-50% = moderate staining; >50% = intense staining. The results obtained, summarized in Fig. 5 showed the absence of GKN1 in tumor tissues (our actual collection of about 30 cases). In fact, the GKN1 staining was intense in normal gastric tissues, low or completely negative in intestinal metaplasia and gastric cancer, respectively (Fig. 5) (Rippa et al., unpublished results).

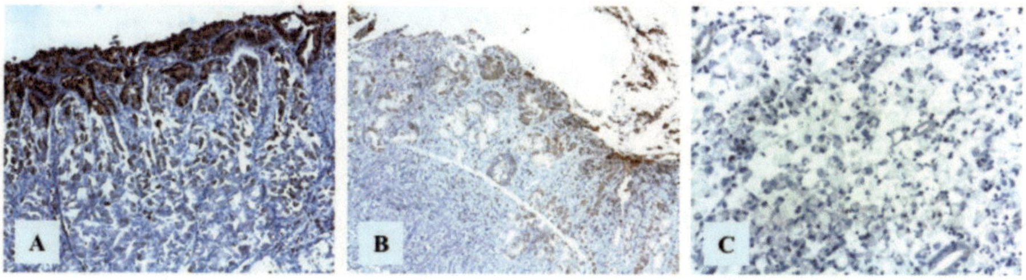

Fig. 5. Representative immunohistochemical images of surgical specimens from: A) Normal gastric tissue (LSAB, orig. magn. X200); B) Intestinal metaplasia (LSAB, orig. magn. x100); C) Intestinal type gastric cancer (LSAB, orig. magn. X200).

In addition, the hystopathological aspect of the tumor specimens correlated to the GKN1 expression with tumor subtype. This observation suggested that GKN1 could play an important role in normal gastric function thus and strongly suggested that GKN1 could be a biomarker for gastric cancer (Yoshihara et al., 2006; Moss et al., 2008).

3. Functional role of GKN1

Regarding the functional role of GKN1, there are two questions that are still to be clarified. The first important question is whether GKN1 is secreted from gastric cells. Although data from bioinformatics analysis and the presence in the protein of a leader peptide sequence, there is not a conclusive answer to this point. If GKN1 is secreted from the gastric mucosa cells, other questions will raise up concerning the sequence of the secreted protein and how it interacts with its target cells. The second question is whether and how the GKN1 protein modulates the behavior of gastric cells. To this aim, we started to elucidate the role of the protein in the processes of proliferation and signalling transduction analyzing the expression of GKN1 in gastric carcinoma cells and its effects on apoptosis.

3.1 Over-expression of GKN1 in gastric cancer cell lines

The knowledge about the biological function of GKN1 is not completely clarified. What is known at the moment is that GKN1 appears to be important in maintaining mucosal integrity and could play a role in cell proliferation and differentiation. In fact, GKN1 might have a protective effect by increasing accumulation of specific tight and adherens junction proteins and also protecting their loss after injury (Walsh-Reitz et al., 2005). The presence in GKN1 of the BRICHOS domain might explain its protective role. In fact, the BRICHOS is present also in another gastric protein GKN2, known also TFIZ1, because of its homology to GKN1. This protein is involved in the binding of tumor suppressor proteins such as the trefoil protein 1 (TFF1). Such interaction could be important in the regulation of the integrity of the mucosa (Bruce et al., 2005; Otto et al., 2006; Baus-Loncar et al., 2007).

The strong down-regulation of GKN1 expression in patients with *H. pylori* infection (Nardone et al., 2007) its absence in gastric cancer (Nardone et al., 2008; Moss et al., 2008) and its absence in human gastric cancer cell lines (AGS and MKN28) (Motoyama et al., 1986; Segal et al., 1996; Oien et al., 2004) are factors that suggest the participation of GKN1 in the host response to *H. pylori* and suggest also that GNN1 can act as gastric tumor suppressor gene (Du et al., 2003). Regarding this point, since GKN1 is highly down-regulated or absent in gastric cancer, one possible explanation of its disappearance could be linked to epigenetic events or loss of heterozygosity, as it was observed for other tumor suppressor genes such as TFF1 (Carvalho et al., 2002). However, as recently reported by Yoon et al., 2010, no significative mutations nor methylation in the GKN1 gene in gastric tumors were found, thus the down-regulation of GKN1 it is likely not depending by epigenetic events.

Toback et al., (2003) proposed that GKN1 could have some mitogenic effects on intestinal epithelial cells (IEC) as compared with EGF 5. Shiozaki et al., 2001, instead found that this protein was able to inhibit proliferation of a human carcinoma cancer cell line (MKN28) cells after transfection. From this finding it emerges that it is important to define the role of GKN1 in the modulation of inflammatory damage or tumorigenesis in the gastric mucosa. Attempts to reduce cancer survival rates include strategies directed towards the identification of specific targets inducing apoptosis in tumor cells.

3.1.1 Evaluation of transient expression of GKN1 in gastric cancer cell

AGS or MKN28 cancer cells (Motoyama, *et al.*, 1986) were transfected with the eukaryotic expression vectors pcDNA 3.1 containing the entire GKN1 cDNA. Cells were grown in 5% CO2 at 37° in DMEM (Dulbecco's modified Eagle's medium) and transfected using lipophectamine 2000. After transfection, cell growth and apoptosis was evaluated by cytofluorimetry.

The overexpression of GKN1 in MKN28 or AGS cells, with respect to control cells, reduced cell growth (Rippa et al., 2010). A similar effect was also reported by Shiozaki et al., 2001, who observed a reduction in MKN28 colony formation in cells transfected with CA11 gene with respect to control cells. Also GKN3, the new gastrokine found in mammals, strongly attenuated the growth of GKN3-overexpressing MKN28 cells (Menheniott et al., 2010). Because tissue repair is determined by many signals coming from the local environment, central to this process is the commitment of gastric cells to undergo apoptosis, survive, or proliferate, following inflammation. Therefore, gastric epithelial cell apoptosis could be influenced by GKN1 during the inflammatory process. The Fas-Fas ligand (FasL) system has been recognized as the major pathway for the induction of apoptosis in a variety of human normal and neoplastic cells (Itoh & Nagata, 1993; Suda et al., 1993; Nagata 1996). The Fas antigen (CD95, APO-1) belongs to a conserved family of membrane receptors known as the tumor necrosis factor receptor or TNFR family (Itoh et al., 1991). Therefore, overexpression of GKN1 could activate Fas, normally expressed at extremely low levels at least in MKN28 cells (Osaki et al., 2001). In fact, the expression of Fas receptor, evaluated by flow cytometry (Figure 6) Western blotting and RT-PCR showed a significant increase.

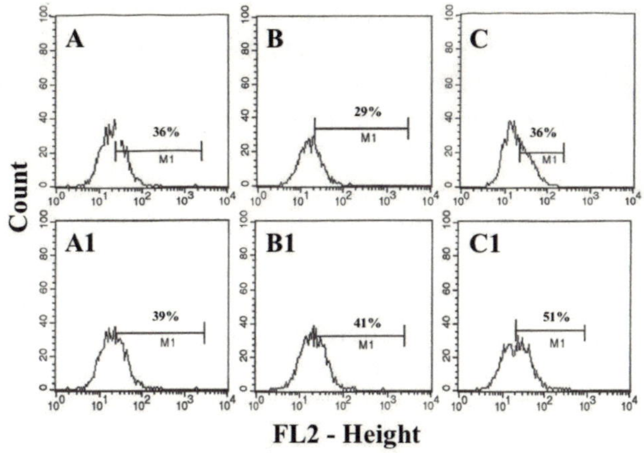

Fig. 6. Flow cytometric analysis of apoptosis in AGS cells. Representative flow cytometry of cells transfected with empty pCDNA 3.1, lipophectamine and GKN1 before (A, B, C) and after (A1, B1, C1) incubation with a monoclonal antibody (IgM) anti-FasL.

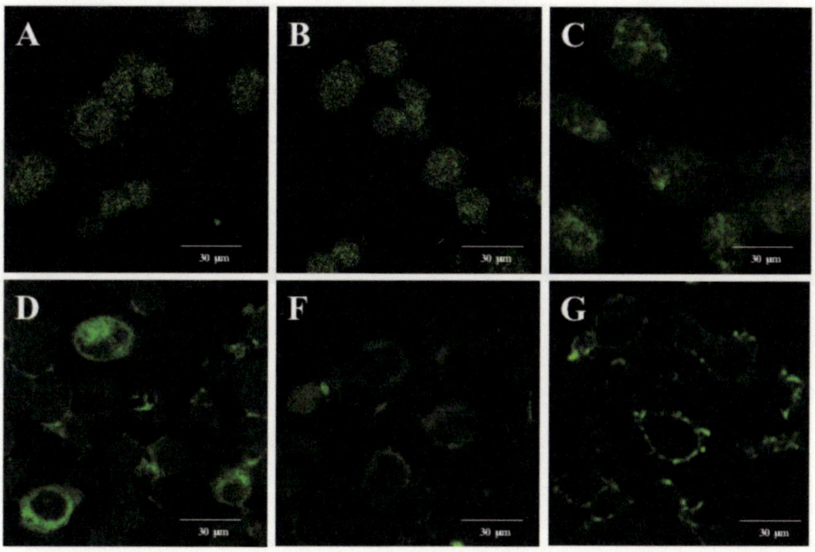

Fig. 7. Confocal microscopy of AGS cells. AGS cells were transfected with pCDNA 3.1 containing the GKN1 cDNA and after 48 hours from transfection cells were analyzed at confocal microscopy in the presence of antibody anti-GKN1 and anti-Fas. A) Untransfected cells. B) Cells treated with lopophectamine. C) Non-premealized transfected cells after incubation with anti-GKN1 antibody. D) Premeabilized transfected cells after incubation with anti-GKN1 antibody. E) Non-premeabilized untransfected cells after incubation with anti-Fas antibody. F) Premeabilized transfected cells after incubation with anti-Fas antibody.

Fas expression was also analyzed by confocal microscopy. As shown in Fig. 7, compared to the control cells, cells treated with lipophectamine and cells transfected with GKN1 showed, exposure of the permeabilized transfected cells to anti-GKN1 antibody showed a gain in the fluorescent signal that indicated mainly a cytoplasmic distribution of GKN1 protein whereas, the exposure of the transfected cells to anti-Fas antibody showed with respect to untransfected cells a gain in the fluorescent signal that was localized mainly at the level of cell membrane.
Therefore, the increase of Fas expression observed in cells transfected with GKN1 appeared to be specific as also demonstrated by the increase of the Fas mRNA transcription evaluated by RT-PCR (not shown). Fas-mediated apoptosis in gastric cells was also described upon infection by *H. pylori*, however in this case other apoptotic factors are involved as well. These include TRIAL and its receptor subtypes (Yang, et al. 2003; Martin et al., 2004). Because the binding of Fas ligand (FasL) to the Fas antigen results in the transduction of a cytolytic signal into the cell followed by apoptosis, cells overexpressing GKN1 showed an increase in apoptosis that is mainly due to the exposure of the MKN28 cells to FasL with respect to that observed in the absence of FasL. In addition, when FasL binds to Fas, intracellular death caspases are activated, resulting in apoptotic demise of the cell (Chen et al., 1999). Also in cells transfected with GKN1, we observed the proteolytic activation of caspase-3, normally present as a 32 kDa inactive precursor (Zou et al., 1997), as evaluated by Western blot and fluorimetric assay, was observed thus indicating that GKN1-transfected cells were signaled to die (Nicholson et al., 1995; Schlegel et al., 1996; Wang et al., 1996).

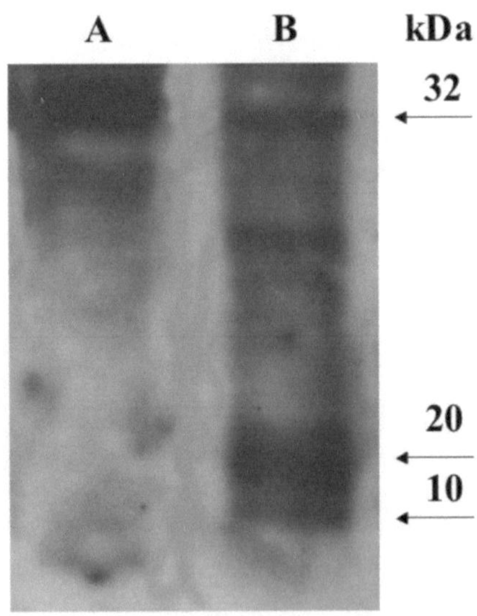

Fig. 8. Western blot of caspase-3. Evaluation of caspase-3 activation in AGS cells before (A) and after (A) 48 h transfection with GKN1 and exposure to FasL.

In addition, Yoon et al., 2011, found that transfection of GKN1 in AGS cells showed activation of apoptosis related proteins, including cleaved caspase 3, caspase 8 and PARP. The GKN1-induced apoptosis is suppressed by the presence of caspase-3 and caspase-8 inhibitors.

4. Conclusion

We have evaluated the expression of GKN1 in normal and unhealthy tissues and found that the GKN1, both at protein and mRNA levels, is down-regulated in human specimens from *H. pylori* infected gastric mucosa or absent in gastric GC tissues or cells. GKN1 is instead normally present in normal tissues and cells or in the peritumoral area of GC. Also the immunohistochemical analysis of human specimens (normal tissues, intestinal metaplasia, GC) showed a progressive decrease of GKN1 expression thus suggesting that GKN1 could be a good biomarker candidate for gastric cancer progression.

In addition, our studies on the overexpression of the protein in gastric cancer cell lines showed that GKN1 could act as modulator of apoptosis and suggested a possible role of GKN1 as a tumor suppressor gene. The modulation of apoptotic signals by GKN1 during the early stages of acute gastric injury may have a profound influence on tissue repair and be instrumental in determining the individual host response.

5. Acknowledgements

This work was supported by funds from the Ministero della Salute, Regione Calabria, 2003.

6. References

Baek, H.Y., Lim J.W., Kim, H., Kim, J.M., Kim, J.S., Jung, H.C. & Kim, K.H. (2004) Oxidative-Stress-Related Proteome Changes In *Helicobacter Pylori*-Infected Human Gastric Mucosa. *Biochemical Journal*, Vol. 379(Pt 2); Apr 15, 2004, pp. 291–299, ISSN 0264-6021.

Baus-Loncar, M., Lubka, M., Pusch, C.M., Otto, W.R., Poulsom, R. & Blin, N. (2007). Cytokine Regulation of the Trefoil Factor Family Binding Protein GKN2 (GDDR/TFIZ1/blottin) in Human Gastrointestinal Epithelial Cells. *Cellular Physiology and Biochemistry*, Vol. 20, No. 1-4, 2007, pp. 193-20, ISSN 1015-8987.

Bruce, R., Westley, S., Griffin, M. & May, F.E.B. (2005). Interaction between TFF1, a Gastric Tumor Suppressor Trefoil Protein, and TFIZ1, a Brichos Domain Containing Protein with Homology to SP-C. *Biochemistry*, Vol. 44, No. 22, pp. 7967-75. ISSN 0006-2960.

Carvalho, R., Kayademir, T., Soares, P., Canedo, P., Sousa, S., Oliveira, C., Leistenschneider, P., Seruca, R., Gött, P., Blin, N., Carneiro, F. & Machado, J.C. (2002). Loss of heterozygosity and promoter methylation, but not mutation, may underlie loss of TFF1 in gastric carcinoma. *Laboratory Investigation*, Vol. 82, No. 10 Oct 2002, pp. 1319-1326. ISSN 0023-6837.

Chen, M.K., Strande, L.F., Beierle, E.A., Kain, M.S., Geldziler, B.D. & Doolin, E.J. (1999). Fas-Mediated Induction of Hepatocyte Apoptosis in a Neuroblastoma and Hepatocyte Coculture Model. *Journal of Surgical Research*, Vol. 84, No. 1, Jun 1999, pp. 82-87. ISSN 0022-4804.

Correa, P. (1992). Human gastric carcinogenesis: a multistep and multifactorial process--First American Cancer Society Award Lecture on Cancer Epidemiology and Prevention. *Cancer Research*, Vol. 52, No. 24, Dec 15, 1992, pp. 6735-6740. ISSN 0008-5472.

Correa, P. (1995). *Helicobacter pylori* and gastric carcinogenesis. *American Journal of Surgical Pathology*, Vol.19, Suppl 1, pp. S37-43. ISSN 0147-5185.

Correa, P. & Piazuelo, M.B. (2008). Natural history of *Helicobacter pylori* infection. *Digestive and Liver Disease*, Vol. 40, No. 7, Jul 2008, pp. 490-6. ISSN 1590-8658.

Du, J.J., Dou, K.F., Peng, S.Y., Wang, W.Z., Wang, Z.H., Xiao, H.S., Guan, W.X., Liu, Y.B. & Gao, Z,Q. (2003). Down-regulated full-length novel gene GDDR and its effect on gastric cancer. *Zhonghua Yi Xue Za Zhi*, Vol. 83, No. 10, Jul 2003, pp. 1166-1168. ISSN 1003-9406.

El-Omar, E.M., Rabkin, C.S., Gammon, M.D., Vaughan, T.L., Risch, H.A., Schoenberg, J.B., Stanford, J.L., Mayne, S.T., Goedert, J., Blot, W.J., Fraumeni, J.F. Jr & Chow, W.H. (2003). Increased risk of noncardia gastric cancer associated with proinflammatory cytokine gene polymorphisms. *Gastroenterology*, Vol. 124, No. 5, May 2003, pp. 1193-1201. ISSN 0016-5085.

Forman, D., Newell, D.G., Fullerton, F., Yarnell, J.W., Stacey, A.R., Wald, N. & Sitas, F. (1991). Association between infection with *Helicobacter pylori* and risk of gastric cancer: evidence from prospective investigation. *British Medical Journal*, Vol. 302, N0. 6788, Jun 1, 1991, pp. 1302-1305. ISSN 09598138

Goldstone, A.R., Quirke, P. & Dixon, M,F. (1996). *Helicobacter pylori* infection and gastric cancer. Journal of Pathology, Vol. 179, No. 2, Jun 1996, pp. 129-137. ISSN 0022-3417.

Holcombe, C. (1992). *Helicobacter pylori*: the African enigma. *Gut*, Vol. 33, No. 4, Apr 1992, pp. 429-431. ISSN 0017-5749.

Huang, Q., Huang, Q., Chenn, W., Wang, L., Lin, W., Lin, J. & Lin, X. (2008). Identification of transgelin as a potential novel biomarker for gastric adenocarcinoma based on proteomics technology. *Journal of Cancer Research and Clinical Oncology*, Vol. 134, No. 11, Nov 2008, pp. 1219-1227. ISSN 0171-5216.

Itoh, N. & Nagata, S. (1993). A novel protein domain required for apoptosis. Mutational analysis of human Fas antigen. *Journal of Biological Chemistry*, Vol. 268, No. 15, May 25, 1993, pp. 10932-10937. ISSN 0021-9258.

Itoh, N., Yonehara, S., Ishii, A., Yonehara, M., Mizushima, S., Sameshima, M., Hase, A., Seto, Y. & Nagata, S. (1991). The polypeptide encoded by the cDNA for human cell surface antigen Fas can mediate apoptosis. *Cell*, Vol. 66, No. 2, Jul 26, 1991, pp. 233-243. ISSN 0092-8674.

Jang, J.S., Cho, H.Y., Lee, Y.J., Ha, W.S. & Kim, H.W. (2004). The differential proteome profile of stomach cancer: identification of the biomarker candidates. *Oncology research*. Vol. 14, N0. 10, pp. 491-499. ISSN 965-0407.

Lands, S.H., Murray, T. & Bolden, S. (1998). Cancer statistics. *Ca Cancer Journal for Clinicians*, Vol. 48, No. 1, Jan/Feb 1998, pp. 6-29. 0007-9235.

Martin, J.H., Potthoff, A., Ledig, S., Cornberg, M., Jandl, O., Manns, M.P., Kubicka, S., Flemming, P., Athmann, C., Beil, W. & Wagner, S. (2004). Effect of *H. pylori* on the Expression of TRAIL, FasL and their Receptor Subtypes in Human Gastric Epithelial Cells and their Role in Apoptosis. *Helicobacter*, Vol. 9, No. 5, Oct 2004, pp. 371-386. ISSN 1083-4389.

Martin, T.E., Powell, C.T., Wang, Z., Bhattacharyya, S., Walsh-Reitz, M.M., Agarwal, K. & Toback, F.G. (2003). A novel mitogenic protein that is highly expressed in cells of the gastric antrum mucosa. *American Journal of Physiology Gastrointestinal and Liver Physiology*, Vol. 285, No. 2, Jul 2003, pp. G332-343. ISSN 0193-1857.

Menheniott, T.R., Peterson, A.J., O'connor, L., Lee, K.S., Kalantzis, A., Kondova, I., Bontrop, R.E., Bell, K.M. & Giraud, AS. (2010). A Novel Gastrokine in Mammals Marks Gastric Atrophy and shows evidence of adaptive gene loss in human. *Gastroenterology*, Vol. 138, No. 5, May 2010, pp. 1823-1835. ISSN 0016-5085.

Moss, S.F., Lee, J.W., Sabo, E., Rubin, A.K., Rommel, J., Westley, B.R., May, F.E., Gao, J., Meitner, P.A., Tavares, R. & Resnick, M.B. (2008). Decreased expression of gastrokine 1 and trefoil Factor Interacting Protein TFIZ1/GKN2 in gastric cancer: influence of tumor histology and relationship to prognosis. *Clinical Cancer Research*, Vol. 14, No. 13, Jul 1, 2008, pp. 4161-4167. ISSN 1078-0432.

Motoyama, T., Hojo, H., & Watanabe, H. (1986). Comparison of seven cell lines derived from human gastric carcinomas. *Acta Pathologica Japonica*, Vol. 36, No. 1, Jan 1986, pp. 65-83. ISSN 0001-6632.

Nabewera, H.M. & Logan, R.P. (1999). Epidemiology of *Helicobacter pylori* infection: transmission, translocation and extragastric reservoirs. *Journal of Physiology and Pharmacology*, Vol. 50, No. 5, Dec 1999, pp. 711-722. ISSN 0867-5910.

Nagata, S. (1996). Apoptosis by death factor. *Cell*, Vol. 88, No. 3, Feb 7, 1996, pp. 355-365. ISSN 0092-8674.

Nardone, G., Martin, G., Rocco, A., Rippa, E., La Monica, G., Caruso, F. & Arcari, P. (2008). Molecular expression of gastrokine 1 in normal mucosa and in *Helicobacter pylori*-related preneoplastic and neoplastic gastric lesions. *Cancer Biology and Therapy*, Vol. 7, No. 12, Dec 2008, pp. 1890-1895. ISSN 1538-4047.

Nardone, G., Rippa, E., Martin, G., Rocco, A., Siciliano, R.A., Fiengo, A. Cacace, G., Malorni, A., Budillon, G. & Arcari, P. (2007). Gastrokine 1 expression in patients with and without *Helicobacter pylori* infection. *Digestive and Liver Disease*, Vol. 39, No. 2, Feb 2007, pp. 122-129. ISSN 1590-8658.

Nicholson, W.D., Ali, A., Thornberry, N.A., Vailancourt, J.P., Ding, C.K., Gallant, M., Gareau, Y., Griffin, P.R., Labelle, M., Lazebnik, Y.A., Munday, N.A., Raji, S.M., Smulson, M.E., Yamin, T.T., Yu, V.L. & Miller, D.K. (1995). Identification and inhibition of the ICE/CED-3 protease necessary for mammalian apoptosis. *Nature*, Vol. 376, No. 6535, Jul 6, 1995, pp. 37-43. ISSN 0028-0836.

Oien, K.A., McGregor, F., Butler, S., Ferrier, R.K., Downie, I., Bryce, S., Burns, S. & Keith, W.N. (2004). Gastrokine 1 is abundantly and specifically expressed in superficial gastric epithelium, down-regulated in gastric carcinoma, and shows high evolutionary conservation. *Journal of Pathology*, Vol. 203, No. 3, Jul 2004, pp. 789-797. ISSN 0022-3417.

Osaki, M., Kase, S., Kodani, I., Watanabe, M., Adachi, H. & Ito, H. (2001). Expression of Fas and Fas ligand in human gastric adenomas and intestinal-type carcinomas: correlation with proliferation and apoptosis. *Gastric Cancer*, Vol. 4, No. 4, pp. 198-205. ISSN 1436-3291.

Otto, W.R., Patel, K., McKinnell, I., Evans, M.D., Lee, C.Y., Frith, D., Hanrahan, S., Blight, K., Blin, N., Kayademir, T., Poulsom, R., Jeffery, R., Hunt, T., Wright, N.A., McGregor, F. & Oien, K.A. (2006). Identification of blottin: A novel gastric trefoil factor family-2 binding protein. *Proteomics*, Vol. 6, No. 15, Aug 2006, pp. 4235-4245. ISSN 1615-9853.

Parsonnet, J., Friedman, G.D., Oremtreich, N. & Vogelman, H. (1997). Risk for gastric cancer in people with CagA positive or CagA negative *Helicobacter pylori* infection. *Gut*, Vol. 40, No. 3, Mar 1997, pp. 297-301. ISSN 0017-5749.

Pisani, P., Parkin, D.M., Bray, F. & Ferlay, J. (1999). Estimates of the worldwide mortality from 25 cancers in 1990. *International Journal of Cancer*, Vol. 83, No. 1, Sep 1999, pp. 18-29. ISSN 0020-7136.

Rippa, R., Martin, G., Rocco, A., La Monica, G., Fiengo, A., Siciliano, R.A., Cacace, G., Malorni, A., Nardone, G. & Arcari, P. (2007). Changes of protein expression in *Helicobacter pylori*-infected human gastric mucosa. *Current Topics in Peptide & Protein Research*. Vol. 8, pp. 35-43. ISSN 0972-4524.

Rippa, E., La Monica, G., Allocca, R., Romano, M.F., De Palma, M. & Arcari, P. (2010). Overexpression of gastrokine 1 in gastric cancer cells induces fas-mediated apoptosis. *Journal of Cellular Physiology*, Dec 28, 2010 [Epub ahead of print]. ISSN 0021-9541.

Sanchez-Pulido, L., Devos, D. & Valencia, A. (2002). BRICHOS: a conserved domain in proteins associated with dementia, respiratory distress and cancer. *Trends in Biochemical Science*, Vol. 27, No. 7, Jul 2002, pp. 329-332. ISSN 0968-0004.

Schlegel, J., Peters, I., Orrenius, S., Miller, D.K., Thornberry, N.A., Yamin, T.T. & Nicholson, D.W. (1996). CPP32/apopain is a key interleukin 1 beta converting enzyme-like protease involved in Fas-mediated apoptosis. *Journal of Clinical Investigation*, Vol. 271, No. 4, Jan 26, 1996, pp. 1841-1844. ISSN 0021-9738.

Segal, E.D., Falkow, S. & Tompkinset, L.S. (1996). *Helicobacter pylori* attachment to gastric cells induces cytoskeletal rearrangements and tyrosine phosphorylation of host cell proteins. *Proceedings of the National Academy of Sciences USA*, Vol. 93, No. 3, Feb 6, 1996, pp. 1259-1264. ISSN 0027-8424.

Shiozaki, K., Nakamori, S., Tsujie, M,, Okami, J., Yamamoto, H., Nagano, H., Dono, K., Umeshita, K., Sakon, M., Furukawa, H., Hiratsuka, M., Kasugai, T., Ishiguro, S. & Monden, M. (2001). Human stomach-specific gene, CA11, is down-regulated in gastric cancer. *International Journal of Oncology*, Vol. 19, No. 4, pp. 701-707. ISSN 1019-6439.

Suda, T., Takahashi, T., Golstein, P. & Nagata, S. (1993). Molecular cloning and expression of the Fas ligand, a novel member of the tumor necrosis factor family. *Cell*, Vol. 75, No. 6, Dec 15, 1993, pp. 1169-78. ISSN 0092-8674.

Toback, F.G., Walsh-Reitz, M.M., Musch, M.W., Chang, E.B., Del Valle, J., Ren, H., Huang, E. & Martin, T.E. (2003). Peptide fragments of AMP-18, a novel secreted gastric antrum mucosal protein, are mitogenic and motogenic. *American Journal of Physiology Gastrointestinal and Liver Physiology*, Vol. 285, No. 2, Jul 2003, pp. G344-G353. ISSN 0193-1857.

Vlahou, A. & Fountoulakis, M. (2005). Proteomic approaches in the search for disease biomarkers. *Journal of Chromatogr B Analytical Technologies in the Biomedical Life Sciences*, Vol. 814, No. 1, Jan 5, 2005, pp. 11-19. ISSN 1570-0232.

Walsh-Reitz, M.M., Huang, E.F., Musch. M.W., Chang, E.B., Martin, T.E., Kartha, S. & Toback, F.G. (2005). AMP18 protects barrier function of colonic epithelial cells: role of tight junction proteins. *American Journal of Physiology Gastrointestinal and Liver Physiology*, Vol. 289, No. 1, Jul 2005, pp. G163-G171. ISSN 0193-1857.

Wang, X., Zelenski, N.G., Yang, J., Sakai, J., Brown, M.S. & Goldstein, J.L. (1996). Cleavage of sterol regulatory element binding proteins (SREBPs) by cpp32 during apoptosis. *EMBO Journal*, Vol. 15, No. 5, Mar 1, 1996, pp. 1012– 1020. ISSN 0261-4189.

Watanabe, T., Tada, M. & Nagai, H. (1998). *Helicobacter pylori* infection induces gastric cancer in Mongolian gerbils. *Gastroenterology*, Vol. 115, No. 3, Sep 1998, pp. 642-648. ISSN 0016-5085.

Westley, B.R., Griffin, S.M. & May, F.E. (2005). Interaction between TFF1, a gastric tumor suppressor trefoil protein, and TFIZ1, a brichos domain-containing protein with homology to SP-C. *Biochemistry*, Vol. 44, No. 22, Jun 7, 2005, pp. 7967-7975. ISSN 0006-2960.

Whary, M.T., Sundina, N., Bravo, L.E., Correa, P., Quinones, F., Caro, F. & Fox, J.G. (2005). Intestinal helminthiasis in Colombian children promotes a Th2 response to Helicobacter pylori: possible implications for gastric carcinogenesis. *Cancer Epidemiology, Biomarkers and Prevention*, Vol. 14, Jun 2005, pp. 1464-1469. ISSN 1055-9965.

Yang, Y., Deng, C.S., Peng, J.Z., Wong, B.C.Y., Lam, S.K. & Xia, H,H.X. (2003). Effect of *Helicobacter pylori* on apoptosis and apoptosis related genes in gastric cancer cells. *Molecular Pathology*, Vol. 56, No. 1, Feb 2003, pp. 19-24. ISSN 1366-8714.

Yoon, J.H., Song, J.H., Zhang, C., Jin, M., Kang, Y.H., Nam, S.W., Lee, J.Y. & Park, W.S. (2011). Inactivation of gastrokine 1 gene in gastric adenomas and carcinomas. Journal of Pathology. Vol. 223, No. 5, Apr 2011, pp. 618-625. ISSN 0022-3417.

Yoshihara, T., Kadota, Y., Yoshimura, Y., Tatano, Y., Takeuchi, N., Okitsu, H., Umemoto, A., Yamauchi, T. & Itoh, K. (2006). Proteomic alteration in gastric adenocarcinomas from Japanese patients. *Molecular Cancer*. Vol. 5, Dec 25, 2006, 75. ISSN 1476-4598

Yoshikawa, Y., Mukai, H., Hino, F., Asada, K. & Kato, I. (2000). Isolation of two novel genes, own-regulated in gastric cancer. *Japanese Journal of Cancer Research*, Vol. 91, No. 5, May 2000, pp. 459-463. ISSN 0910-5050.

Zou, H., Henzel, W.J., Liu, X., Lutschg, A. & Wang, X. (1997). Apaf-1, a Human Protein Homologous to C. elegans CED-4, Participates in Cytochrome c–Dependent Activation of Caspase-3. *Cell*, Vol. 90, No. 3, Aug 8, 1997, pp. 405-413. ISSN 0092-8674.